I0836997

BEASLEY'S PRESCRIPTION-BOOK.

THE BOOK OF PRESCRIPTIONS; containing Two Thousand, Nine Hundred Prescriptions, collected from the Practice of the most Eminent Physicians and Surgeons. By HENRY BEASLEY, Author of "The Medical Formulary," "The Druggists' Receipt-Book," &c., &c. In one volume, duodecimo. Price, $1.50.

The editor, carefully selecting from the mass of materials at his disposal, has compiled a volume, sufficiently comprehensive, and yet sufficiently portable, in which, both *physician* and *druggist, prescriber* and *compounder*, may find, under the head of each remedy, the manner in which that remedy may be most effectively administered, or combined with other medicines in the treatment of various diseases. The alphabetical arrangement adopted renders this easy; and the value of the volume is still further enhanced by the short account given of each medicine, and the lists of doses of its several preparations. This is really a most useful and important publication, and from the great aid which it is capable of affording in prescribing, it should be in the possession of every medical practitioner. Amongst other advantages is, that, by giving the prescriptions of some of the most able and successful practitioners of the day, it affords an insight into the methods of treatment pursued by them, and of the remedies which they chiefly employed in the treatment of different diseases. The volume is small, and its cost trifling.—*Lancet.*

BEASLEY'S FORMULARY.—(New Edition.)

THE MEDICAL FORMULARY; comprising Standard and Approved Formulæ for the Preparations and Compounds employed in Medical Practice. By HENRY BEASLEY. Second American, from the Sixth London Edition. In one volume. Price, $1.50.

The fact that Mr. Beasley's Formulary has reached a sixth edition, is a sufficient proof of the estimation in which it is held by the medical and pharmaceutical public. It is, in fact, a very comprehensive work, containing a great mass of information in a very small compass. The arrangement is alphabetical, as being most convenient. It contains selections from the American, French, German, and other foreign Pharmacopœias, in addition to the Formulæ from the three British ones. The work, however, is so well known, that it is unnecessary to do more than announce the present edition, and to state that the doses of the various medicines have now been added.—*Medical Times and Gazette.*

THE WHOLE ART OF PERFUMERY.—With Illustrations.

THE ART OF PERFUMERY, AND METHOD OF OBTAINING THE ODOURS OF PLANTS, with Instructions for the Manufacture of Perfumes for the Handkerchief, Scented Powders, Odorous Vinegars, Dentifrices, Pomatum, Cosmetiques, Perfumed Soap, &c. With an Appendix, on the Colours of Flowers, Artificial Fruit, &c., &c. By G. W. SEPTIMUS PIESSE, Author of "The Odours of Flowers," &c., &c. Duodecimo. Price, $1.25.

"The volume is replete with valuable information, conveyed in a plain, succinct manner, free from any technicalities, and, we believe, covers the entire ground of the subject. It is valuable to almost every one, giving, as it does, simple formulas whereby any lady can keep her toilet laden with luxurious perfumes at a merely nominal cost, and by which also she can prepare choice syrups, ratifias, and many other articles of which elegant cookery involves the use. The book is well illustrated, and we think would be an acceptable gift to every lady, housekeeper or otherwise, as well as to all who seek information upon such subjects."—*Evening Journal.*

KURTEN ON SOAPS AND CANDLES.

THE ART OF MANUFACTURING SOAPS, including the most recent discoveries, and the best methods for making all kinds of Hard, Soft, and Toilet Soaps. Also, Olive Oil Soap, and others, necessary in the manufacture of Cloths; with Receipts for making Transparent and Camphene Oil Candles. By PHILIP KURTEN, Practical Soap and Candle maker at Cologne on the Rhine. 1 vol., 12mo. Price $1.

"Mr. Kurten's book is offered as a Manual of Scientific, yet simple preparations for the article in every condition, variety, and quality; and if practical experience and careful observation give him any claims to the favourable considerations of manufacturers, his book should be found in the hands of all Soap dealers."—*Journal of Useful Knowledge.*

THE DRUGGIST'S
GENERAL RECEIPT BOOK:

COMPRISING A COPIOUS

VETERINARY FORMULARY,

AND TABLES OF

VETERINARY MATERIA MEDICA;

NUMEROUS RECIPES IN

PATENT AND PROPRIETARY MEDICINES,

DRUGGISTS' NOSTRUMS, ETC.:

Perfumery and Cosmetics;

BEVERAGES, DIETETIC ARTICLES, AND CONDIMENTS;

TRADE CHEMICALS, &c.

WITH AN APPENDIX OF USEFUL TABLES.

BY HENRY BEASLEY,

AUTHOR OF "THE MEDICAL FORMULARY" AND "THE BOOK OF PRESCRIPTIONS."

Third American Edition,

WITH NUMEROUS ADDITIONS.

PHILADELPHIA:
LINDSAY & BLAKISTON.
1857.

ADVERTISEMENT.

In preparing this Third Edition of the Druggist's General Receipt Book, the whole has undergone a careful revision. While the addition to the work of upwards of two hundred new forms, receipts, and processes, collected from the most approved authorities, will, it is hoped, establish for it a further claim to that public approbation which it has already confessedly gained.

CONTENTS.

VETERINARY

MATERIA MEDICA.

A Table of the Properties and Doses of the Principal Medicinal Substances used in Veterinary practice.

N. B.—Where the doses are given without mentioning the animal intended, it must always be understood to refer to the Horse.

Acacia Gummi. See Gum Arabic.

Acetate of Ammonia. Spirit of Mindererus. Diaphoretic and diuretic. It is also regarded as antiseptic. Dose, for horses and cattle, from 4 to 8 oz. For smaller animals, from 2 to 8 dr. Externally, in strains, ophthalmia, &c.

Acetate of Copper. See Verdigris and Copper.

Acetate of Lead. Astringent and sedative; in doses of 30 to 40 grains with opium, in internal hemorrhage, chronic diabetes, and diarrhœa: but chiefly used externally, in cooling lotions, eye-waters, ointments, &c. (For Diacetate of Lead, see Goulard's Extract.) As antidotes for an overdose give Epsom or Glauber's Salts, with opiates if required.

Acetate of Potash. Diuretic and cooling: dose for horse and cattle, 2 oz. In much larger doses it is a laxative, but not to be depended on.

Acetate of Soda. Similar in properties and uses to Acetate of Potash.

Acetic Acid.—Strong acetic (or pyroligneous) acid acts as a rubefacient and caustic, but is rarely employed for this purpose. In the weaker forms of common, or dis-

2

tilled vinegar, or diluted wood vinegar, it is frequently used. See Vinegar.

ACIDS. See Muriatic Acid, Nitric Acid, Prussic Acid, Sulphuric Acid, &c.

ACUPUNCTURATION. Used in some spasmodic and paralytic affections.

ÆGYPTIACUM. A preparation of verdigris and honey. A mild caustic, used as a local application to ulcers of the mouth, running thrush, grease, &c. Internally poisonous.

ÆTHER. See Ether.

ALCOHOL. Poisonous to all animals—2 drachms will kill a dog. See Spirits, Ardent.

ALLSPICE. *Pimento.* A useful stimulant and carminative; used in cordial balls and drinks, and to correct the action of purgatives. Dose for horses, 2 to 4 dr.: cattle, $\frac{1}{2}$ oz. to 1 oz. Dose of the Tincture, 4 ounces, in gripes.

ALOES. The most valuable purgative for the horse, but not to be depended on for cattle and sheep. A horse requires from 4 to 8 dr. of Barbadoes aloes, from 5 to 9 dr. of Socotrine, and from 6 to 10 of Cape. Mr. Youatt says 3 dr. of Barbadoes are equal to 4 of Cape. Mr. Morton considers a mixture of equal parts of Cape and Barbadoes aloes to be quite as efficacious as the latter alone. But the fine-ground Barbadoes aloes are the most certain in their operation. If the animal be prepared by previous mashes, 5 dr. are generally, and 6 dr. almost always sufficient. Mr. BLAINE recommends 2 dr. every 6 hours till 8 dr. have been taken, as a nauseant and purgative: but Mr. YOUATT strongly disapproves of this plan, particularly in inflammation of the lungs. Aloes require from 18 to 36 hours to produce their effect, during which time the horse should not be ridden far or fast. Though not to be depended on for cattle, 4 to 6 dr. are sometimes added to the purgative salts. Large doses, (in some cases sufficient to destroy life) have been given to sheep without purging. Small dogs require from 15 to 30 gr., medium sized ones, a dr.; some larger ones require 2 dr., or more. Hogs can bear but a few grains. Externally, in the form of tincture, aloes is used as a stimulating application to wounds.

ALUM. Astringent and styptic. Given in doses of 2 to 4 dr. to horses in diabetes and diarrhœa; but BOURGELAT says that its too frequent use induces a phthisical condition. A dose of alum whey, consisting of 2 dr. of the powder in a pint of hot milk, may be given after excessive purging. Cattle require from 2 to 6 or 8 drachms in diabetes and red water; and from 2 to 4 oz. are given to cows, to dry their milk. To calves and lambs it is given in dr. doses, in warm milk, for diarrhœa, &c. Dogs, 10 to 15 gr. Externally it is applied to cracked and greasy heels, joint wounds, sore mouths, inflammation of the eye, chronic discharges from the nostrils, and to arrest bleeding from wounds. *Burnt* alum is more powerful, and is used as a mild caustic, mixed with honey, to fungous growths, sore mouths, &c.

ALTERATIVES. Medicines, which without producing any considerable or immediate sensible operation, and without interfering with food or work, effect a slow change in the diseased action of certain parts, so as gradually to restore a healthy state.

AMMONIA, CARBONATE OR SESQUICARBONATE OF. *Volatile Salts.* Stimulant and antacid. Dose, 1 dr. to 2 dr. [MOIROUD says from 2 to 8 dr.] to horses in tympanitis, and the last stage of pneumonia. To cattle, in hoven (distention from the fermentation of green food,) 1 to 4 dr. [MOIROUD says to 12 dr.] The solution of carbonate of ammonia has the same properties as the spirit of hartshorn, which see.

AMMONIA, AROMATIC SPIRIT OF. Properties as the last. Dose, ½ oz. to 1 oz.; or to cattle in hoven, 2 to 4 oz.

AMMONIA, LIQUID. Water of ammonia is more pungent and stimulant than the carbonate, and is used for the same purposes, particularly in tympanitis and hoven, largely diluted with water or some aromatic infusion; but it is chiefly used externally in stimulating liniments; also both internally and outwardly as an antidote to the bite of vipers. The dose of common water of ammonia may be from 2 to 6 dr.; or for cattle to 2 ounces. For small animals from ½ dr. to 1½. The vapour from the liquid ammonia (applied by holding an open bottle containing it to the eye) is used for the relief of amaurosis and other chronic affections of the eye.

AMMONIA, ACETATE OF. See Acetate of Ammonia.

AMMONIA, MURIATE OF. See Muriate of Ammonia.

ANALEPTICS. Medicines or food which restore exhausted strength.

ANGELICA. The root in powder or infusion, is a warm tonic. Dose ½ oz. to 2 oz.

ANISEED. This warm seed is used as a cordial, carminative, and pectoral. Dose for the horse, ½ oz. to 1 oz.; or ½ dr. of the essential oil. The latter is often added to purgatives to prevent griping. Cattle take 1 or 2 oz. of the powdered seeds. The oil is said to be poisonous to pigeons.

ANODYNES. Medicines which alleviate pain. Opium is chiefly employed for this purpose.

ANTIMONIALS. The preparations of antimony (besides their effect in producing vomiting in carnivorous animals) are considered to have a special action on the skin and lungs. They are also termed resolvent, and purifiers of the blood, and are supposed to be useful in visceral and glandular obstructions, farcy, &c. MR. BLAINE says "they lessen arterial action without operating very sensibly either in nauseating the stomach or greatly relaxing the skin." Some writers attribute diuretic effects to them. They are also said to promote *condition*. Pigs are supposed to fatten under their use. The principal preparations employed in veterinary practice are mentioned below.

ANTIMONY, CRUDE. *Black or (sesqui-) Sulphuret of Antimony*. Diaphoretic and alterative. The levigated (prepared) antimony is to be preferred. Given to horses in doses of from 2 to 6 dr., with nitre and sulphur, in surfeit, hide bound, and other skin diseases; and to improve the coat. MR. YOUATT says the dose should not exceed 4 dr. For cattle, the dose is sometimes increased to 2 or 3 oz. Dogs take from 10 to 30 grains. Hogs a drachm or more daily.

ANTIMONY, LIVER OF. (Hepar Antimonii,) and Crocus of Antimony (Crocus Metallorum,) are occasionally used in veterinary practice; but are uncertain in their composition and action. Dose, 1 or 2 drs. MR. CLARK says these compounds, and the glass of antimony, derange the stomach, but that it is doubtful if they have any other effect.

ANTIMONY, CALX OF. Diaphoretic. Dose 2 to 4 dr.

ANTIMONIAL POWDER. Similar to James' powders. Diaphoretic. In colds, fevers, inflammation, &c. Dose for horses or cattle, 1 or 2 dr; swine, 6 grains; dogs, from 2 to 5 grains. Less efficient than Emetic Tartar.

ANTIMONY, PRECIPITATED SULPHURET OF. Dose, ½ dr. to 2 dr. in obstinate skin diseases.

ANTIMONY, TARTARIZED. *Emetic Tartar.* Diaphoretic, expectorant, and reduces arterial action. It is also regarded as diuretic and vermifuge. Dose, ½ dr. to 1½ dr. in gruel, 3 times a day, in fevers, in inflammation of the lungs, and catarrhal affections. To destroy worms, 2 dr. may be given with powdered tin, or some other mechanical vermifuge, fasting, and followed by aloes; or 1 dr. for 6 mornings, followed on the 7th by a dose of physic. Mr. WHITE says he has not seen any good effect from it as a vermifuge. Cattle require from ½ dr. to 1 dr. Sheep from 10 to 20 gr. To swine and dogs it is emetic; the former require from 2 to 5 gr.; the latter, from 1 to 3 gr. Externally it produces an eruption on the skin. Formed into an ointment with lard, it has been rubbed on externally in chest affections, but it is dangerously irritant.

ANTIMONY, BUTTER OF. *Muriate or Chloride of Antimony.* Used externally only, as a caustic in canker, &c.

ANTIPERIODICS. Remedies against those diseases which return at regular intervals, as agues.

ANTISEPTICS. Remedies which counteract putrefaction.

ANTISPASMODICS. Medicines which relieve spasm, as opium, ether, camphor, ammonia, ardent spirits, &c.

ARNICA. Nervine, sedative, and diaphoretic. 40 to 60 gr. of the powdered plant (the flowers in preference) have been given twice a day for paralysis, amaurosis, rheumatism, blows or falls, &c. A decoction may be used outwardly as a fomentation to bruises, wounds, &c.

ARISTOLOCHIA. See Birthwort.

ARSENIC. *White Arsenic, or Arsenious Acid.* Very poisonous to all animals. In small doses, tonic and alterative,—but its operation requires to be carefully watched. It has been given, in doses of 2 gr., gradually increased to 20, in farcy and glanders. Externally, as a caustic, but dangerous and unmanageable. Used in solution to destroy vermin in cattle and sheep; but it is not free from danger. Mr. YOUATT remarks —"We have better and safer tonics, and better and safer caustics." The best antidotes are, hydrated oxide of iron, and calcined magnesia, in very large quantities, or a mixture of lime water and linseed oil.

ASSAFŒTIDA. Stimulant, antispasmodic, and expectorant. It is prescribed in nervous affections and chronic coughs; also in farcy and worms; and to increase the appetite and digestion. The dose is ½ dr. to 2 dr.; but according to MOIROUD, may be carried to 2 oz. for the horse, and 2 or 3 oz. for horned cattle. Externally it is applied to indolent tumours, &c.

ASTRINGENTS. Medicines which produce a more obvious and decided constriction of the muscular fibres than the simple tonics.

BALSAMS. Natural balsams appear to act on the mucous membrane generally; but are chiefly given as diuretics and expectorants. See Balsam of Canada, copaiva, Peru, &c.

BALSAM OF CANADA. Diuretic. Dose ½ oz. to 1 oz.

BALSAM OF COPAIVA. As a diuretic to horses, ½ oz. to 1 oz. as an expectorant in chronic coughs, 1 or 2 dr. For dogs, ½ dr. to 1 dr.

BALSAM, FRYAR'S. Comp. Tincture of Benzoin. It is sometimes given in ½-oz. doses to horses, in chronic coughs, mixed with yelk of egg, gruel, or linseed tea. But more frequently applied to wounds, indolent ulcers, &c.

BALSAM OF LUCATELLI. Dose, ½ oz. in old coughs.

BALSAM OF TOLU, AND OF PERU. 2 dr. in old coughs; but too expensive.

BALSAM OF SULPHUR. A stimulating expectorant in old coughs, in doses of ½ oz. to 1 oz. Sometimes used as an outward application.

BARBADOES TAR. Stimulant, diuretic, and expectorant. Dose, 1 to 4 dr. or more (2 to 4 ounces—MORTON,) in old coughs, and chronic chest affections. Externally in skin diseases, wounds, grease, &c.

BARK, PERUVIAN. Tonic, astringent, antiseptic, and antiperiodic. Dose for a horse, 6 or 8 dr. [to 2 or 3 oz. —MOIROUD] in diabetes, general weakness, a tendency to gangrene, &c. To small animals, 1 or 2 dr. Applied also to indolent and foul ulcers.

BARLEY. The decoction (of Scotch or pearled barley in preference) is given as an emollient, demulcent, or diluent drink in inflammatory diseases; more frequently as a vehicle for more active remedies.

BARYTES. All its compounds are poisonous. The following doses have been given in farcy and glanders:—Muriate of barytes, 20 gr. gradually increased to 60; pure barytes, 10 to 20 gr.; carbonate 1 to 4 gr. A dog was killed by 15 gr.

BASILICON, YELLOW AND BLACK. *Resin Cerate.* See V. Formulary (Digestive Ointments.)

BAY BERRIES. Stomachic and carminative. An ingredient in diapente, but rarely given alone. Dose of the powdered berries, ½ oz., or of the oil of bays, ½ dr. to a dr. The leaves are used in fomentations.

BELLADONNA. *Deadly Nightshade.* Narcotic and sedative. Dose, of the extract from 1 to 4 dr., in diseases where there is undue action of the nervous and vascular systems, [MAVOR.] M. MOIROUD directs from 6 to 8 dr. of the powder. For dogs, from 2 to 8 gr. of the powder. The extract is also applied to the eye, to dilate the pupil.

BENNET, HERB. *Avens.* Tonic and astringent. Dose, of the powdered root ½ oz. to 1 oz or more.

BENZOIN. Stimulant and expectorant. Dose, 1 to 3 dr. But seldom used. Externally it is applied, in balsamic tinctures, to wounds, ulcers, &c. See Tincture of Benzoin.

BIRTHWORT. A gentle stimulant, supposed to act especially on the uterine system. Dose, ½ oz. It is given to cows in cleansing drinks, but it is of doubtful utility.

BISTORT ROOT. Astringent. Dose, 4 to 8 dr. [or 2 oz., MOIROUD.] The decoction is used also as an astringent and cleansing lotion.

BITTER-SWEET. *Dulcamara.* Diuretic, narcotic, and alterative. Dose, ½ oz. in decoction.

BITTER APPLE. See Colocynth.

BLEEDING. The quantity of blood usually abstracted from the horse is from 2 to 4, or, in some cases, 6 or 8 quarts; or until faintness is produced. From cattle, from 2 to 6 quarts, or till faint. Sheep, 16 ounces. Lambs, 4 oz. Dogs, in the proportion of 1 oz. for every 3 lb. weight. [Or 1 or 2 oz. from a very small dog; 7 or 8 oz. from a larger one.—Mr. YOUATT.]

BLISTERING FLY. See Cantharides. BLISTERS are applied in the form of ointments, or liniments, to excite superficial inflammation, followed by vesication; and are intended to draw away inflammatory action from more deeply-seated, but not distant parts. Also to excite the action of the absorbents, and to promote suppuration. See Blistering Ointment, and Liquid Blister, in the Formulary.

BLUE VITRIOL. See Copper, Sulphate of.

BOLE, ARMENIAN. Slightly astringent, and absorbent. Dose, ½ oz. to 2 oz., in diarrhœa, bloody urine, &c. A common ingredient in drenches to dry the milk of cows; dose, 1 to 3 oz. It is also used outwardly as an astringent and desiccative.

BORAGE. A decoction of the plant is pectoral and demulcent.

BORAX. Detergent. Applied to sore mouths, mixed with honey. It is supposed to be a uterine stimulant, but is not often used in veterinary practice as an internal remedy.

BOX LEAVES. They are given, chopped with corn, as a vermifuge. They are also used as a preventive of hydrophobia. (See the V. Formulary.) The rasped wood is considered sudorific, and prescribed in rheumatic and skin diseases, and even in farcy and glanders.

BRAN. Mucilaginous, and slightly laxative: given in mashes.

BRANDY. See Spirits, Ardent.

BRIONY. White briony root is poisonous. ½ oz. killed a dog.

BROMINE. Poisonous. 5 gr. killed a dog. Its medical use is not well ascertained, but appears analogous to that of iodine.

BROOM. The Spanish broom, and particularly the seeds, are supposed to produce inflammation of the bladder in sheep and cattle.

BUCKBEAN. A bitter tonic and purgative. The powdered plant has been given to sheep for rot, in 1-dr. doses.—[Dr. PARIS.]

BUCKWHEAT. Slightly laxative, but chiefly used to fatten poultry.

BUCKTHORN. Purgative; principally administered to dogs. Dose of the juice, 2 or 3 dr.; but it is usually given in the form of Syrup. See Syrup of Buckthorn. The berries are more active, but seldom employed.

BURDOCK. Diuretic and sudorific. Used, but rarely, in rheumatism, and skin diseases.

BURGUNDY PITCH. Similar to resin in its properties. It is chiefly used outwardly, in charges, &c.

BUTTER OF ANTIMONY. *Chloride of Antimony.* See Antimony, Muriate of.

CABBAGE TREE BARK. Vermifuge. Dose for a horse, 2 to 4 dr. But rarely used.

CALAMINE, OR LAPIS CALAMINARIS. Slightly astringent, drying, and healing. Sprinkled on excoriations and sores; and used in ointments, lotions, eye-waters, &c. The greater part of what is sold is factitious, and only calculated to do harm.

CALAMUS AROMATICUS. *Sweet flag.* A warm stomachic. Dose, from 1 oz. to 2 or 3 oz. in infusion.

CALOMEL. Alterative, vermifuge, sialogogue, purgative; it also increases the action of diuretics and diaphoretics. In doses of 1 or 2 dr., [20 to 60 grains, YOUATT,] combined with or followed by aloes, it is given to horses for worms; or from 10 to 20 gr. as an alterative, in skin diseases, grease, farcy, constitutional affections, &c. If too often repeated, it salivates. It does not agree with cattle (see Mercury,) but is sometimes given, in doses of from 10 to 20 gr., in inflammation of the liver, and jaundice. Some writers mention much larger doses. On dogs it acts as a purgative, and often as an emetic, and it is very apt to salivate. The same applies to swine. Dose for dogs, 1 or 2 gr. [Never exceeding 3.—YOUATT.] Many dogs are destroyed with calomel.

Hogs require 3 to 5 gr. Poultry should not have more than a grain, in divided doses, in the day,

CALUMBA. Tonic. Dose of the powdered root, from 2 to 4 dr.

CAMPHOR is reputed antispasmodic, narcotic, and diuretic. It assists the action of diaphoretics; is frequently added to fever medicines to allay irritation; and is used as an antiseptic in malignant epidemics, &c. Mr. SPOONER combines it with opium in cases of lock-jaw. Dose, 1 or 2 dr. MOIROUD says 2 to 12 dr. Its use is questionable where active inflammation exists. Externally it is used as a discutient and anodyne, in embrocations, eye-waters, &c. Its vapours are thought to act favourably on old coughs.

CANELLA BARK. A warm tonic. Dose, for horses, 2 to 4 dr.; for cattle, 2 to 6 dr.

CANTHARIDES. Stimulant and diuretic. Mr. VINES says, "Of all medicines given for farcy and glanders none equal cantharides;" but they should not be given too early, nor without due caution. [Mr. BLAINE.] Dose, in debility, 3 to 5 gr.; in dropsy, farcy, and glanders, 5 to 8 gr. daily, gradually increasing the dose to 15 grs., suspending their use for a time when their diuretic effect is manifest. Of the tincture, 2 to 3 dr. in incontinence of urine; and from ½ oz. to 2 oz. in red water. The practice of giving cantharides as a venereal stimulant is reprobated by the best authorities. Externally it is used in blistering and stimulating ointments and liniments. It does not permanently blemish, but this effect is often produced by other ingredients combined with it in blistering ointments.

CAPSICUM. Cayenne pepper. A hot stimulant. From 10 to 20 grs. may be given in weakness of the stomach, and from 20 to 60 grs. in flatulent colic, or in severe colds. It is also used externally as a stimulant.

CARBONATE OF AMMONIA; Carbonate of potash; and carbonate of soda. See Ammonia, carbonate; potash, subcarbonate; soda, subcarbonate.

CARAWAY SEEDS. Carminative and stomachic. Dose, ½ oz. to 1 oz.; or double that quantity to cattle. Used in cordial balls and drenches; and often added to purgatives, to prevent griping. The essential oil is used for the same purposes, in doses of 10 to 30 drops. Mr. YOUATT considers caraway and ginger the only cordials required for the horse.

CARDAMOM SEEDS. Carminative. Dose, 1 to 4 dr.

CARMINATIVES are stimulants which by their rapid impression on the stomach, &c., occasion the expulsion of wind, and relief of pain.

CARROTS. Restorative and alterative. Given to horses as food after severe illnesses; and in coughs, grease, foul humours, &c. Externally in poultices.

CASCARILLA. A warm, bitter tonic. Dose, 2 or 3 dr.

CASSIA. A warm stimulant. Dose, 1 to 2 dr.

CASTOR. Antispasmodic. ½ oz. has been given in locked jaw. But rarely used.

CASTOR OIL. Laxative. It is uncertain as a purgative for the horse, and sometimes produces much irritation in large doses. ½ pint may be given every six hours till it operates, with watery solution of aloes. Cattle require a pound, or pint; calves, 2 to 4 oz.; sheep and swine, 1 to 2 oz.; dogs, 2 to 4 dr., with syrup of buckthorn. The seeds are more active: from 2 to 6 are sometimes given to swine and dogs, crushed and mixed with food; but from their effects on man, their use would seem to require caution.

CATECHU. *Terra Japonica.* Astringent. Dose for a horse, in diabetes, diarrhœa, &c., 1 or 2 dr. [YOUATT,] or to 1 oz. [BLAINE;] cattle, 2 to 4 dr. in gruel. [It is usually combined with chalk, opium, and gum.—YOUATT.] Dogs require from 10 to 40 gr. In India it is said to be given in doses of 2 oz., for the purpose of taming vicious horses. The tincture is useful in promoting the healing of wounds.

CATHARTICS. Purgatives (which see.)

CAUSTICS. Solid or liquid substances which burn or destroy the part to which they are applied. The *actual cautery* consists in burning with an iron heated to whiteness.

CHALK. Antacid and astringent. Horses require from ½ oz. to 1 oz.; cattle, 1 or 2 oz.; sheep and swine, 1 dr.; dogs, 10 to 20 gr. It is often combined with catechu. Externally it is sprinkled on sores.

CHAMOMILE. A mild tonic, stomachic, and febrifuge. Dose, 1 to 4 dr. of the powdered flowers, or an infusion of ½ oz. of the flowers in a quart of water, in debility of the stomach, flatulence, and in the last stage of fevers, and influenza. It is the first tonic that should be used in convalescence. Ginger, or some other aromatic, is usually joined with it.

CHARCOAL. Antiseptic. Used as an application to foul ulcers, either sprinkled on them, or mixed with poultices.

CHARGES. Compositions of an adhesive nature, usually mixed with tow, which adhere to the part to which they are applied for some time. See V. Formulary.

CHLORATE OF POTASH. Mr. MORTON states that Mr. SIMONDS found it useful in hoven and tympanitis. Dose, 1 to 2 dr.

CHLORIDE OF LIME. Antiseptic and disinfectant. From 2 to 4 dr. in a quart of water, given to horses in flatulent colic, and to cattle in hoven; and in putrescent diseases. Externally, as a wash for mange, foul ulcers, &c., and as a disinfectant, ½ oz. to be well mixed with a pint of water, and after a time decanted or strained.

CHLORIDE OF POTASH. *Eau de Javelle.* Recommended by French authors for the same purposes as the chlorides of lime and soda. Dose, for hoven or tympanitis, ½ oz. to 1 oz.; for sheep, ¼ oz., in water, with or without the addition of ether.

CHLORIDE OF SODA. Labarraque's Disinfecting Solution. The properties and uses are the same as chloride of lime; it is perhaps better adapted for internal use. Dose, 2 to 4 dr. of the solution, gradually increased to 1 oz. or more, largely diluted. It has been tried in glanders. As a lotion, about 1 oz. to a pint of water.

CHLORINE. Antiseptic. A strong watery solution of chlorine gas is antiseptic—in large doses poisonous. It is used for the same purposes as the chlorides of lime, potash, and soda, but the latter are preferable.

CHLORIDE OF ANTIMONY. See Antimony, Butter of.

CHLORIDE OF ZINC. It is a powerful caustic. A diluted solution is used as a disinfectant.

CHLOROFORM. Used to produce insensibility to pain in the same manner as ether; and as a remedy for Tetanus.

CINCHONA. See Bark, Peruvian.

CINNABAR AND VERMILION. Native and factitious red sulphuret of mercury. Alterative and vermifuge? Dose, $\frac{1}{2}$ oz. daily to horses, in skin diseases and obstinate coughs. Formerly given in larger doses, as a vermifuge. Cinnabar of Antimony, so called from the mode of preparation, does not differ from common vermilion in its properties. Care must be taken to get pure vermilion, as this compound, being used as a pigment, is sometimes adulterated with red-lead and other poisonous matters.

CINNAMON. Stimulant and carminative. Dose, 2 dr.; but cassia is usually substituted for it.

CLOVES. A hot stimulant, cordial, and carminative. Dose, 1 to 3 drachms in powder; or from 10 to 20 drops of the oil; the latter is a frequent adjunct to purging balls, to prevent griping. Cloves are also an ingredient in Masticatories.

CLYSTERS. These are injected into the rectum by a proper syringe, or a bladder and pipe, either to unload the bowels, abate inflammation and pain, or to act on the system generally, when medicines cannot be given by the mouth. See V. Formulary.

COLCHICUM. Poisonous to most animals. A diuretic and drastic purgative, chiefly used in rheumatic affections. Dr. LEMANN found it useful in constitutional ophthalmia, and in pneumonia, in doses of a drachm, twice a day, with nitre. According to M. MOIROUD, the dose for larger animals is from 1 to 2 dr. For smaller 6 or 8 gr.

COLOCYNTH. Bitter apple. It has little effect on the horse. It is purgative to dogs, and in large doses poisonous.

CONFECTION OF OPIUM. Anodyne and carminative. Dose, 4 to 6 dr., in flatulent colic.

CONFECTION OF ROSES. Slightly astringent; but only used to form astringent powders, &c., into balls. Masses formed with it retain their consistence well.

COPAIVA. See Balsam of Copaiva.

COPPER. All the compounds of this metal are poisonous. In small doses they are tonic. The antidotes are white of eggs, milk, iron filings, or hydrated sulphuret of iron.

COPPER, ACETATE OF. Crystallized (commonly called *dis-*

tilled) verdigris. Caustic and cleansing. Stronger than common verdigris.

COPPER, DIACETATE OF. See Verdigris.

COPPER, DINIODIDE OF. Tonic, and promotes absorption. Dose, 1 or 2 dr. daily, in farcy, glanders, swelled legs, &c., and topically, to ill-conditioned ulcers.

COPPER, NITRATE OF. Sometimes used as a caustic.

COPPER, SULPHATE OF. *Blue Vitriol.* Tonic and styptic. In doses of ½ dr. gradually increased to 2 dr. or more daily, it is given in diabetes, farcy, &c. Small doses may be given in balls with gentian and ginger; larger doses in gruel. It has been thought useful in glanders; but Mr. YOUATT says it is only proper in nasal discharges without fever. Dose for cattle, 1 to 2 dr., Sheep, 20 to 40 gr., Rabbits (in sniffles,) 1 or 2 gr. twice a day. Externally the solution is used for the foot-rot of sheep: and as a cleansing wash for foul ulcers in horses and cattle. Used also in the solid state to destroy proud flesh.

COPPER, AMMONIO-SULPHATE OF. Tonic and astringent; dose, 1 to 2 dr. twice or thrice a day.

CORDIALS. Warm stimulating medicines, such as spices, and the aromatic seeds, fermented liquors and spirits, &c., which temporarily restore exhausted strength, revive the spirits, and rouse the system generally. The best modern practitioners condemn their indiscriminate employment as the source of much mischief. For cordial balls, &c., see V. Formulary.

CORIANDER SEEDS. A mild aromatic stimulant and carminative, used in cordial balls and drinks. Dose, ½ oz. to 1 oz.

CORROSIVE SUBLIMATE. One of the most virulent poisons. In small doses it is alterative and diuretic. It has been tried, in doses of 2 to 5 gr., gradually increased to 10 or 20, in farcy and glanders, but rarely with lasting benefit. Externally it is used as a powerful caustic. A dilute solution is employed as a wash for scab and lice in sheep, but the practice is not free from danger. Applied to wounds in cattle it has proved as fatal a poison as when swallowed. The antidote for an overdose is white of egg, or milk, or the hydrated sulphuret of iron; with demulcent drinks.

COWHAGE. Vermifuge; but has little effect on the horse.

CREAM OF TARTAR. Cooling, laxative, and diuretic. Seldom given alone; but combined with antimonials, mercurials, or sulphur, as an alterative in skin diseases; and used as an adjunct to aloes in purging balls. Cattle require 2 or 3 oz.; when given in larger doses it should be given in plenty of warm water. Sheep require ½ oz. to 1 oz. Dogs, 5 to 20 grains.

CREASOTE. Tonic, stimulant, and antiseptic. Dose, 20 to 30 drops daily, in gruel or linseed tea, in glanders. Externally in lotions and ointments, to fistulous wounds, unhealthy ulcers, &c.

CROCUS OF ANTIMONY. See Antimony, liver of.

CROTON SEEDS AND OIL. Purgative. The oil produces great irritation in the horse. Dose, about 20 drops: 30 drops have proved fatal. The powdered seeds, and the meal or ground cake left after expressing the oil, are also used; 3 gr. of the former and 5 of the latter being considered equivalent to 1 dr. of aloes. It operates with less certainty, and produces more debility, than aloes, but is sometimes preferred on account of its more speedy action. It is usually given in the form of a ball, 20 or 30 gr. being mixed with 1 oz. linseed meal. Mr. NORTON gives from 12 to 24 grains of the seed. Mr. YOUATT prescribes 30 gr. of the powdered seeds in a drink, in tetanus and brain fever, followed by smaller doses (10 gr.) every 6 hours. It will purge rapidly when placed upon the tongue, but is then likely to inflame the mouth. From 10 to 20 gr. are sometimes added to salts in purging drenches for cattle, in extreme cases. One drop of the oil purges a dog freely.

CUMMIN SEED. A warm carminative. Dose, from 1 to 4 dr. of the powdered seeds; or from 6 to 20 drops of the oil.

CUSPARIA, OR ANGUSTURA BARK. An aromatic bitter tonic. Dose, 1 to 4 dr. in debility, diabetes, diarrhœa, &c.

CYANIDE OF POTASSIUM. It possesses the same poisonous and medicinal properties as prussic acid. M. LAFORE has given it with success in a case of idiopathic tetanus of the horse; but it failed to cure traumatic tetanus. Dose, 4 gr.

DAFFY'S ELIXIR. Sometimes given in colic or gripes.

DALBY'S CARMINATIVE. Given to calves, in diarrhœa. Dose, ½ a bottle.

DETERGENTS, OR DETERSIVES. Remedies which cleanse foul ulcers.

DIAPENTE. A compound powder, reputed cordial and stomachic. Too much of what is sold in the shops is almost worthless. Dose, ½ oz. to 1 oz.

DIAPHORETICS. Medicines which promote perspiration.

DIGESTIVES. Mildly stimulating applications, which excite healthy action in indolent ulcers, wounds, &c.

DIGITALIS. *Fox-glove.* Sedative and diuretic. It reduces the frequency of the pulse and diminishes irritability. It is poisonous to animals generally; 6 gr. will kill a dog. It is asserted, however, that it produces no effect on poultry. The common dose of the powdered leaves, for a horse, is from 10 to 30 gr. Mr. YOUATT prescribes 60 gr., with emetic tartar and nitre, in inflammation of the chest; but its effect on the pulse must be carefully watched. To cattle, ½ dr. to 1 dr. Sheep, 5 to 15 gr. Dogs, 1 to 2 gr. An infusion of the leaves is applied to inflamed eyes.

DIURETICS. Medicines which increase the flow of urine. Some of them, juniper, capivi, squills, broom, &c., appear to carry off water only; while the alkaline salts remove solid matters also, and thus purify the blood. Diuretics are employed to lessen the quantity of the circulating fluid in fevers and inflammations. The legs of many horses cannot be kept fine, nor the grease be subdued, without the use of diuretics. Plenty of water should be allowed with them. But their too frequent use is injurious.

DOG-GRASS. It is emetic to dogs.

DOVER'S POWDER. Sudorific to cattle in rheumatism. Dose, 1 dr.

EGGS. Nutritive and demulcent. Sometimes given in diarrhœa. They constitute the best antidote to poisoning by corrosive sublimate.

ELATERIUM. It has little effect on the horse.

ELDER. An infusion of the flowers is given in catarrhal complaints. The leaves boiled with lard form an emollient ointment, which is a common application to sore udders. The fresh leaves of the dwarf elder are given (according to BOURGELAT and MOIROUD) with some success as a deobstruent and aperient, in swelled legs, dropsy, and farcy.

ELECAMPANE. The root is reputed stimulant, diaphoretic, diuretic, stomachic, and expectorant. Dose, 4 to 8 dr. in chronic catarrh, dropsical swellings, indigestion, &c.

EMETIC TARTAR. See Antimony, Tartarized.

EMETICS. Medicines which excite vomiting. It is scarcely possible to produce this effect in herbivorous animals.

EMOLLIENTS. Medicines which soften and relax the tissues of the organs.

EPSOM SALT. A cooling laxative. It is not to be depended on as a purgative for the horse; but in doses of 4 or 5 oz., in a large quantity of water, repeated 3 times a day, it is useful as a laxative and diuretic in inflammatory diseases. Cattle require from 12 to 20 oz., with ginger or any of the warm seeds. It is sometimes rendered more active by aloes or gamboge. Calves require from 1 to 2 oz., according to their age and strength. Sheep, ½ oz. to 2 oz. Dogs, from 1 to 3 dr. wrapped in tissue paper. A large elephant takes a pound and a half, preceded by a dr. of calomel.—YOUATT.

ERGOT OF RYE. It promotes parturition. Dose for a mare, 2 or 3 dr. A cow, 2 dr. repeated at intervals of half an hour. An ewe, 20 to 40 gr. Bitch, 5 to 10 gr. [Mr. SPOONER says from 2 to 4 gr.,] or an infusion of a scruple given at three times, at intervals of half an hour. Larger doses than the above are indicated by M. MOIROUD.

ERRHINES. Remedies which excite a discharge from the nostrils.

ESCHAROTICS. Caustics. Substances which destroy the surface to which they are applied.

ETHER. A diffusible stimulant and antispasmodic; used chiefly in colic. Dose, ½ oz. to ¾ oz.; cattle, ½ oz. to 1 oz.; dogs, 7 to 14 drops. It is used outwardly in cooling lotions and eye-waters. The vapour, inhaled by means of a proper apparatus, produces insensibility to pain;

but some of the early experiments with this agent have proved most unfortunate.

ETHIOPS MINERAL. The mildest of the mercurial compounds. Alterative and vermifuge. Dose, 2, to 4 dr. daily in farcy, glanders, grease, skin diseases, and worms, alone, or with cream of tartar. For cattle, 1 dr.; swine, 3 to 10 gr.; dogs, 5 gr. in mange. With an equal weight of prepared antimony it forms Antimonial Ethiops —a more efficient preparation.

EUPHORBIUM. Very acrid and poisonous. Used in blisters, chiefly to economize the more expensive flies; but irritates extremely. It is employed in the form of tincture and ointment as a local stimulant.

EXCITANTS. Medicines which quicken the circulation, produce warmth, and render the organs more active.

FENNEL SEEDS. A weak carminative and diuretic. Dose, ½ oz. to 2 oz.

FERN. Powdered male fern is given in doses of 6 dr., followed by a mercurial purgative, for expelling worms. M. MOIROUD carries the dose to 4 oz.; or 5 or 6 dr. for smaller animals.

FŒNUGREEK SEEDS. Emollient, nutritive, and stomachic. Dose, 1 oz. daily, to promote condition in horses, and in diseases of the chest. It is also added to the food of swine, to promote their fattening. Used also externally in fomentations.

FORGE WATER. The water of the blacksmith's forge is sometimes given as a tonic, or applied as a wash to ulcerated and cankered mouth.

FOXGLOVE. See Digitalis.

GALANGAL ROOT. A warm aromatic; similar in properties to ginger. Dose, ½ oz. of the powder, or 1 oz. in infusion.

GALBANUM. Stimulant, expectorant, and antispasmodic. Dose, 2 to 4 dr. But rarely used, assafœtida being stronger and cheaper.

GALL NUTS. Astringent; in diarrhœa. Dose of the powder for horses and cattle, 2 to 4 dr. Calves, ½ dr. to 1 dr., Dogs, 4 to 8 grains.

GAMBOGE. A drastic purgative. The dose for a horse is said to be from 2 to 6 dr., but its purgative effect cannot be depended on, and it gripes. 3 dr. have been known to cause great prostration, and the horse being killed, marks of intense inflammation were found in its stomach and bowels. It is a bad medicine for herbivorous animals. 2 dr. are sometimes added to salts and other purgatives for cattle. Sheep have been killed by 2 dr. A few grains are given to dogs, to destroy and expel worms.

GARLIC. A stimulating expectorant. Dose, 1 oz. in chronic coughs and asthmatic complaints, made into balls with liquorice powder; or boiled in milk. It is a common remedy for coughs and chest affections in all domestic animals. It is also reputed vermifuge. For the roup in fowls it is given in doses of 5 gr.

GENTIAN ROOT. Tonic and stomachic; in debility, after severe illness, &c. Dose for a horse, 2, 3, or 4 dr. of the powder; or from ½ dr. to 1 dr. of the extract. (See V. Formulary, Tonic Balls.) Cattle, 2 to 4 dr. or more. Sheep, 20 to 60 gr. Generally joined with ginger. An infusion is recommended as a wash to ulcers.

GINGER. Stimulant and carminative: a general ingredient in cordial and tonic medicines. Dose, 1 to 3 dr., or in flatulent colic, 2 to 6 dr. Cattle, 2 to 6 dr. Calves, 20 to 30 gr. Sheep, 30 to 60 gr. The smaller of the above doses may be added to all aperient medicines. It is also used as a masticatory. Dose of the tincture, ½ oz. to 2 oz.

GLASS, POWDERED. Used to destroy worms in dogs. Mr. BLAINE recommends as much as will lie on a sixpence, with butter.

GLAUBER'S SALT. *Sulphate of Soda.* Aperient and diuretic. Seldom given to horses as a purgative (Mr. CLARKE says 1 ℔. produces scarcely any effect;) but is said to be useful, in doses of 6 oz. 3 times a day, in epidemic catarrh. To cattle the usual dose is 16 oz., or from 12 to 20 oz., with ginger or caraway. It is considered more diuretic than Epsom salt.

GOULARD'S EXTRACT OF LEAD. *Solution of Diacetate of Lead.* Cooling and astringent. Used externally only, in lotions, &c., in the same cases as sugar of lead. (See Lead, Acetate of.) For inflamed eyes, 1 dr. or 1½ to a pint of water: for other purposes it is made stronger.

GRAINS OF PARADISE. A warm stimulant; chiefly used in cattle medicines. Dose, 3 to 6 dr.

GRUEL. A decoction of oatmeal. Nutritive and demulcent.

GUAIACUM [GUM.] Sudorific and expectorant. It has been given to horses, in doses of 4 dr., in chest affections, farcy, rheumatism, &c.; and to cattle in doses of 4 or 6 dr. But its utility is doubted. The guaiacum wood is given to the amount of 4 oz., in decoction, repeated 2 or 3 times in 24 hours.

GUM ARABIC. Emollient and demulcent. Used in inflammatory affections of the bowels, or of the respiratory or urinary organs. Dose, for horses and cattle, 1 to 4 oz., dissolved in water. For smaller animals, from $\frac{1}{4}$ oz. to 1 oz. It is also used to suspend in water insoluble powders and oils. Gum senegal and gum tragacanth are used for the same purposes. The latter will thicken twenty times as much water as Gum Arabic. [For Gum Ammoniac, Benzoin, &c., see Ammoniacum, Benzoin, &c.]

HARTSHORN, SPIRIT OF. See Ammonia. It is chiefly used in stimulating liniments, and for the bites and stings of venomous reptiles and insects. For salt of hartshorn, see Ammonia, Carbonate of.

HELLEBORE, WHITE. Poisonous to all classes of animals. In small doses, it has been strongly recommended as a nauseant and diaphoretic, in inflammatory diseases; but it requires to be very carefully watched, otherwise a fatal collapse may be induced. The usual dose is 20 gr. every four or six hours till nausea is produced, or the pulse affected. Mr. YOUATT says it cannot safely be given in doses of a drachm, but that it is given with advantage in ounce doses in chronic grease. Externally, it is used in ointments and washes for the mange; but even in this way its use requires caution. It is also blown into the nostrils as a sternutatory.

HELLEBORE, BLACK. The root is used as an irritating seton for cattle, and introduced into fistulous sores of the horse.

HEMLOCK, SPOTTED. A narcotic poison. In doses of a drachm of the powdered leaves, or the extract, gradually increased, it is sometimes given to quiet obstinate coughs. It is also an ingredient in some old remedies for farcy, scirrhous tumours, and cancer. For dogs, from 1 to 4 gr., in coughs and cancerous diseases. A decoction of the herb is used as a fomentation to painful tumours. Water hemlock is a more virulent poison, and often destroys cattle. M. MOIROUD says that ruminants bear hemlock better than other animals. Mr. YOUATT considers both common and water hemlock harmless to the horse, though he admits that cows have been poisoned by the latter.

HENBANE. Narcotic and sedative. Dose, 15 to 20 gr. of the powder [1 to 2 dr. of the extract, MORTON] twice or three times a day, to allay arterial action. On dogs it acts as on man: dose, 3 to 5 gr. German horse-dealers are said to give a plump appearance to diseased horses by mixing henbane seeds with their corn.

HONEY. Demulcent, emollient, and slightly laxative. Used in cough medicines, and to make up balls. Horses are fond of it. Externally, it is detergent, and is perhaps useful in defending ulcers from the air.

HOPS. Tonic and slightly anodyne, but chiefly used in fomentations.

HOREHOUND. Sometimes given in coughs; a quart of the decoction, or 1 oz. of the powder.

HORSERADISH. Stimulant and diuretic. Said to be useful in dropsical complaints, and in recent epidemics attended with chronic inflammation. The fresh root is rasped and mixed with barley meal.

IODINE. Alterative, and promotes absorption. Used externally and internally to reduce glandular swellings, and scirrhous and other tumours. 5 gr. of iodine, or 1½ or 2 dr. of the compound tincture, may be given twice a day in farcy. Cattle take from 5 to 10 gr., and from 1 to 2 dr. of the compound tincture. Dogs, ¼ to 1 gr. twice daily. The compound iodine ointment is used to disperse glandular enlargements. It is rapidly superseding cantharides.

IODIDE OF IRON. Tonic and alterative, promoting the action of the absorbents. Dose, ½ dr. to 1 dr.

IODIDE OF POTASSIUM, OR HYDRIODATE OF POTASH. It possesses the same properties as iodine, but irritates less.

It is often combined with iodine, which it renders soluble in water. The dose by itself, is rather larger than of iodine—from 15 to 30 gr. twice a day: to cattle, 5 to 10 grains.

IPECACUANHA. Little used in veterinary practice, except as a sudorific, in combination with opium (Dover's powder.) A drachm or two may be given to horses in asthmatic affections. It purges sheep, purges or vomits the pig and dog. Dose for the latter, 4 to 20 gr. [From 2 to 30 gr.—MOIROUD.] 3 oz. killed a horse [Mr. B. CLARKE.]

IRON. The preparations of this metal are tonic; some of them (as the sulphate or muriate) astringent and styptic. The usual doses for a horse are, 2 oz. of iron filings, once or twice a day, with corn, or in a mash; 1 to 3 or 4 dr. of the sulphate; 2 to 6 dr. of the sesqui-oxide or carbonate, or of rust of iron, or of the powdered scales; 1 to 3 dr. of tartarized iron; and ½ to 1½ dr. of the iodide. Cattle, 2 to 4 dr. of the sulphate in chronic diarrhœa. For sheep, a sixth or eighth of the above doses. [M. MOIROUD prescribes much larger doses of the above.] The muriated tincture of iron is prescribed in doses of 2 or 3 dr. for incontinence of urine. The sulphate is sometimes used externally in astringent lotions.

JALAP. Purgative, but has little or no such effect on the horse, or other herbivorous animals. It is sometimes added to other purgatives, but probably without any benefit. Dose for swine, ½ dr. to 2 dr. Dogs, 15 to 40 gr. Cats, 10 to 20 gr.; but it is rather uncertain.

JAMAICA PEPPER. See Allspice.

JAMES'S POWDER. Similar to antimonial powder, but considered more certain and uniform in its operation. Dose, 20 to 30 gr., in fevers and inflammatory complaints. It is also given to dogs as a remedy for distemper, 4 gr. twice a day.

JATROPHA SEEDS. The seeds of the physic nut (J. curcas) are given as croton seeds, doubling the dose.

JUNIPER BERRIES. Diuretic and slightly stimulant. Dose for a horse, 1 to 2 oz., or 1 to 2 dr. of the essential oil; for cows, 2 or 3 oz.; sheep, ¼ to ½ oz. An extract from the berries (prepared by evaporating a clear decoction, or rather a cold infusion of the berries, to the consistence of treacle) is much used on the Continent as a vehicle for various remedies.

KERMES' MINERAL. A preparation of antimony, similar to the precipitated sulphuret, not much used in this country, but highly esteemed in France. Dose for horses, 1, 2, or 3 dr. For cattle, 4 dr. or more. For a good-sized dog, 1½ gr., gradually increased.

LARD. Half a pound, with warm water, is laxative and emollient. It is also used to make up balls, and is thought to prevent griping, as well as to preserve their consistence. It forms a common basis for ointments.

LAUDANUM. *Tincture of Opium.* See Opium.

LAVENDER. The compound spirit is carminative and cordial. Dose, ½ oz. in peppermint water.

LEAD. The preparations of this metal are poisonous. See Acetate of Lead, and Goulard's Extract of Lead.

LEAD, WHITE AND RED. Common ingredients in ointments and plasters. Also sprinkled on sores as desiccatives. They are likewise used for dusting sheep for the fly.

LIME. Quicklime is sometimes used as a caustic; the powder dusted over foul ulcers, greasy heels, &c.

LIME WATER. Antacid and tonic. Sometimes given in diabetes, from 2 to 4 quarts. Used also as a wash for sores, and as an injection into the nostrils in glanders and chronic discharges. Mixed with linseed oil, it forms a liniment for burns.

LIME, CHLORIDE OF. See Chloride of Lime.

LINSEED. Demulcent and pectoral. A decoction of the seeds is very mucilaginous, and is used in colds, sore throats, and internal inflammations; also to counteract the effects of corrosive and irritant poisons, and as a vehicle for more active medicines. Linseed meal is used for poultices. Linseed oil is laxative. Dose for a horse, a pint, or a pint and a half; for cattle, 1 or 2 pints; sheep, 2 or 3 oz.

LIQUORICE. Demulcent and pectoral, in coughs, &c. Dose, ½ oz. to 2 oz. of the powdered root; or ½ oz. of the foreign extract (Spanish or Italian juice.)

LIVER OF SULPHUR. See Sulphuret of Potassium.

LOBELIA INFLATA. It is poisonous to horses, and produces salivation in cattle; but its remedial powers have not been ascertained.

LOGWOOD. Astringent. 2 or 3 dr. of the extract, or a decoction of 3 or 4 oz. of the wood, may be given in diarrhœa, &c.

LOTIONS. Washes. Liquid applications, with which external parts are bathed.

MADDER. Formerly supposed to be useful in glanders and farcy, and as a preventive of the effects of the bites of venomous reptiles; but it is nearly discarded from modern practice. It is sometimes given to pigs, but with what specific intention it is difficult to say. It colours the bones of animals fed with it.

MAGNESIA. Antacid and laxative. From ½ oz. to 3 oz. to horses and cattle, with some warm carminative in flatulent distention. To calves in diarrhœa, ½ oz. Either the common or the calcined magnesia may be used.

MAGNESIA, SULPHATE OF. See Epsom Salt.

MALLOW. Demulcent. A handful of the leaves is boiled in a quart of water. More frequently used as a lavement. The *root* of the *marshmallow* is preferred; a decoction of 2 or 4 ounces is given as a drink in both coughs and internal inflammations, and used as a clyster, and as a fomentation.

MALT. Nutritive, pectoral, and alterative. It is given, in the form of mashes, in chest affections, when no inflammation is present, and in grease, farcy and mange.

MANNA. Slightly laxative and pectoral. Dose, 2 oz. with honey, or dissolved in water, in inflammatory diseases and chronic coughs.

MASHES. See Bran Mash, &c., in V. Formulary.

MERCURY, OR QUICKSILVER. The preparations of this metal are alterative, most of them purgative, and all apt to produce salivation. Dogs may easily be salivated, but graminivorous animals with greater difficulty. The editor of "Clater's Cattle Doctor" says, "Mercury does not seem to agree with herbivorous animals, in any form, or in any disease." The preparations in use are indicated below.

MERCURIAL OINTMENT. Applied to callous swellings, enlarged joints, mange, scab in sheep, &c. The weaker ointment is generally sufficient.

MERCURY WITH CHALK. Alkalized Mercury. A mild preparation. Dose, from 1 to 3 dr., in farcy, glanders, &c.

MERCURY, SUBMURIATE, OR CHLORIDE OF. See Calomel.

MERCURY, BICHLORIDE. See Corrosive Sublimate.

MERCURY WITH SULPHUR. Black Sulphuret of Mercury. See Ethiops Mineral.

MERCURY, RED SULPHURET OF. See Cinnabar.

MERCURY, NITRIC OXIDE. See Red Precipitate.

MERCURY, BLACK OXIDE. Dose, 1 to 2 dr. [MORTON.]

MERCURY, AMMONIO-CHLORIDE. See White Precipitate.

MERCURY, NITRATED OINTMENT OF. See Ointment, Citrine.

MERCURY, ACID NITRATE OF. Used as a Caustic. See Caustics, V. Formulary.

MILK. Sometimes given in quantities of 1 to 3 quarts, in acute inflammations, coughs, and all internal irritations, especially those occasioned by acrid and corrosive poisons. It is a convenient vehicle for administering medicines to the dog or cat.

MINDERERUS' SPIRIT. See Acetate of Ammonia.

MINT, AND PEPPERMINT. Carminative, cordial, and sudorific. A strong infusion of the plant, or the distilled water, may be given in flatulent colics. Dose, 1 or 2 pints; but chiefly as vehicles for more active remedies. Dose of the oil of peppermint, 20 to 30 drops, or to 60 drops of oil of spearmint. A few drops of the oil are added to purgative medicines, to prevent griping. The other mints have similar properties.

MITHRIDATE. Cordial and anodyne. ½ oz. to 1 oz. may be given in flatulent colic, but would be injurious in inflammation.

MULLEIN. An infusion of the flowers is given as a demulcent for the same purpose as linseed tea. A decoction of the leaves is used in emollient fomentations and cataplasms.

MURIATIC (OR HYDROCHLORIC) ACID. *Spirit of salt.*

Tonic and antiseptic; but principally used to dissolve calcareous concretions in the bladder. It has been used in the pestilent epidemics of cattle. Dose for a horse, 1½ to 2 or 3 dr., in plenty of water, twice a day. Externally as a caustic, strongly recommended by YOUATT.

MURIATE OF AMMONIA. *Sal Ammoniac.* Formerly used in influenza or epidemic catarrh. It is said also to have proved useful in farcy, and perhaps deserves trial in other chronic diseases. It renders the blood more fluid. Its use requires caution. 2 oz. produced inflammation of the mucous membrane of a horse; 2 drachms killed a dog, and ½ dr. a rabbit. M. MOIROUD states the dose to be from 2 to 8 dr. for horses and cattle, and for small animals from a scruple to a drachm largely diluted. Externally it is a frequent ingredient in discutient lotions to splints, old strains, bruises, indolent tumours, &c. in horses and cattle. It is also employed as an embrocation to sore teats.

MURIATE OF ANTIMONY. See Antimony, butter of.

MURIATE OF BARYTES. Poisonous; in small doses, alterative. It has been tried in glanders and farcy, with the usual ill success. Dose, ½ dr. in milk.

MURIATE OF COPPER. Used externally only as a mild caustic.

MURIATE OF LIME. *Chloride of Calcium.* Alterative and resolvent, in glandular diseases; but rarely used in veterinary practice. It has been proposed in glanders and farcy. In an overdose it is poisonous. We have not met with any specific statement of doses. 3½ drachms killed a dog.

MURIATE OF SODA. *Chloride of Sodium.* See Salt, common.

MUSTARD. Stimulant; but little used as an internal remedy. Flour of mustard, with or without vinegar, is applied externally as a rubefacient, to relieve internal inflammation.

MYRRH. Tonic, expectorant, antiseptic, and balsamic. From 1 to 3 dr. to a horse in chronic cough. To cattle 2 to 4 dr. or more. The tincture is used for ulcers of the mouth in all animals, and to indolent sores.

NAPHTHA. Rectified wood naphtha is used instead of spirit of wine, for making tincture of myrrh and aloes.

NAPHTHALINE. A stimulating expectorant. It possesses many of the properties of camphor, and a solution of it in spirit may be substituted for camphorated spirit, and with oils, &c., for liniments and ointments. The ointment is substituted for tar ointment.

NARCOTICS. Medicines which induce stupor or sleep, and ease pain.

NAUSEANTS. Medicines which produce nausea, diminish arterial action, and thus abate inflammation.

NETTLE SEED. It is said to be given with the horse's corn, to give a smooth coat, and an appearance of condition and liveliness.

NITRE. *Nitrate of Potash.* Cooling and diuretic. In colds, fevers, and inflammatory complaints of the horse, from 2 to 4 dr. may be given daily, in plenty of water, or linseed tea, till the desired effect is produced. An ounce is often given, but smaller doses repeated are better. Cattle 2 to 4 dr. [1 oz. in 24 hours for some days.—MOIROUD.] Swine and sheep, 30 to 40 gr.: dogs, 4 to 10 gr. A strong solution is applied to gangrenous wounds.

NITRIC ACID, NITROUS ACID, AND AQUAFORTIS. Used externally only, as a strong caustic; or largely diluted (2 dr. to a pint of water) as an antiseptic wash to foul ulcers.

NITRATE OF SILVER. *Lunar Caustic.* Tonic; but rarely given to animals, except to dogs in chorea, in doses of $\frac{1}{8}$th to $\frac{1}{4}$ of a gr. Externally caustic. It is the best caustic that can be applied to the bites of rabid animals. A weak solution (10 gr. to 1 oz. rain water) is used to excite sluggish wounds, and to remove opacity from the cornea of the eye.

NUX VOMICA. Poisonous to all animals. Given in doses of 8 or 10 gr., gradually increased to 30 gr., in paralysis of the horse; but its effect requires to be carefully watched. It has been tried in glanders and farcy, but without much success. In small doses it invigorates the digestive functions. A few grains will destroy a dog. A drachm has killed a horse. See Strychnine.

NUTGALLS. See Gall-nuts.

NUTMEGS. Stimulant, and perhaps narcotic. Sometimes given in colic, but not much in use.

OAK BARK. Astringent and tonic. Dose, ½ oz. to 2 oz., in powder, or boiled in water, for diarrhœa, diabetes, and debility in horses. To cattle, in dysentery, and in red-water (after purgatives,) ½ oz. or 1 oz. The powdered bark and the decoction are applied to unhealthy wounds, &c. In France, a mixture of oak-bark, gentian, and chamomile is used as a substitute for Peruvian bark.

OIL, FISH. Common whale oil is a good preventive of the fly, and does not injure the wool.

OIL OF SPIKE. As sold for veterinary purposes it consists of turpentine, coloured, and merely scented with foreign oil of lavender. It is used in warm liniments.

OIL OF TURPENTINE. See Turpentine.

OIL OF TAR. See Tar.

OILS, EXPRESSED. Olive, almond, and linseed oils are laxative, demulcent, and emollient. Dose, 3 to 16 oz., or a pint. In the latter dose they are given (especially linseed oil) as a substitute for castor oil; they are harmless, but rather uncertain in their operation. (See Castor Oil.) They are useful in poisoning by acrid and corrosive poisons. Olive oil is used, both inwardly and outwardly, as a remedy for the bites of reptiles and stings of insects. Externally they are used in liniments and ointments. Oil of bays is gently stimulant and antispasmodic, but chiefly used outwardly.

OILS, ESSENTIAL OR VOLATILE. The essential oils of peppermint, cloves, aniseed, caraway, &c., possess in a concentrated state the warm carminative properties of the drugs from which they are distilled. They are frequently added to purgative medicines to prevent griping. Oil of juniper is diuretic, in doses of 1 to 3 dr. Oil of origanum is almost exclusively used outwardly in stimulating liniments. Oil of bitter almonds is poisonous.

OILS, EMPYREUMATIC. Oil of amber and other empyreumatic oils are antispasmodic; but mostly used in outward applications. The fœtid oil called Dippel's Animal Oil (or oil of hartshorn) is sometimes given as a worm medicine, in doses of 1 oz. (sometimes increased to 2 oz.) to horses, or a drachm to small animals. As an outward application it is sometimes added to powders against the fly in sheep; but injures the wool. Oil of paper or rag is an empyreumatic fluid obtained by burning these substances. Mixed with water it is used in inflammation of the eyes, mouth, &c.

OILS, COMPOUND. See Oils and Liniments in the Veterinary Formulary.

OINTMENTS. See V. Formulary.

OLIVE OIL. See Oils, expressed.

ONIONS. Stimulant and diuretic. They are said to be useful in colic and gripes. Externally used in poultices to promote suppuration.

OPIUM. Anodyne, antispasmodic, sedative, indirectly astringent, and in large doses narcotic or stupefactive, and capable of destroying life. In combination with ipecacuanha and tartarized antimony it is sudorific. The dose for horses in ordinary cases is from ½ dr. to 1 dr. But in locked-jaw, spasmodic colic, and other urgent cases, it may safely be given in doses of 2 dr., and even (according to MOIROUD) to 4 dr. YOUATT states the dose as 1 dr. to 3 dr. In inflammation of the bowels, after bleeding, it is recommended to give 2 dr. at once, and 1 dr. every hour afterwards until it take effect. To cattle, the dose is from 10 to 40 gr.; or in lock-jaw, &c., 1 dr. Calves, 10 gr. Sheep, 2 to 4 gr. Much larger doses have been given with impunity. Dogs require from ½ gr. to 2 gr., according to size and case. M. MOIROUD says the dose for dogs should not exceed that prescribed for man. Mr. BLAINE thinks they are much less affected by it than men. The dose of tincture of opium is (for horses) from 1 to 2 oz.; of the extract, 20 to 30 gr. Externally, opium is used in anodyne liniments, and is useful in inflammation of the eye. See Eye-waters, Liniments, &c., in Vet. Formulary.

OPODELDOC. Soap liniment. Used externally only, in stimulating liniments.

ORIGANUM. Wild Marjoram. Stimulant. The essential

oil is hot and pungent, and a frequent ingredient in liniments for old strains, and in blisters.

ORPIMENT. Yellow Arsenic. Poisonous. Used, mixed with lard, for fistulous sores, warts, &c., but is not free from danger.

OXYMEL. Cooling and pectoral. Used in catarrhal affections. Dose, 3 or 4 oz.

OXYMEL OF SQUILLS. A stimulating expectorant. Seldom used in veterinary practice.

PALM OIL. Emollient. Used in compounding ointments and liniments; and of late much commended as a basis of aloetic and other balls. It has also been given as a laxative; dose, 12 oz. or more.

PEPPERMINT. Carminative. The distilled water and the essential oil are chiefly used. See Mint.

PEPPER, BLACK, WHITE, AND LONG. Warm stimulant cordials. The latter kind is chiefly used in veterinary practice. It must be carefully avoided in inflammatory complaints. Dose for horses and cattle, 2 to 4 dr. For Jamaica Pepper, see Allspice.

PEPPER, CAYENNE. The ground pods of some species of capsicum. See Capsicum.

PERIWINKLE. The plant, in decoction, or chopped up in a mash, is said to relieve quinsy. Pulverized and mixed with Ethiops Mineral, it has been vaunted as a remedy for glanders.

PERUVIAN BARK. See Bark.

PETROLEUM. See Barbadoes Tar.

PEWTER. The scrapings are given to dogs for worms. Dose, ½ dr. to 1 dr. Tin filings are safer. See Tin.

PHELLANDRIUM. The seeds of water-fennel (Ph. aquaticum) are used in Germany in chronic catarrhal affections. Dose, ½ oz. to 1 oz.

PHYSIC. In veterinary practice this term is applied to purgatives. See Physic or Purging Balls, V. Formulary.

PIMENTO. See Allspice.

PITCH. Stimulant, balsamic, probably diuretic: but rarely given internally. It is more frequently used externally in charges and warm plasters. For liquid pitch, see Tar.

PITCH, BURGUNDY. Stimulant. Used in charges, and warm and strengthening plasters.

POMEGRANATE. The rind of the fruit is given (in decoction or powder) as an astringent to cattle in diarrhœa. Dose, from ½ oz. to 1 oz. The bark of the root is used to destroy worms. MOIROUD directs 5 or 6 oz. to be boiled in water for some hours, and the decoction given in divided doses.

POPPY HEADS. Anodyne; but principally used in fomentations. (See also Syrup of Poppies.) An extract prepared by evaporating the expressed juice of the ripe capsules and tops is said to be nearly half the strength of opium. Of the ordinary extract (from the decoction) 5 gr. are said to equal 2 of opium.—LEBAS.

POTASH, CAUSTIC. *Fused Hydrate of Potash.* A powerful caustic.

POTASH, SUBCARBONATE. *Salt of Tartar or prepared Kali.* Antacid and diuretic. Dose for a horse from 2 to 4 dr. or more. It is seldom given alone, but sometimes joined with tonics, stomachics, purgatives, and with other diuretics. The bicarbonate is milder, and may be given in larger doses.

POULTICES. Are useful in relieving inflammation and pain. See V. Formulary.

PRECIPITATE, RED. A mild caustic, and detergent to indolent and foul ulcers.

PRECIPITATE, WHITE. Principally used to destroy vermin in the horse and other animals.

PRUSSIATE OF POTASH. Ferro-prussiate of potash may probably be found useful in veterinary practice; but its properties and uses are not yet precisely ascertained. It must not be confounded with the simple prussiate of potash (cyanide of potassium,) which is an energetic poison. See Cyanide of Potassium.

PRUSSIC ACID (Medicinal.) A strong poison to all animals. Rarely used in veterinary practice. May be given by enema in Tetanus. The dose Mr. MORTON states to be from ½ dr. to 1 dr. Mr. YOUATT recommends a lotion composed of a drachm of the medicinal acid to a pint of water, to allay cuticular irritation in dogs.

PULSE. The following table, from VATEL, is inserted as a useful remembrancer to the practitioner:—

Table of the Number of Pulsations in a Minute in various Animals.—In the horse, 32 to 38 [36 to 40—WHITE;] ox or cow, 35 to 42 [42 to 45—CLATER; 50 to 55 SPOONER;] ass, 48 to 54; sheep, 70 to 79; goat, 72 to 76; dog, 90 to 100; cat, 110 to 120; rabbit, 120; guinea-pig, 140; duck, 136; hen, 140; heron, 200.

PURGATIVES. *Cathartics or Laxatives.* Medicines which more or less actively promote evacuations from the bowels. Aloes is almost the only purgative for the horse that is at once certain and safe. For cattle, Epsom or Glauber's salt is the most preferable. Aloes, gamboge, or linseed or castor oil is sometimes combined with them. Sulphur is used when a very strong purgative is not required; yet this requires some caution. See those various articles.

QUASSIA. A bitter tonic. Dose, 1 or 2 dr., with a little ginger, in debility of the stomach. Its poisonous effects on insects and small animals suggest caution in its use.

QUICKSILVER. See Mercury.

QUININE, SULPHATE OF. Tonic. Dose, ½ dr. to 1 dr. Recommended by Mr. MORTON in the prostration which follows influenza. But too expensive for general use. It is given to dogs in chorea, in doses of 2 to 5 gr.

RAGWORT. The herb is said to produce a kind of lethargy or staggers in horses and cattle. Externally it is used as a poultice in quinsy.

RAKING. Removing hardened fæces from the lower bowel by the hand.

RANUNCULUS REPENS. Acrid stimulant. It is poisonous to sheep.

REED. The great reed (arundo donax,) and the Bankside reed (arundo phragmitis) are reputed diuretic. The former is supposed to have the property of diminishing the secretion of milk.

REFRIGERANTS. Cooling Medicines. See Temperants.

RESIN OR ROSIN. Diuretic. ½ oz. to 1 oz. may be given daily to horses in their corn, for swelled legs. The yellow or amber resin is preferable. Externally it is adhesive and gently stimulating; and is a common ingredient in digestive ointments, and in plasters and charges.

RHODODENDRON. Supposed to be useful in the rheumatism of cattle. Dose, ½ oz. to 1 oz., boiled in water.

RHUBARB. Tonic and stomachic. Scarcely laxative to large animals. From ½ oz. to 1 oz. is given in jaundice to horses and cattle. On dogs it acts as a purgative, but an uncertain one, in doses of ½ dr. to 1 dr.

ROSEMARY. A mild stimulant and carminative. The essential oil is chiefly used in warm liniments and ointments; but is sometimes given in doses of ½ dr. to 1 or 2 dr. in colic.

RUE. Stimulant, uterine, antispasmodic, and vermifuge. It is also supposed to resist contagion and poisons. A decoction or infusion of 2 to 4 oz. of the fresh herb in water or beer is given for worms; as an antidote to the bite of vipers; with diuretics in farcy; with box leaves as a preventive of hydrophobia; and with camphor and opium in locked-jaw. The bruised leaves are put into horses' ears for the staggers. It is given to poultry for the cure of roup. Externally rue is used in fomentations as a stimulant, antiseptic, and discutient.

SAFFRON. Cordial, antispasmodic, and uterine; but too weak and expensive for veterinary use.

SAGE. Stimulant and tonic. In habitual relaxation of the bowels. The powder may be given in a ball, or the herb infused. The infusion is used as a mouth wash.

SAGO. Nutritive and demulcent. Used in the form of gruel.

ST. JOHN'S WORT. Vulnerary. The flowers were formerly an ingredient in FRYAR'S Balsam and other similar compounds. An infused oil of the plant is sometimes used in liniments.

SAL AMMONIAC. See Muriate of Ammonia.

SAL PRUNELLA. *Fused Nitre.* Its uses and doses are the same as nitre.

SALICINE. Tonic. Dose, 10 to 30 gr.

SALT, COMMON, OR CULINARY. In small doses it is tonic, digestive, and alterative: in large doses purgative and vermifuge. As a digestive, 1 oz. may be sprinkled on the horse's corn. As a purgative, or to expel worms, the dose may be from 4 to 6 oz. It is also a common ingredient in laxative clysters. For cattle, an ounce or more may be sprinkled on the hay, to assist digestion: as a purgative, 4 to 8 oz. may be given, but it is not suitable in inflammatory or febrile diseases. Sheep require 2 oz. as a purgative; or smaller doses daily as a preventive of the rot. To dogs, a teaspoonful or one and a half will act as an emetic; smaller doses as a vermifuge. Half a teaspoonful of a solution of salt, as strong as it can be made, is given to poultry as an emetic in roup. Externally, salt dissolved in water is used as a discutient, as a stimulant to old strains, and as a collyrium in chronic ophthalmy.

SALTS, EPSOM AND GLAUBER'S. See Epsom Salts, and Glauber's Salts.

SARSAPARILLA, AND CHINA ROOT, are diaphoretic and alterative; but seldom used in veterinary practice.

SAVIN. An acrid stimulant. The powder is given in doses of 1 or 2 dr. (with or followed by aloes) for worms, but its efficacy is doubtful. Long continued use of savin is reported to have occasioned the hair to fall off. Externally it is applied, in powder or ointment, to warts.

SCAMMONY. An uncertain as well as expensive purgative, far inferior to aloes.

SCUTELLARIA. *Skull-cap.* Mr. YOUATT and others regard this plant as a preventive of hydrophobia. Dose, 40 gr. daily, gradually increased.

SEA WATER. Laxative. Dose, 2 or 3 pints.

SEDATIVES. Medicines which produce quiet, and relieve pain.

SENNA. Purgative; but rarely used in veterinary practice. 5 or 6 oz. are required to purge a horse.

SERPENTARY. Stimulant, tonic, diaphoretic, and antiseptic. It is also supposed to resist the effects of the bites of serpents, &c. Dose, from ½ oz. to 1 oz. or more; but rarely used.

SETONS. These consist of cord, tape, or a mixture of horsehair and hemp twisted together; they are inserted through a portion of the skin to excite irritation and discharge. Mr. MORTON uses cotton cord soaked in a cantharidal liquid. See No. 15, Blistering Solutions, V. F.

SIMARUBA. Tonic and stomachic, for the same purposes as gentian. Seldom used.

SOAP. Antacid and diuretic. Dose, ½ oz. to 2 oz.

SODA. Prepared natron, carbonate or subcarbonate of soda. The common washing soda is generally sufficiently pure. Antacid and diuretic. Dose, 2 to 4 dr. It is sometimes added to aloes as a corrective, and to tonics in weakness of the stomach. The bicarbonate of soda is milder, and may be given in larger doses.

SODA, CHLORIDE OF. See Chloride of Soda.

SODA, SULPHATE OF. See Glauber's Salt.

SODIUM, CHLORIDE OF. The modern name of common salt. See Salt, common.

SOOT. Some French veterinarians prescribe from 2 to 3 oz. of soot as a vermifuge. Also used externally in mange, &c. We presume *wood*-soot is intended.

SPERMACETI. Demulcent and pectoral. Dose, ½ oz. to horses in cough; and to cows, after calving. Externally emollient, in ointments.

SPIDERS' WEB. Externally, styptic. Internally, has been given to dogs in convulsive fits, in ½-grain doses.

SPIRIT OF HARTSHORN. This ammoniacal liquor is stimulant, antacid, and antispasmodic. Dose, ½ oz. But more frequently used in stimulating liniments, and as an application to the bites and stings of venomous reptiles and insects.

SPIRIT OF SAL VOLATILE. This also owes its pungency to ammonia. Dose, ½ oz.

SPIRITS, ARDENT. Brandy, gin, and rum are given as stimulants and antispasmodics, especially in colic. Dose, from 2 to 4 or 5 oz. with warm water. Rectified spirit of wine may be given in the same way, in smaller doses (1 to 2 oz.;) but is more commonly employed for making tinctures; and externally in lotions.

SPIRIT OF MINDERERUS. See Acetate of Ammonia.

SPIRIT OF NITRE, SWEET. *Spirit of Nitric Æther*. Diuretic, diaphoretic, and antispasmodic. Dose for horses, in fever, ½ oz. 3 times a day. In colic, from ½ oz. to 2 oz. Cattle, ½ oz. to 1 oz. in low fevers. Sheep, 1 dr. Dog, from 10 to 20 drops.

SQUILL. A stimulating expectorant. Dose for a horse, 1 dr.; for cattle, 1½ to 2 dr. It is also applied in frictions to the abdomen. MOIROUD has seen it remove ascites.

STARCH. Demulcent. Chiefly used in clysters, but sometimes also in drinks. Dose, 1 to 2 oz., rubbed smooth with a little cold water, and then boiled in 3 or 4 pints of water. It is occasionally used in fomentations.

STAVESACRE SEEDS. Poisonous. 2 dr. will destroy a horse. Only used outwardly to destroy vermin, either powdered and mixed with grease, or infused in vinegar.

STEEL, SALT OF. See Iron, Sulphate of. For the other preparations (so called) of steel, see *Iron*.

STIMULANTS. See Excitants. Diffusible stimulants are those which produce a sudden and temporary excitement of the circulation, and on the nervous system.

STOMACHICS. Medicines which invigorate the stomach and promote digestion.

STOPPINGS. Compositions employed to keep the feet moist and supple. The term is also applied to mechanical plugs for the feet when they are dry and diseased, as cow-dung, clay, tar, &c.

STORAX. Balsamic and expectorant. Dose, ¼ oz. But rarely used.

STRYCHNIA. The active principle of nux vomica: chiefly used in paralysis. Dose, 1 to 3 grains; to be very cautiously increased if necessary: 15 grains have proved fatal. Dose for the dog, 1-16th to ⅛th of a grain.

STYPTICS. Astringent applications employed locally to stop bleeding.

SUBLIMATE, CORROSIVE. *Bichloride of Mercury.* See Corrosive Sublimate.

SUGAR, SYRUP, AND TREACLE. These are used to sweeten drinks; and to give form to balls and other compounds.

SUGAR OF LEAD. See Lead, Acetate of.

SULPHATE OF COPPER. *Blue Stone.* See Copper. Sulphate of.

SULPHATE OF IRON. See Iron, Sulphate of.

SULPHATE OF MAGNESIA. See Epsom Salts.

SULPHATE OF POTASH. Purgative; but seldom used. Dose, 2 to 4 ounces, in colic, &c.

SULPHATE OF QUININE. Tonic. Dose, ½ dr. to 1 dr.

SULPHATE OF SODA. See Glauber's Salt.

SULPHATE OF ZINC. *White Vitriol.* See Zinc, Sulphate of.

SULPHUR, OR BRIMSTONE. It is in 3 forms—roll brimstone, flowers of sulphur, and black brimstone or sulphur vivum. The flowers are generally used. The black is very impure, and sometimes contains arsenic. Sulphur is laxative, alterative, and pectoral. Dose, to horses, as an alterative in skin diseases, grease, want of condition, &c., 1 oz. As a laxative, 4 or 5 oz., but it is rarely employed with this view, and very large doses are not always safe. To cattle, as a laxative, 6 or 8 oz. Sheep, 2 or 3 oz. Dogs, 1 dr. in milk. Swine, 2 dr. It is used outwardly in ointments for mange in all animals. As an alterative it is usually combined with antimonials and nitre.

SULPHURET OF IRON. It has been used in hemorrhage, dysentery, and worms. The hydrated persulphuret (see Ferri persulphuretum hydratum, Pocket Formulary) is strongly recommended by BOUCHARDAT as an antidote for metallic poisons; also as a remedy for incipient farcy. Dose, 1½ oz. to 8 oz.

SULPHURET OF MERCURY. See Ethiops Mineral, and Cinnabar.

SULPHURET OF POTASH. Mr. Blaine prescribes 2 dr. with astringents, in diabetes. In large doses it is poisonous.

SULPHURIC ACID. Poisonous. The strong acid (*oil of vitriol*) is used as a powerful caustic. It is also used in ointments, or mixed with tar, to form an external application. In small doses, about 1 to 2 dr., plentifully diluted, it is, rarely, given as a tonic. The diluted acid (1 oz. to a pint) is used as a lotion in grease, foul ulcers, &c.

SUPERTARTRATE (BITARTRATE) OF POTASH. See Cream of Tartar.

SYRUP OF BUCKTHORN. Purgative. Seldom given to

5

horses, except when used in forming powders into balls. Dose for cattle, 2 to 4 oz. with castor oil. A common physic for dogs; dose 2 to 4 dr.

SYRUP OF POPPIES. A mild anodyne and sedative. Dose for dogs, 1 dr. Seldom given to large animals.

TANNIN (OR TANNIC ACID.) The astringent principle of nutgalls. A powerful astringent in diarrhœa, &c. Dose, 5 to 10 gr. Catechu is more generally used.

TANSY. Tonic and vermifuge. Externally in fomentations.

TAR, BARBADOES. See Petroleum.

TAR. Internally, in old coughs, from 2 to 4 dr. Externally it is cleansing and gently stimulating. It is particularly used in thrushes and all diseases and wounds of the feet, both of horse and cattle, to punctured wounds, and for the cure of mange and other skin diseases. Mixed with fish oil, it is applied with a brush to hard, brittle feet. Tar water (see Formulary) is also given in chronic coughs. Oil or spirit of tar is used in mange ointments, and as a dressing for sheep. The latter requires some caution: sheep have been killed by it.

TARTAR EMETIC. See Antimony, Tartarized.

TEA. Tonic, in simple indigestion, or when connected with staggers [DELAFOND.] Dose, 4 to 6 dr., infused in 3 or 4 pints of water.

TEMPERANTS. Medicines which moderate the circulation, and reduce animal heat.

TIN. Vermifuge. A drachm of the filings daily to dogs. A horse requires from 1 to 3 oz.

TOBACCO. An acro-narcotic poison. In small doses, diuretic and emetic. Principally used as a wash for the mange, and to destroy lice and fly in sheep. But it is not altogether safe, as it is apt to be absorbed. It vomits the dog, pig, and cat: but there are safer emetics. Herbivorous animals are less readily affected by it, but instances of its having proved fatal to them are recorded. In some parts of France, jockeys are said to stupify vicious horses for sale by tobacco diffused in spirits.

TONICS. Medicines which give tone to the fibres, and invigorate the system when relaxed and debilitated. The principal tonics used in veterinary medicine are gentian,

Peruvian bark, chamomile, and other vegetable bitters and astringents; and the preparations of iron, copper, arsenic, zinc, &c. The over free use of them, particularly when fever and inflammation are present, is a frequent source of mischief.

TORMENTIL ROOT. Astringent. Dose, 1 oz. to 1½ oz. Its presence in pastures is supposed to prevent the rot in sheep.

TURBITH MINERAL. *Subsulphate of Mercury.* An irritating purgative, and, in large doses, poisonous. Dose, ½ dr. in farcy. Given to dogs as an emetic: dose, 1 gr. to 3 gr.

TURMERIC. A weak aromatic stimulant. Supposed to be useful in jaundice, or yellows. Dose, 1 oz.

TURPENTINES. They are all stimulant, diuretic, and expectorant; and in larger doses, vermifuge and purgative. Dose of common turpentine, ½ oz. to 1 oz. They are used in digestive ointments. Oil or spirit of turpentine is a more stimulating diuretic, in doses of 2 to 4 dr.; it is also considered efficacious as an antispasmodic in colic (gripes,) and as a remedy for worms. Dose for the latter purposes, from 2 to 4 oz., or sometimes still larger doses for worms. To cattle (in hoose, from worms in the bronchial passages) about 2 oz. To sheep in rot, 1 dr. It is not a safe medicine for dogs; but is sometimes given in doses of 2 dr. with olive oil. Externally, it is used in stimulating liniments, embrocations, ointments, &c. It is very irritating to the skin of the horse, and also of the dog, instantly producing great excitement. Like the common and Venice turpentine, it enters into the composition of some digestive ointments.

UVA URSI. *Bearberry.* Astringent. Dose, 4 to 6 dr., in diabetes. But GIRARDI says it inflames the stomach.

VALERIAN. A stimulant, acting chiefly on the nervous system. Dose, for horses and cattle, 1 to 4 oz. in powder. 2 oz. twice a day have been given to a horse without any observable effect. In dogs it is said to act as a vermifuge. Dose, 1 to 4 dr.

VERDIGRIS. *Subacetate (or Diacetate) of Copper.* Tonic, caustic, poisonous. It has been given in doses of 1 dr. to 2 dr. daily, in farcy and glanders. Externally, detergent and caustic, in ointments, and in the form of Ægyptiacum. The crystallized acetate of copper is more powerful in its action.

VERJUICE. Properties and uses the same as of vinegar; but preferred by some for outward use.

VERMILION. See Cinnabar.

VINEGAR. Diaphoretic, cooling, and antiseptic. In combination with honey, it is used in coughs. In large quantities, it irritates the stomach; a pint is said to have destroyed a horse. It should always be plentifully diluted. Vinegar which contains much sulphuric acid should be avoided. It is chiefly used as an external application as a lotion for strains, bruises, sprains, and inflammations; and hot as a revulsive. The vapours are thought to possess disinfecting properties, but are less effectual than chlorine.

VITRIOLATED ZINC. *White Vitriol.* See Zinc, Sulphate of.

VITRIOL, BLUE. See Sulphate of Copper.

WALNUT. The green shells are astringent, and sometimes applied, bruised as a cataplasm, or in decoction as a lotion.

WATER. Besides its use as a drink, and as a vehicle for medicines, water is used remedially, on the hydropathic system. Rugs wetted with cold water, and well covered with dry ones, are used to produce perspiration, assisting their operation by copious draughts of cold water, adding 4 oz. of sweet spirit of nitre to each pailful. This treatment is said to have succeeded in the recently epidemic pleuro-pneumonia.

WAX. Chiefly used in making cerates, plasters, charges, &c.

WHEY. A cooling and nutritive drink in inflammatory diseases, and during convalescence from them.

WILLOW BARK. Possesses in some degree the same properties as Peruvian bark. Dose, in powder or decoction, 1 to 4 oz.

WINE. Stimulant. In wine countries it is frequently given as a restorative. Port wine has been given as an astringent in obstinate diarrhœas. Dose for horses and cattle, ½ pint to a bottle.

WINTER BARK. A warm tonic and stomachic. Dose, 2 to 6 dr.

WOLFSBANE. *Aconite.* A virulent poison.

WORMWOOD. A bitter tonic and vermifuge. An infusion of from 2 to 4 oz. of the dry, or twice as much of the fresh herb, may be given in dropsy, and diseases of general debility; or from 2 to 4 dr. of the powder may be given in a ball. A few drops of the essential oil are often added to aloes, &c., for worms.

WORT. See Malt.

YEW. It is not used medicinally. The leaves are poisonous to horses and cattle, producing symptoms which resemble those of apoplexy. To counteract its effect, it is recommended to give 10 gr. of croton meal, and afterwards drenches of gruel with vinegar. The croton to be repeated in 6 hours, if it has not operated.

ZEDOARY. A weak aromatic stimulant, formerly prescribed in jaundice; but now rarely employed. It is weaker than ginger.

ZINC, CHLORIDE OF. In solution this constitutes Sir W. Burnett's disinfecting fluid. Much diluted it is applied as a detergent lotion to foul ulcers. The dry salt is a powerful caustic.

ZINC, OXIDE. *Flowers of Zinc.* A mild astringent and tonic; dose, ½ oz.; but chiefly used in dusting ulcers and excoriations, to promote skinning.

ZINC, SULPHATE OF. *White Vitriol.* Tonic. Dose, for the horse, 1 to 4 dr., frequently combined with cantharides. Externally, astringent, detersive, styptic, and healing; in lotions and ointments, to indolent ulcers, grease, &c. It is a frequent ingredient in eye-waters,—about 3 gr. to an ounce of water. A saturated solution is used as an injection for quitters.

VETERINARY FORMULARY.

Medicines for Horses.

BALLS AND BALL MASSES.

THE roots, seeds, and other dry substances are to be reduced to powder; and it is of importance that the aromatic seeds, especially, should have been recently powdered. The drugs should be of good quality. It is hoped that the trash sold as horse-powders will not much longer be known in establishments which have any pretensions to respectability. After this general notice, it will be unnecessary to occupy the space by repeating the words, "powdered," "freshly powdered," "genuine," &c. Balls should not be too hard, but merely stiff enough to retain their form, and should be wrapped in soft paper.

[*Mode of Administering Balls.*—The horse should be backed into the stall, the tongue drawn gently out with the left hand on the off side of the mouth, and then fixed by pressing the fingers against the side of the lower jaw. The ball, being now taken between the tips of the fingers of the right hand, must be passed rapidly up the mouth, as near the palate as possible, until it reach the root of the tongue; it must then be delivered with a slight jerk, so that, the hand being immediately withdrawn, and the tongue liberated, the ball may be forced through the pharynx into the œsophagus. A slight tap under the chin may then be given, or a draught of water to assist in carrying it down.]

COMMON MASS, as a basis for balls in general. Mix with the hands equal weights of linseed meal and treacle, and add a little palm oil.—CHERRY.

ALTERATIVE BALLS. The term *alterative* is applied to medicines which, without any sensible operation, or with a laxative or diuretic operation so gradual as not to interfere with the usual work or diet, produce a favourable change in the system, and, in common language, "purify the blood." Alterative balls are given in skin diseases, swelled legs, grease, foul humours, &c.; usually 1 daily, or every other day.

Diuretic Alterative Balls. 1. Dried common soda 1 oz., Castile soap 6 dr., rosin 2 oz., liquorice powder ½ oz., Barbadoes tar to form 6 balls; 1 daily.—WHITE.

2. Acetate of potash ½ oz., rosin ½ oz., fenugreek 1 oz., treacle enough to form a mass for 2 balls; 1 daily.

Laxative Alterative Balls. 1. Aloes 4 oz., soft soap 4 oz., common mass 24 oz.; mix; dose, 1 oz.—V. C.

2. Socotrine aloes 8 oz., soft soap 8 oz., common mass 16 oz; mix; dose, 1 oz.—V. C.

3. Aloes 10 dr., soap 12 dr., caraways 12 dr., ginger 4 dr., treacle q. s. for 4 balls; 1 daily.—WHITE.

4. Aloes 1 dr., diuretic mass (No. 1 or 3) 9 dr.

5. Antimonial powder 1 dr., aloes 1 or 2 dr., diuretic mass (No. 1 or 3) 1 oz.

Antimonial or Diaphoretic Alterative Ball. 1. Levigated antimony 2 to 4 dr., caraway seeds 4 dr., treacle q. s. to form a ball.—WHITE.

2. Prepared antimony 2 dr., nitre 3 dr., sulphur 2 dr., linseed meal 2 dr., palm oil to form a mass; one every night, in megrims.—CLATER.

3. Tartarized antimony 2 dr., elecampane 2 oz., guaiacum 6 dr., sulphur 1 oz., treacle and flour to form 6 balls; one daily.

4. Tartarized antimony 3 dr., ginger a scruple, soap 1 oz. For 3 balls: one every other morning.—VINES.

5. Emetic tartar 5 oz., ginger 3 oz., opium 1 oz., and syrup to make 16 balls.

Mercurial Alterative Balls. 1. Ethiops mineral 4 oz., sulphur, prepared antimony, cream of tartar, cinnabar, of each 5 oz., honey to form a mass for 12 balls; 1 every morning for a month in farcy.—TAPLIN.

2. Calomel ½ dr., aloes 1 dr., Castile soap 2 dr., oil of juniper 30 drops, syrup to form a ball.—WHITE.

3. Blue pill 1 dr., black antimony 2 dr., diuretic mass 4 dr., aloes 1 dr., for a ball, daily.

4. In Grease: prepared antimony, sulphur, nitre, Ethiops mineral, of each 3 oz., Castile soap 10 oz., oil of juniper 3 dr., syrup or honey q. s. for 12 balls; 1 every morning for 2 or 3 weeks.—TAPLIN.

5. Quicksilver 2 parts, sesquioxide of iron 1 part, confection of roses 3 parts. Rub together till the quicksilver disappears. Dose, ʒss to ʒij, with common or other mass q. s.—DR. COLLIER'S Blue Pill.

6. Strong mercurial ointment ¼ ℔, powdered ginger 3 oz., liquorice powder 10 oz., treacle to mix for 12 balls. —FRANCIS.

Alterative Tonic Balls. See Tonic Balls.

ASTRINGENT BALLS. These are given in diarrhœa, diabetes, &c.

1. (V. C. Astringent Mass.) Catechu 1 oz., cinnamon 1 oz., common mass 6 oz.; mix; dose, 1 ounce.

2. Peruvian bark 12 oz., grains of paradise, 2 oz., gentian 3 oz., honey q. s. for 16 balls; 1 every morning; for diabetes.—RYDING.

3. Catechu ½ oz., alum 3 dr., cascarilla 2 dr., flour 2 dr., treacle q. s.—WHITE.

4. Catechu 2 dr., opium ½ dr., linseed meal 2 dr., treacle to form a ball. For profuse staling, 1 night and morning; if they confine the bowels, add 1 dr. of aloes. —CLATER.

5. Peruvian bark 1½ oz., alum ½ oz., treacle q. s. For the same purpose.—LAWRENCE.

6. Oak bark 1 oz., (or Peruvian bark ½ oz.,) opium 1 dr., ginger 2 dr., syrup to form a ball; for diarrhœa.—WHITE.

7. Opium ½ dr., prepared chalk 6 dr., cassia 1½ dr.,

tartarized antimony 2 dr., syrup to form a ball; for the same.—WHITE.

8. Nut-galls 2 dr., cassia ½ dr., conserve of roses to form a ball.

9. Burnt rhubarb 1 dr., compound powder of chalk 3 dr., common mass 6 dr.; for diarrhœa.

10. Tormentil or bistort 1½ dr., marshmallow root ½ oz., chalk 2 dr., syrup to form a ball.

11. For bloody urine. Acetate of lead 10 gr., sulphate of zinc 40 gr., catechu 4 dr., conserve of roses to form a ball; once daily.—BLAINE.

12. Powdered opium ½ dr., soda 1 dr., powdered cassia or ginger 1½ dr., flour and syrup to form a ball.

13. For Diabetes. Catechu ½ oz., alum ½ dr., sugar of lead 10 gr., with conserve of roses to form a ball. See also Tonic Balls.

COUGH BALLS; Expectorant Balls. The following formulæ are chiefly intended for chronic coughs and thickness of wind. The bowels should be kept open by mashes and an occasional laxative. Coughs occasioned by worms require a different treatment. In coughs connected with inflammation of the chest, and epidemic catarrh, see Balls for Inflammation of the Lungs.

1. Aloes 2 oz., digitalis (powdered) 1 oz., common mass 13 oz.; dose 1 oz. twice a day.—MORTON.

2. Emetic tartar ½ dr., digitalis ½ dr., nitre 1½ dr., tar enough to form a ball; every night.—YOUATT.

3. Powdered squill 1 dr., gum ammoniac 3 dr., opium ½ dr., syrup to form a ball.—WHITE.

4. Ipecacuanha 1 dr., camphor 2 dr., liquorice powder 1 dr., honey to form a ball; to be given every morning.—BLAINE.

5. Sulphur ½ oz., assafœtida 1 oz., liquorice powder 1 oz., Venice turpentine, 1 oz., for 4 balls; one every night for 4 times.—HINDS.

6. Calomel 20 gr., gum ammoniacum 2 dr., balsam of Peru 1 dr., p. squill 1 dr., honey to form a ball; one every morning.—BLAINE.

7. P. marshmallow root and liquorice, of each 1 dr.,

elecampane, sulphur, and Kermes mineral, of each ½ dr., honey to form a ball; twice a day.—LEBAS.

8. Squill 2 dr., gum ammoniac 4 dr., ipecacuanha 4 dr., opium 4 dr., pimento 1 oz., balsam of sulphur 4 oz., Castile soap 2 oz., treacle to form a mass for six balls; one twice a day.—HINDS.

9. Spermaceti 1 oz., balsam of copaiva 1 oz., benzoin 2 dr., sulphur 2 oz., elecampane 2 oz., p. squill 4 dr., emetic tartar 2 dr., syrup of poppies to form a mass for 8 balls.—B. CLARKE.

10. Liquorice powder ½ oz., linseed or barley meal 1 oz., tar 1 dr., honey to form a ball.

11. Castile soap, aniseed, liquorice, of each 5 oz., Barbadoes tar 6 oz., ammoniacum 3 oz. balsam of Tolu 1 oz., honey q. s. to make a mass for 12 balls; one every morning for a fortnight.—TAPLIN.

12. Digitalis 1 dr., nitre 2 dr., liquorice 4 dr., tar enough to form a ball.—CLATER. See also Mixed Balls (Pectoral Cordial.)

BALLS FOR INFLAMMATION OF THE LUNGS, BRONCHITIS, &c.

1. Antimonial powder 2 dr., digitalis 3 dr., nitre 3 dr., cream of tartar 3 dr., honey to form a ball; one every 4, 6, or 8 hours, in inflammation of the lungs.—BLAINE.

2. Digitalis 1 dr., emetic tartar 1½ dr., nitre 3 dr., honey q. s.; when the pulse intermits, reduce the dose to half.—YOUATT.

3. Nitre 6 dr. emetic tartar 2 dr., flour and syrup to form a ball; twice a day.—WHITE.

4. Digitalis 1 dr., emetic tartar 1 dr., nitre 3 dr., sulphur 1 dr. linseed meal 2 dr.; beat together with palm oil.—CLATER.

5. In epidemic catarrh. To the last add 2 dr. of the Physic Mass (No. 10;) repeat this twice.

6. In the advanced stage when suppuration has taken place. Carbonate of ammonia 1½ dr., opium 1 dr., aniseed ½ oz., syrup to form a ball.—SPOONER.

7. *Cough Ball.* Digitalis ½ dr., camphor and emetic tartar each 1 dr., nitre 3 dr., and linseed meal 1 dr., to be made up with Barbadoes tar.

CORDIAL BALLS. For exhaustion from over-exertion, and as a stimulus to weak stomachs. But their frequent and unnecessary use is hurtful.

1. Ginger and gentian, equal parts, treacle to form a mass; dose, 1 oz. to 1½ oz.—V. C.

2. Caraway, bruised raisins, of each 4 parts, ginger and palm oil, of each 2 parts.—YOUATT.

3. Aniseed, caraway, cardamom, each 1 oz., saffron 2 dr., sugar candy 4 oz., liquorice powder 1½ oz., Spanish juice (softened with water) 2 oz., oil of aniseed ½ oz., wheat flour q. s.; dose, 1 oz. to 1½ oz.—BRACKEN.

4. Aniseed, caraway, sweet fennel, liquorice, of each 4 oz., of ginger and cassia, each 1½ oz., honey to form a mass.—WHITE.

5. Ginger, caraway, each 4 ℔, gentian 1 ℔, palm oil 4½ ℔, beat together; dose, 1 oz. to 1½ oz.—CLATER.

6. Gentian 8 oz., ginger 4 oz., coriander 8 oz., caraway 8 oz., oil of aniseed ½ oz., treacle q. s.; dose, 1½ oz.—BLAINE.

7. Aniseed, caraway, ginger, each 8 oz.; gentian, grains of paradise, cummin, and turmeric, each 4 oz.; cassia 2 oz., oil of caraway 2 dr., treacle to form a mass; dose, 1½ oz. To keep it moist, add 2 oz. of acetate of potash.

8. Cummin, aniseed, caraway, each 4 oz.; ginger 2 oz., treacle q. s.; dose, 1½ oz. to 2 oz.—WHITE.

9. Pimento 1 ℔., sifted barley meal 2 ℔., treacle q. s. —B. CLARKE.

MIXED BALLS. *Cordial Astringent Ball.* Cordial ball (No. 2) 1 oz., catechu 1 dr., opium 10 gr.; to washy horses, before or after a journey.—YOUATT.

Cordial Anodyne Balls. 1. Cordial mass (No. 6) 10 dr., camphor 1 dr., opium 20 gr.—BLAINE.

2. Opium ½ dr. to 2 scruples, soap 2 dr., ginger 1 dr., aniseed 4 dr., oil of caraway ½ dr., treacle q. s.—WHITE.

Balsamic Cordial Ball. Cordial mass (No. 6) 1 oz., myrrh 1 dr., balsam of Tolu 1 dr.—BLAINE.

Pectoral Cordial Balls. 1. For old coughs. Fenugreek, aniseed, cummin, safflower, elecampane, coltsfoot, sulphur, of each 3 oz., liquorice juice 1 oz., olive oil 8 oz., honey 8 oz., Genoa treacle 12 oz., oil of aniseed 1 oz., wheat meal 1½ ℔., or q. s.; one ball, or 2 oz. (dissolve in water or warm wort) every day for 12 or 15 days, if required.—QUINCY.

2. Elecampane ½ oz., ginger 1½ dr., squill 1 dr., oil of aniseed 20 drops, syrup of Tolu q. s.—WHITE.

Diuretic Cordial Balls: to fine the legs of debilitated and overworked horses; and sometimes given in old coughs, &c. 1. Resin 2 oz., soap, nitre, caraway, of each 2 oz., ginger 1½ oz., sulphur 2 oz., oil of caraway ½ dr., oil of juniper ½ dr., syrup to form a mass.

2. Soap and common turpentine each 4 dr., ginger 1 dr., opium ½ dr., caraway seeds q. s. for 1 dose.—WHITE.

3. Strained turpentine 8 oz., resin 4 oz., olive oil 2 oz., soap 8 oz., melt together and add powdered ginger 6 oz., pimento 6 oz., liquorice powder q. s. to form a mass.

4. Resin 4 dr., nitre 2 dr., and ginger 1 dr., with sufficient soap to form a ball.—SPOONER.

DIURETIC BALLS. For swelled legs, grease, &c., for carrying off bad humours. And in many chronic diseases. The too free use of diuretics injures the kidneys, and weakens the system. See Alterative Balls (Diuretic,) page 55.

1. Resin, soap, nitre, of each equal parts, beaten together into a mass; dose, 1 oz. to 1½ oz.—V. C.

2. Common turpentine 4 oz., Castile soap 4 oz., caraway 8 oz., ginger 1 oz., flour q. s.—WHITE.

3. Resin 16 oz., white soap 16 oz., nitre 8 oz., dried common soda 2 oz., oil of juniper 4 oz.; beat together, adding flour, if required; dose, 1 oz. to 1½ oz.

4. Nitre 1 ℔., Castile soap ½ ℔., common turpentine 1 ℔., barley meal 2½ ℔., or sufficient; dose, about 1 oz. —B. CLARKE.

5. White soap 8 oz., nitre 3 oz., resin 3 oz., camphor 3 dr., oil of juniper 3 dr. For 6 balls, 1 every, or every other morning.—TAPLIN.

6. Common turpentine 16 oz., sulphur 24 oz., nitre

8 oz., honey 8 oz., flour or linseed meal q. s.; dose, 1½ oz.

7. Camphor 2 dr., nitre 1 oz., flour and syrup to form a ball; for stoppage of water.—WHITE.

8. Yellow resin 4 ℔, common turpentine 2 ℔, yellow soap 1 ℔; melt together, and add nitre 1 ℔.—BLAINE.

9. Common turpentine (or powdered resin) ½ oz., linseed meal ¼ oz., ginger ½ dr., palm oil q. s.—YOUATT.

10. Yellow resin 2 oz., common turpentine 4 oz., soap 3 oz.; melt together, stir in 1 oz. sweet oil, add oil of aniseed ½ oz., oil of juniper ½ oz., ginger 2 dr., linseed meal q. s.; mix, and divide into 8 balls; 1 a day till the water is affected.—HINDS.

11. Resin 2½ ℔, cream of tartar ½ ℔, sulphur ½ ℔, linseed meal 1 ℔, palm oil 1 ℔; dose, 1 oz. to 2 oz.—CLATER.

12. Nitre 1 oz., vermilion ½ oz., resin 1 oz., camphor ½ oz., honey q. s. for 4 balls.—LEBAS.

13. Nitre 8 oz., oxysulphuret of antimony 1 oz., sulphur 8 oz., resin 8 oz., oil of juniper 1 oz., yellow soap 8 oz., treacle to form a mass; dose, 1½ oz.

14. White soap 1 oz., extract of juniper berries q. s. for 2 balls.—BOURGELAT.

Tonic Diuretic Ball. Gentian 1 dr., ginger ½ dr., sulphate of iron 2 dr., diuretic mass (No. 11) ½ oz., oil of juniper 10 drops, syrup of squills ½ oz.; twice a day in dropsy of chest; less frequently in swelled legs.—CLATER. See also Leicester Red Balls. (Miscellaneous Balls.)

FEVER BALLS.

1. Emetic tartar ½ dr., camphor ½ dr., nitre 2 dr., common mass 6 dr., or q. s. for 1 ball; to be given once or twice a day.—MORTON.

2. Camphor 1 dr., nitre 6 dr., antimonial powder 2 dr., flour and syrup to form a ball.—WHITE.

3. Antimonial powder 2 dr., nitre 3 dr., cream of tartar 2 dr., honey to form a ball; in influenza, twice a day after a mild laxative.—BLAINE.

4. See Balls for Inflammation of Lungs, No. 4.—CLATER.

BALLS FOR FARCY AND GLANDERS. Mr. COLEMAN says he has tried the various preparations of arsenic, antimony, copper, mercury, zinc, aconite, digitalis, hemlock, henbane, hellebore, nightshade, &c., in glanders, without any specific or curative effect. Mr. YOUATT considers it useless to attempt the cure of glandered horses; but that farcy in its early stage and mild form may be successfully treated. Mr. BLAINE says, "All the mercurials have been used with benefit in farcy; but they must be discontinued as soon as the mouth is affected, or sickness, loss of appetite, &c., produced.

1. Æthiops mineral 2 dr., blue pill 1 dr., prepared antimony 3 dr., diuretic mass 4 dr. One every morning.

2. Strong mercurial ointment 2 to 3 dr., guaiacum 3 dr., soap 4 dr., fenugreek 12 dr., treacle to form a mass, for 6 balls. [See Mercurial Alterative Balls, page 56.]

3. Sulphate of copper 1 dr., corrosive sublimate 8 gr., linseed powder ½ oz.—WHITE.

4. Corrosive sublimate 10 gr., gradually increased to 20, gentian 2 dr., ginger 1 dr., syrup to form a ball; to be given night and morning till some effect is produced; when the mouth is affected, the sublimate may be exchanged for 1 dr. sulphate of copper.—YOUATT.

5. Corrosive sublimate 10 to 20 gr., opium ½ to 1 dr., powdered aniseed ½ oz., with syrup to make a ball.

6. Sulphate of copper 1 dr., calomel 20 gr., common turpentine 3 dr., liquorice powder and syrup q. s. for one ball.—COLEMAN.

7. Sulphate of copper 1 dr., white arsenic 8 gr., corrosive sublimate 8 gr., linseed powder ½ oz., syrup to form a ball.—WHITE.

8. Æthiops mineral 2 dr., opium 10 gr., liquorice powder and mucilage to form a ball; to be given twice a day till the breath or urine is affected.—HINDS.

9. Sulphate of iron 2 dr., Peruvian bark 1 oz., opium ½ dr., syrup to form a ball.—SMITH.

10. Cantharides 4 gr., gradually increased to 6 or 8 gr., gentian, ginger, and caraway, each 1 dr., syrup q. s.; every or every other day.—VINES.

11. Sulphate of iron 2 dr., iodide of potassium 10 gr.,

ginger 1 dr., gentian 2 dr., made into a ball with treacle. —SPOONER.

12. Diniodide of copper 1 dr., gentian 1½ dr., pimento 1 dr., cantharides 5 gr.; for one ball.—MORTON.

13. Sulphate of zinc 15 gr., cantharides 7 gr. pimento or ginger 15 gr., treacle and oatmeal to form a ball; 1 daily.—BRACY CLARK.

14. Sublimate, arsenic, verdigris, each 8 gr., sulphate of copper 20 gr.; for one ball (with common mass q. s.;) the dose may be gradually increased, carefully watching its effects, but should never exceed 15 gr. of sublimate and arsenic.—BLAINE.

15. Sublimate 10 gr., gentian 2 dr. ginger 1 dr., linseed meal ½ oz., palm oil to form a ball; night and morning for a fortnight; for farcy.—CLATER.

16. Sulphate of copper ½ dr. to 1 dr., ginger and gentian, each one dr., linseed meal and palm oil to form a ball; morning and night for a fortnight, then daily as long as necessary; in glanders.—CLATER.

17. Strong mercurial ointment 3 oz.; white soap 2 oz., starch 2 oz.; form a mass, and divide into 12 balls; 1 every morning.—MOIROUD.

18. Assafœtida 3 oz.; vermilion 2 oz., muriate of lime 3 dr., galangal 1 oz., strong mercurial ointment 2 oz.; beat together into a uniform mass, and divide into 6 balls; one every other morning.—LEBAS.

19. Æthiops mineral 8 oz., powdered burdock root 16 oz., treacle q. s.; make into 32 balls.—MOIROUD.

20. Antihecticum Poterii 2 dr., with 6 dr. of cordial ball; every other day.—Mr. LAWRENCE.

21. Calomel 1 oz., assafœtida 4 oz., galangal powder 1 oz., mercurial ointment 2 oz. Mix and form six balls. One every other morning.—LEBAS.

22. Hydrargyro-iodide of potassium (see Hydrargyri et Potassii iodidum, Pocket Formulary) 3 oz., powdered althæa root and honey, q. s. to make 100 balls. Give from 1 to 8 daily, gradually increasing the dose to the latter number.—BOUCHARDAT.

BALLS FOR GREASE. See Diuretic Balls, and Alterative Balls.

BALLS FOR YELLOWS, OR JAUNDICE, AND INFLAMMATION OF LIVER (HEPATITIS.)

1. For Hepatitis without purging; calomel 1 dr., antimonial powder 2 dr., aloes 3 dr., syrup to form a ball; one every 4 or 5 hours, till the bowels are opened.—BLAINE.

2. Calomel ½ dr., aloes 1 dr., soap 2 dr., rhubarb ½ oz., syrup to form a ball; to be given every 12 hours, till it purges moderately.—WHITE.

3. Aloes 2 dr., calomel 1 dr., syrup to make a ball, twice a day.—YOUATT.

4. Opium 1 dr., calomel 1 dr., emetic tartar 2 dr.; liquorice powder 3 dr., syrup to form a ball; once every 12 hours.—WHITE.

Yellows (*Jaundice*) *without Fever.* 1. Calomel 1 dr., aloes 2 dr., soap 2 dr.; for one ball; night and morning till purged, then so as to keep them lax.—BLAINE.

2. Calomel ½ dr., aloes 1½ dr., Castile soap 2 dr., rhubarb 3 dr. syrup to form a ball.—WHITE.

3. In the latter stage when not costive, calomel 12 gr., sulphate of copper 1 dr., gentian 3 dr., oak bark 3 dr., chamomile 3 dr., syrup to form a ball; once or twice a day.—BLAINE.

PHYSIC OR PURGING BALLS. The animal should be prepared by bran mashes for two days, and the ball given, fasting in the morning. Gentle exercise with a ball is useful, but not after it begins to operate. Genuine Barbadoes aloes should be used (from the gourd, not melted,) and the dose seldom need exceed 6 dr. A week should be allowed after the operation of one ball before another is given. See Aloes, in the Veterinary Materia Medica.

1. (V. C. Cathartic mass.) Bruised B. aloes 8 oz., olive oil 1 oz.; melt together in a vessel placed in hot water; remove it from the fire, add 3 oz. treacle, and stir all together; dose, 6 to 12 dr., equal to 4 to 8 dr., of aloes.

2. (V. C. Stronger.) To each dose of the last add from 4 to 8 drops of croton oil.

3. B. aloes 4 to 8 dr., soap 3 to 4 dr., ginger 1 dr.,

oil of cloves 10 drops, (or oil of caraway or aniseed 20 drops,) water 1 dr. or q. s.; beat together into a mass. —WHITE. Mr. W. says this is the best that can be employed.

4. B. aloes 15 oz., ginger 1 oz.; mix and beat up 8 oz. of palm oil. Dose, 1 oz. to 1½.—Mr. YOUATT.

5. Barb. aloes 24 dr., Cape aloes 12 dr., olive oil 4 dr., treacle 12 dr.; dose, 7 to 14 dr.; mix as No. 1.—MORTON.

6. B. aloes 5 dr., 7½ dr., or 9 dr., oil of caraway 10 drops; made up with palm oil or lard.—Mr. BLAINE'S Nos. 1, 2, and 3.

7. Melt Barb. aloes (in a tin vessel immersed in boiling water) with a fifth of its weight of treacle, and, while soft, pour it into paper moulds; 1 oz. is a full dose for a large sized saddle or coach horse.—B. CLARK. (For a convenient apparatus for melting and casting these balls, see Mr. BRACY CLARK'S Pharmacopœia Equina; or Vol. V. of the Pharmaceutical Journal.

8. B. aloes 5 to 8 dr., cream of tartar 2 dr., oil of cloves 10 drops; treacle to form a ball.—PEALL.

9. Aloes 7 dr., Castile soap 4 dr., aromatic powder 1 dr., oil of caraway 6 drops; mucilage to form a ball —HINDS.

10. Barb. aloes 7½ parts, socotrine aloes 7½ parts, ginger 1 part; mix the powders, add 7½ parts of palm oil, and beat to a mass, keep it in a jar closely covered; dose, 1¼ oz. to 1¾ oz.—CLATER.

11. B. aloes 13½ oz., lard 6 oz., treacle 1½ oz., water 1½ oz.; put them in an earthen vessel, placed in boiling water; mix, and form the mass into 18 balls.—McEWEN.

12. Aloes and hard soap each 5 oz., pearl ashes 1 oz., powdered ginger 2 oz. Melt in a ladle, and divide, while warm, into 8 balls.

Mercurial Physic Balls. 1. Cathartic mass (No. 10 above) 10 to 14 dr., calomel 1 dr. to 1½ dr.; mix.—CLATER.

2. For stomach staggers: Aloes 1 oz., calomel ½ oz., cascarilla 3 dr., syrup to form a ball.—WHITE.

LAXATIVE BALLS.

1. Ipecacuanha 1 dr., aloes 3 to 4 dr., liquorice powder and mucilage to form a ball.—HINDS.

2. Aloes 3 to 4 dr., soap 3 dr., oil of caraway 20 drops, syrup q. s.—WHITE.

3. Aloes 3 to 4 dr., soap 4 dr., emetic tartar 2 dr., mucilage to form a ball—HINDS.

For other Formulæ, see Alterative Balls (laxative.)

NAUSEATING BALLS. These are given in inflammatory diseases.

1. Powdered white hellebore ½ dr., linseed meal 4 dr., treacle to form a ball; one night and morning till some effect is produced in inflammation of the kidneys.—CLATER.

2. White hellebore 20 gr., common mass or other proper material to form a ball: give one every 4, 6, or 8 hours, till symptoms of nausea appear, taking care not to carry it too far.—Mr. PERCIVAL. See Fever balls. See Hellebore, in Veterinary Màteria Medica.

STOMACHIC BALLS. For indigestion. and during recovery from debilitating diseases which have impaired the appetite. A mild purge should be previously given.

1. Gentian, quassia, grains of paradise, of each 3 dr., Venice turpentine q. s. for one ball.—BLAINE.

2. Gentian 2 or 3 dr., carbonate of soda 1 dr., ginger 1 dr., treacle to form a ball.—WHITE.

3. Chamomiles 2 dr., calumba 2 dr., common salt 1 dr., fenugreek 2 dr., syrup to form a ball.

4. Myrrh 1½ dr., cascarilla 2 dr., Castile soap, 1 dr. syrup to form a ball.—WHITE.

5. *Laxative Stomachic Ball.* Aloes 3 dr., rhubarb 3 dr., subcarbonate of soda 2 dr., ginger 1½ dr., treacle to form a ball.—WHITE.

6. Calumba and chamomile in powder, each 2 dr., Venice treacle ½ oz., oil of caraway 25 drops, honey q. s.—LAWRENCE. See Tonic Balls, for other formulæ.

TONIC BALLS. In diseases attended with general debility, and to restore strength after a tedious illness.

Vegetable Tonics. 1. Peruvian bark 1 oz., opium ½ dr., ginger 1½ dr., oil of caraway 20 drops, treacle to form a ball.—WHITE.

2. Sulphate of quinine 1 dr., gentian, oak bark, and honey to form a ball.—MOIROUD.

3. Gentian 1 dr., ginger ½ dr., cascarilla 1 dr., treacle and linseed meal to form a ball.—CLATER.

4. Myrrh 2 dr., mustard flour 1 dr., cantharides 5 gr., chamomile 4 dr., Venice turpentine q. s. for one ball.—BLAINE.

5. Gentian 4 dr., chamomile 2 dr., carbonate of iron 1 dr., ginger 1 dr., syrup q. s. for one ball.—YOUATT.

6. Quassia 2 dr., canella 2 dr., opium ½ dr., ginger 1 dr., treacle q. s.—WHITE.

Mineral Tonics. 1. Sulphate of iron 4 oz., ginger 4 oz., common mass 10 oz.; beat together to form a mass; dose, 1 oz. to 1½ oz.—V. C.

2. Sulphate of iron ½ oz., aromatic powder 2 dr., mucilage q. s. to form a ball.—WHITE.

3. Scales of iron 12 oz., gentian 8 oz., honey to form a mass.—MOIROUD.

4. Myrrh 3 dr., sulphate of iron 2 dr., chamomile 3 dr., ginger 1 dr., Venice turpentine or palm oil to form a ball.—BLAINE.

5. Gentian 4 dr., chamomile 2 dr., carbonate of iron 1 dr., ginger 1 dr., syrup for one ball.—YOUATT.

6. Sulphate of iron 2 dr., carbonate of potash 2 dr., cascarilla 2 dr., caraway 4 dr., treacle q. s.—WHITE.

7. Sulphate of iron 1 dr., carbonate of soda 2 dr., myrrh 1 dr., ginger 1 dr., cantharides 6 gr., caraway ½ oz., treacle q. s.—WHITE.

8. Tonic mass. Sulphate of copper 2 oz., ginger 2 oz., common mass 12 oz.; beat together; dose 1 oz. to 1½ oz. —V. C.

9. Sulphate of copper and ginger, of each 1 dr., canella 4 dr., conserve of roses q. s. for one ball.—BLAINE.

10. White arsenic 5 to 10 gr., aniseed ½ oz., opium ½ dr., treacle q. s.; sometimes 2 dr., of sulphate of zinc may be added.—WHITE.

11. Arsenic 10 gr., gentian and cascarilla, of each 3 dr., conserve of roses q. s.—BLAINE.

Mild Alterative Tonics. To promote condition; a mild dose of physic should be previously given,

1. Aloes 1 dr., Winter's bark 2 dr., verdigris 1 dr., treacle or honey q. s.

2. Arsenic 8 gr., pimento 1 dr., extract of gentian 4 dr.; daily

3. Nitre 1 oz., sulphur 6 dr., physic mass ½ oz., gentian 6 dr., ginger ½ oz., palm oil q. s. for 4 balls. One daily, after an attack of stomach staggers.—CLATER.

WORM BALLS.

1. Calomel 1 or 2 dr. at night, and an aloetic ball in the morning.—CLATER.

2. Emetic tartar 2 dr., ginger a scruple, linseed meal and treacle to form a ball; one every morning an hour before feeding.—YOUATT.

3. Calomel 8 gr., arsenic 8 gr., tin filings 1 oz., Venice turpentine ½ oz.; mix; and give every morning fasting, for a fortnight.—BLAINE.

4. Common salt ½ oz., gentian 2 dr., rust of iron 2 dr., savin 1 dr., treacle to form a ball, to be given every morning for a week; then a purging ball.

5. B. aloes 6 dr., ginger 1½ dr., oil of wormwood 20 drops, subcarbonate of soda 2 dr., syrup to form a ball; ½ dr., or 1 dr., of calomel may be added, or given the previous night; to be repeated at intervals of 10 days if required.—WHITE.

6. Emetic tartar 2 dr., common mass 6 dr.; to be given for 6 mornings, and a purging ball on the 7th.

7. Assafœtida 2 dr., calomel 1 or 2 dr., savin 1½ dr., oil of wormwood 20 drops, syrup q. s.; at night, and a physic ball in the morning.

8. Emetic tartar 1 dr., sulphur 1 dr., linseed meal 4 dr., palm oil to form a ball; one every morning after a mercurial physic ball.—CLATER.

9. For long round worms. Emetic tartar 2 dr., ginger ½ dr., tin filings 6 dr., linseed meal 1 dr., palm oil to form a ball.

10. Assafœtida 4 oz., gentian 2 oz., strong mercurial ointment 1 oz., honey to form a mass, for 16 balls; one or more every morning.—LEBAS.

MISCELLANEOUS BALLS.

Garlic Ball. Beat garlic to a paste with enough linseed or liquorice to form a mass; dose, 10 dr.

Camphor Ball. Mix into a ball 2 dr. of camphor with liquorice powder and syrup enough to give it a proper consistence.

Iodine Ball. Iodine 5 gr., linseed meal 5 dr., palm oil to form a ball.

Ball to prevent Hydrophobia. Skull-cap 2 scruples, belladonna 2½ gr., form them into a ball, to be given night and morning; the second week two balls, the third 3 balls, and this continued for six weeks.—YOUATT.

Leicester Red Balls. Nitre 1 ℔., resin 1 ℔., common soda 2 oz., Castile soap ½ ℔., ginger 2 oz., oil of juniper 2 dr., cinnabar ½ oz.; dose, 1½ oz.

Balls for Appetite. Equal weights of assafœtida, saffron, bay-berries, and aloes, made into a mass with extract of gentian; dose, 1 oz.—LEBAS.

Anodyne Ball. Opium ½ dr. to 1 dr., camphor 1 dr., aniseed ½ oz., soft extract of liquorice q. s.—WHITE.

Antispasmodic Ball. Opium 1 dr., powdered belladonna 10 gr.; linseed meal 3 dr., palm oil or treacle q. s.; twice or thrice a day, in spasm of the neck of the bladder. —CLATER.

Ball for Roaring. The cough Ball, No. 12, may be tried; and the compound iodine ointment rubbed on the throttle for some weeks or months.

Stimulating Diaphoretic Ball. Emetic tartar 1½ dr., ginger 2 dr., camphor ½ dr., opium 2 scruples, oil of caraway 15 drops, honey to form a ball; for hide-bound and unhealthy coat without any other disease.—WHITE.

BARTLETT'S *Perspiration Ball.* Dover's Powder 3 dr., camphor 1 dr., treacle q. s.

HINDS' *Sweating Ball.* Emetic tartar 1 dr., assafœtida 1 dr., liquorice powder and syrup to form a ball; repeat in 12 hours if required.

Grease Ball. Liver of antimony 16 oz., salt of tartar 16 oz., gum guaiacum, fenugreek, parsley seed, of each 4 oz., treacle to form a mass; dose, 1½ oz.

Sedative Ball. In slight colic. Assafœtida 4 dr., opium

4 dr., syrup and liquorice powder to form 4 balls.—HINDS.

Cordial and Anodyne Ball. Castile soap 3 dr., camphor 2 dr., ginger 1½ dr., and Venice turpentine 6 dr., into 1 ball.

Stimulating Diuretic Balls. Cantharides 1 dr., aloes 2 dr., strained turpentine 1 oz., honey q. s.; make 4 balls, and roll in elecampane powder.—M. GOHIER, *in dropsy.*

Stimulating Expectorant Ball. Assafœtida 3 dr., galbanum 1 dr., carbonate of ammonia ½ dr., ginger 1½ dr., honey q. s.—WHITE.

Sedative Aperient Ball. In epidemic catarrh or distemper. Balls for inflammation of the lungs (No. 4) 6 dr., physic ball (No. 10) 2 dr.; one at night and another in the morning.—CLATER.

Zinc and Valerian Ball. Oxide of zinc 1 oz., valerian 2 oz., oil of hartshorn 1 oz., soft extract of juniper berries q. s. to make 4 balls, one, twice a day.—ECKEL.

CHEWING BALLS, *or* MASTICATORIES. The ingredients are to be tied in a piece of a rag, and fixed by a string so that it may be kept in the mouth and chewed.

1. *Emollient Masticatory.* Marshmallow root, liquorice, gum Arabic, of each (in powder) 1 oz., honey 1 oz., or q. s.—LEBAS.

2. *To promote appetite.* Assafœtida, liver of antimony, juniper berries, bay-wood, pellitory, made into a mass with verjuice, tied as above.—SOLLEYSELL.

3. Assafœtida, common salt, mastic, galangal, each 1 oz.—LEBAS.

4. Assafœtida 2 oz., salt 1 oz.—BOURGELAT.

5. Angelica ½ oz., assafœtida 1 oz., vinegar 2 dr.—SOLLEYSELL.

6. Flour of mustard ½ oz., sal ammoniac 2 dr., powdered pellitory 1 oz.,—MOIROUD.

ELECTUARIES & CONFECTIONS.

Electuaries are compound medicines in the state of a soft paste. When the paste is hard enough to be formed into balls, the compound resembles ball masses or balls, under which we have placed them. French pharmaciens often use the term *opiates* as nearly synonymous with electuaries; but we only apply the name (opiates) to compounds containing opium.

OPIATE CONFECTION. (*Veterinary.*) Opium 1½ oz., macerate in a little hot water till soft, and rub it to a paste; then add ginger 3 oz., caraway 6 oz., treacle 1½ ℔; dose, 1½ to 2 oz.—WHITE.

DEMULCENT AND PECTORAL ELECTUARIES.

1. Marshmallow root and liquorice (in powder) of each 2 oz., honey 10 oz.: mix; to be given at twice, with a spatula. MOIROUD.

2. Melt ½ oz. spermaceti with 2 oz. of olive oil, add 6 oz. of honey, and mix in 1½ oz. p. marshmallow root; to be given daily.—MOIROUD.

3. (*With Opium.*) Powdered gum 2 oz., marshmallow 1 oz., extract of opium 2 dr., honey 3 oz.; for 2 doses.

4. *Cough Electuary with Manna.* Manna 2 oz., honey 6 oz.; in the morning; said to have cured acute bronchitis, &c.

5. Powdered liquorice 8 oz., elecampane 4 oz., sulphur 2 oz., honey of squill 32 oz.; mix; for 8 doses.

STIMULANT AND CORDIAL ELECTUARIES.

[M. LEBAS gives a form for an electuary (*Thériaque*) of many ingredients, the first of which (cordial powder) itself contains 26 different substances. We only insert here the simpler formulæ of the French veterinarians.]

1. Powdered angelica root 2 oz., masterwort 1 oz., muriate of ammonia ½ oz., honey 8 oz.—MOIROUD.

2. *Stimulant and Expectorant.* Assafœtida 4 oz., elecampane 8 oz., honey 32 oz. for 6 doses.—MOIROUD.

3. Powdered cassia and ginger, each 1 oz., honey 6 ounces.—MOIROUD.

TONIC AND ASTRINGENT ELECTUARIES.

1. Red oxide of iron 8 oz., gentian 12 oz., extract of juniper-berries 32 oz. MOIROUD prescribes 6 oz. for a horse, or 1 oz. for a sheep; but these are larger doses than are customary in England.

2. Peruvian bark 6 ounces, nitre 1 oz., camphor ½ oz., honey 16 oz.—LEBAS.

3. Powdered bistort 1 oz., calcined magnesia 4 dr., honey 4 oz.—MOIROUD.

PURGATIVE AND LAXATIVE ELECTUARIES. Aloetic compounds are usually made stiff enough to form into balls. See Physic Balls.

1. Oil of croton 20 drops, powdered senna 4 dr., honey q. s.—MOIROUD.

2. Sulphate of magnesia 4 oz., honey 16 oz., bran a quart; infuse the bran in sufficient hot water, and add the salt and honey; twice a day till the bowels are relaxed.—BOURGELAT.

3. Sulphate of soda or magnesia 5 oz., manna 4 oz., bran 1 quart; as the last.—MOIROUD.

DIURETIC ELECTUARIES. 1. Acetate of potash 2 oz., oxymel of squills 4 oz.; oatmeal or flour to give a soft consistence.—MOIROUD.

2. Nitre 1 oz., camphor 2 dr. (rubbed with yolks of 2 eggs,) oxymel 4 oz.; flour or liquorice powder, to give a suitable consistence.—MOIROUD.

DIAPHORETIC ELECTUARIES.

1. Sulphur 1 oz., powdered angelica 1½ oz., honey 5 oz.—MOIROUD.

2. Prepared antimony 1½ oz., elecampane 2 oz., treacle 4 oz.

3. Kermes mineral 1 oz., powdered sassafras and elecampane, each 2 dr., honey 6 oz.

VETERINARY POWDERS.

MR. B. CLARK'S PULVIS UTILIS, *as a vehicle for other powders.* Turmeric ½ ℔., oat-meal or sifted barley-meal 4 ℔.; mix.

AROMATIC POWDER, OR HORSE SPICE.

1. WHITE'S *Aromatic Powder.* Caraway 6 oz. pimento 4 oz., ginger 2 oz., liquorice 2 oz.; mix; dose, 6 to 8 dr.

2. *Common Horse Spice.* Caraway, aniseed, coriander seeds, of each 16 oz.; turmeric 32 oz., cummin seeds, liquorice, and ginger, of each 8 oz.; mix.

3. This is inserted, not as a desirable form, but as a specimen of what is used in the trade. Cayenne 2 oz., bean flour 45 ℔, mustard hulls 45 ℔, cummin seed 15 ℔, caraway 15 ℔, turmeric 9 ℔, bay-berries 3 ℔, ivory black 1 ℔.—GRAY'S SUPPLEMENT. The cordial powder of LEBAS contains 26 ingredients.

ABSORBENT POWDERS.

1. Carbonate of soda 2 to 4 dr., ginger 1 dr., calumba 2 to 4 dr.—WHITE.

2. Prepared chalk 4 dr., gentian 2 to 4 dr., aromatic powder (above) 1 or 2 dr.

ALTERATIVE DIURETIC, AND DIAPHORETIC POWDERS. For swelled legs, grease, foul humours, hide-bound, mange, surfeit, old coughs, and to render the skin fine. They are usually given with moistened corn. Too free use of these powders may prove injurious.

1. Sulphur 2 parts, black antimony 1, nitre, 1; mix; dose ½ oz. to 1 oz.—V. C.

2. Sulphur 4 dr., levigated antimony 2 dr., nitre 3 dr., mix; in *hide-bound* and unthrifty coat every night. —YOUATT.

3. Æthiop's mineral ½ oz., cream of tartar 1 oz.; mix; give every night, in a mash; *for grease.*—BLAINE.

4. Sulphur 12 oz., antimony (black) 12 oz.; mix, and divide into 24 powders; *for mange,* &c.—TAPLIN.

5. Nitre 16 oz., resin 16 oz., prepared antimony 4 oz., flowers of sulphur 24 oz.; mix; dose 1 oz. every evening, with moistened corn for 6 or 8 times.

6. Equal weights of antimony, nitre and cream of tartar; dose 6 to 9 dr.—BLAINE.

7. Nitre 6 oz., vermilion ½ oz., resin 6 oz., tartarized antimony 2 dr.; for 12 doses.

8. Sulphur ½ oz., prepared antimony 1 dr.; once a day in the food, for 10 or 14 days.—CLATER.

9. TAPLIN'S *Alterative Powders.* Levigated anti-

mony 8 oz., sulphur 8 oz., Æthiop's mineral 4 oz., cream of tartar 4 oz.; in 12 doses.

10. Cream of tartar 2 dr., nitre 2 dr., sulphur 4 dr., for one dose.—BLAINE.

11. Nitre 1 oz., resin 1 oz., rust of iron 1 oz., emetic tartar 15 grains; dose 1 oz.—LEBAS.

12. *In Farcy.* Prepared antimony 12 oz., sulphur 12 oz., cream of tartar 8 oz., cinnabar 6 oz.; mix, and divide into 20 doses; one every night, in corn.—TAPLIN.

CONDITION POWDERS. A want of condition is generally indicated by, and connected with the unthrifty state of the coat, which the above (alterative) powders are supposed to remedy. Sometimes warm and bitter tonics are added to those ingredients which promote the action of the skin and kidneys, to increase the appetite and promote nutrition; but the most scientific practitioners condemn these additions; and particularly when the animal is changing its coat.

1. Black antimony 4 oz., flowers of sulphur 2 oz., bean flour or barley-meal ½ ℔; a table-spoonful with corn.—Mr. B. CLARK.

2. Sulphur 2 ℔, fenugreek 4 ℔, cream of tartar 1 ℔, liquorice 1 ℔, nitre 1 ℔, black antimony ½ ℔, gentian ¼ ℔, aniseed ¼ ℔, common salt 1 ℔; dose, 1 oz., daily for 2 or 3 weeks.

3. Gentian 4 oz., liquorice 4 oz., fenugreek 16 oz., diapente 6 oz., nitre 4 oz., salt 4 oz.; to promote appetite.

4. Aromatic powder 2 oz., assafœtida ¼ oz., cream of tartar ¾ oz., crocus metallorum ½ oz.; for 2 doses.—LEBAS.

DIAPENTE. This should be made with equal parts of myrrh, gentian, ivory-dust, bay-berries, and birthwort. But a worthless compound is commonly sold for it. The following is one of the least objectionable substitutes:—Equal parts of gentian, turmeric, bay-berries, and mustard. Another form in use is—Bay-berries 2½ ℔, guaiacum wood 2 ℔, gentian 14 ℔, bole 2 ℔, bark which has been used for the tincture 2 ℔.

Fever Powders. 1. Nitre 1 oz., camphor 2 dr., tartarized antimony 2 dr.—WHITE.

2. Nitre 6 dr., camphor 2 dr., calx of antimony 1½ dr.—HINDS.

3. Nitre 1 oz., unwashed calx of antimony 2 dr., antimonial powder 3 dr., camphor 1 dr.—WHITE.

Pectoral Powder. Powder of gum tragacanth 6 oz., nitre 1 oz.; give a tablespoonful in their mashes or food, in coughs.

Purgative Powder. Epsom salt 8 oz., aloes 10 oz., aniseed 3 oz.; dose, 2 oz.—LEBAS.

Powder for the Gripes. Aloes, senna, ginger, cream of tartar, of each 1 ℔; mix. This was formerly honoured with the title of Pulvis Sanctus.

Worm Powders. 1. Sulphur 12 parts, quicksilver 4 parts; triturate together till the mercury is extinct; then add male fern, rhubarb, tansy, gentian, of each 4 parts, wormwood, savin, aloes, castor seeds, of each 1 part; dose, 1½ oz. to 2 oz.—LEBAS.

2. Fern root 4 parts, tansy 2, assafœtida and aloes, each 1 part; dose, as the last.—MOIROUD.

3. Sulphur 1 oz., emetic tartar 4 dr., common salt 8 oz., liver of antimony 1 oz; mix; for 6 doses; one daily in wetted corn.—HINDS.

Mr. WHITE'S *Compound Arsenical Powder.* White arsenic 1 dr., cream of tartar 9 dr.; mix carefully; give 10 gr. 3 times a day.

HAYNE'S *Bitter Powder*, for loss of appetite. Sulphate of potash 2 oz., gentian 1 oz., flour q. s. To be given twice a day.

MEDICATED PROVENDER. Bruised oats 4 ℔, bruised juniper berries 2 oz., common salt 1 oz.; mix. Nourishing and stimulant.—DELAFOND.

Liquid Medicines for Horses.

DRINKS, DRENCHES, MIXTURES, MASHES, ETC.

Drinks, properly speaking, are liquids which the horse will take willingly; *Drenches* are those liquid medicines which must be administered by a horn, bottle, or funnel. But this distinction is not always observed.

MILD DRINKS. Demulcent, pectoral, cooling, and diuretic.

Barley Water. Barley 1 ℔, water 2 gallons; boil to 6 quarts, strain, and add 1 ℔ of honey. If common barley is used, it should be first boiled with a little water, and this thrown away. If pearled barley is used, this will be less necessary. In inflammatory and catarrhal complaints.

Oatmeal Gruel. 1. Mix gradually 4 oz. of sweet oatmeal with as much cold water as will form a smooth mixture. Put 2 quarts of water in a saucepan over a clear fire, and before it gets very hot, add in the mixture of oatmeal and water; stir the whole till it boils, and let it simmer a little while. Take care not to smoke it.

2. Mix half a pint of oatmeal with the same measure of water; triturate them in a marble mortar with a wooden pestle, for some time; then add 1 gallon of boiling water, and boil for a few minutes.—Mr. B. Clark.

Blanche Water. Wet 3 or 4 handfuls of bran with scalding water, and work it with the hands till it becomes clammy; then add as much more water as may be desired. A mixture of oatmeal and cold water is also called white water, and in France potato or other starch is used for the same purpose.

Linseed Tea. 1. Infuse 4 oz. of linseed in 3 pints of boiling water for several hours near the fire, stirring occasionally; then strain off, and add 4 oz. of honey; for 2 doses; in coughs, &c.

2. Pour 1 gallon of boiling water on ½ lb of linseed; let the infusion stand till nearly cold, then pour off the clear liquid.—YOUATT.

Compound Decoction of Linseed. Linseed 4 oz., liquorice root 4 oz., mallows 2 handfuls; boil in 6 quarts of water for half an hour. Let the horse drink it freely.—BLAINE.

Cooling and Refreshing Drink. Barley water, linseed tea, or blanche water, 8 quarts, simple oxymel 16 oz.—MOIROUD.

Cooling and Diuretic Drink. Dissolve 1 oz. of nitre in a pail of water.

Camphorated Diuretic Drink. Water 10 quarts, nitre 1 oz., camphor (rubbed with yolks of 2 or 3 eggs) ½ oz.; mix, and let the animal drink when thirsty.—MOIROUD.

MASHES.

Bran Mash. Bran or pollard ½ peck; put it in a bucket, and pour on it enough scalding water to wet it thoroughly; let it be well stirred with a stick, or worked with the hands, and let it stand, covered up, till new-milk warm. Emollient and slightly laxative. When intended to be nutritive, oats should be scalded with the bran.—B. CLARK.

Malt Mash. Upon a peck of ground malt pour a gallon and a half of boiling [better not quite boiling] water. Stir frequently, and give when new-milk warm. Nutritive, in diseases attended with great debility.—MARKHAM.

Linseed Mash. HINDS' *Cooling Decoction.* Linseed 2 quarts, coarse sugar 2 oz., boiling water 6 quarts; simmer for 3 or 4 hours.

DRENCHES.

DRENCHES FOR DIARRHŒA, DYSENTERY, AND DIABETES.

For Diarrhœa. 1. Restringent Draught. Opium 1 dr., prepared chalk 1 oz., compound powder of tragacanth 1 oz., mint water 1 pint.—WHITE.

2. Prepared chalk 2 oz., gum arabic ½ oz., catechu 2 dr., thin starch ½ pint.—BLAINE.

3. Prepared chalk 1 oz., catechu 2 dr., p. opium 1 dr., p. ginger 1 dr.; rub together with contents of one egg and add ½ pint of thin gruel.—CLATER.

4. For purging from corrosive sublimate. Powdered opium 2 dr.; rub down with the yolk and white of one egg, add the contents of two more eggs, and gradually stir in ½ pint of thin gruel.—CLATER.

For Dysentery or Molten Grease. 1. Castor oil 8 oz., ipecacuanha 1 dr., opium 20 gr., liquid arrow-root 8 oz. Repeat once or twice at intervals of 6 hours; then substitute boiled starch for the castor oil.—BLAINE.

2. Opium 2 dr., nux vomica ½ dr., ipecacuanha 1 dr., red wine 1 quart; mix; morning and evening.

For Diabetes. 1. Opium 1 dr., ginger 2 dr., p. oak bark 1 oz., decoction of oak bark, 1 pint.—WHITE.

2. Sulphuret of potash 2 dr., uva ursi 4 dr., oak bark 1 oz., catechu 2 dr., opium ½ dr. In strong chamomile tea.—BLAINE.

3. Calomel 3 dr., cascarilla 2 dr., salt of steel 2½ dr., salt of tartar 1½ dr., tincture of opium ½ oz., strong beer q. s.—WHITE.

CARMINATIVE AND ANTISPASMODIC DRENCHES for spasmodic and flatulent colic, or gripes.

[N. B. As most of these drenches would be injurious in *inflammation of the bowels* (Enteritis,) care should be taken to distinguish between these diseases. Inflammation is known by the quick but small pulse, redness of the inside of the eyelids, coldness of the ears and legs, and scanty and high-coloured urine. In colic, the attacks and remissions of pain alternate; in inflammation the pain and distress continue. In colic, the pain is relieved by friction and motion; in inflammation, it is increased. Colic is sudden in its attack; inflammation, more gradual in its approach.]

1. Brandy, rum, or gin from 4 to 6 oz., hot water 12 oz. Mr. CLARK directs a wineglassful of spirits to half

a pint of warm water. A pint of ale is sometimes substituted.—WHITE.

2. Half a large bottle of Daffy's Elixir, with hot water.

3. Tincture of Pimento 4 oz., warm water half a pint.—B. CLARK.

4. Anodyne carminative tincture (WHITE'S, see below) 2 to 4 oz., hot water half a pint.—WHITE.

5. *Antispasmodic Draught.* Spirit of nitric ether 2 oz., tincture of opium 1 oz., solution of aloes (see below) 4 oz.—V. C.

6. Spirit of nitric ether ½ oz., tincture of opium ½ oz., oil of turpentine 3 oz., gruel 1 pint.—BLAINE.

7. Rectified oil of turpentine 3 oz., tincture of opium 1 oz., warm ale 1 pint. If it does not relieve, repeat half the quantity with 1 oz. aloes dissolved in warm water.—YOUATT.

8. Strong ether 1 oz., laudanum 2 oz., oil of peppermint 1 dr., ale and gin, each a ¼ of a pint.—BLAINE.

9. Camphor 2 dr., tincture of opium 1 oz., oil of peppermint 30 drops, warm water 1 pint. In a violent attack, add 1 oz. of spirit of turpentine.—PEALL.

10. The juice of 3 or 4 onions, with half a pint of sound ale.

11. Pepper ½ oz., oil of turpentine 3 oz., laudanum 1 oz., ale ¼ pint.—BLAINE.

12. Pepper a teaspoonful, juice of 2 or 3 large onions, gin ¼ of a pint.—BLAINE.

13. Laudanum 1 oz., sweet spirit of nitre 4 oz., oil of juniper, 1 oz., tincture of benzoin 2 oz., spirit of sal volatile 1½ oz., oil of peppermint 1 dr.; mix; give a fourth part in warm water or gruel, and repeat in 3 or 4 hours, if necessary.—HINDS.

14. Heat ½ ℔. of common salt, and quench it in a quart of good ale. Give it new-milk warm.—DOWNING.

15. In flatulent colic, when there is an evident distention of the abdomen with gas: chloride of lime ½ oz. (or solution of chlorinated soda 1 oz.,) water 1 quart; repeat in half an hour if necessary.

16. Ginger, caraway, nutmeg, pimento, of each 1 oz.,

bruise, and boil them in ¾ of a pint of ale for a few minutes, and add a gill of any spirits.—TAPLIN.

Cordial Antispasmodic Drink, for Spasm of the Diaphragm. Ginger 1 dr., caraway 2 dr., laudanum 1 oz., sweet spirit of nitre 1 oz., warm ale ½ pint.—CLATER.

Antispasmodic Drench for Suppression of Urine. Nitre 1 oz., camphor 2 dr., linseed tea 1 pint.—WHITE.

Diuretic Camphor Drink. Camphor 2 to 3 dr., olive oil 1 oz., carbonate of soda 1 dr.; rub together, and add tincture of opium 1 dr., warm water 2 pints.

Antispasmodic Drenches for Locked Jaw. 1. Opium 1½ dr., camphor 2 dr., ginger 3 dr., brandy-and-water 8 oz.—WHITE.

2. Ether ½ oz., tincture of opium 2 oz., camphor 1 dr., peppermint water ½ pint.

CORDIAL AND STIMULANT DRENCHES. These are used in the same cases as the cordial balls, but are preferred where a more quick and powerful operation is required. Some of them are used in indigestion and slight attacks of colic.

1. Cloves and black pepper (bruised) ½ oz., boiling water a quart; infuse and give warm.—MOIROUD.

2. Any of the cordial balls may be dissolved in warm ale or water, or peppermint water, and given as a drench.

3. A bottle of wine, 1 oz. of extract of juniper-berries, and ½ oz. of cinnamon in powder.—M. LEBAS.

4. Peppermint 2 oz., chamomiles ½ oz.; infuse in 2½ pints of water, and give it before it is cold; in slight colic and indigestion.

PECTORAL AND EMOLLIENT (or DEMULCENT) DRENCHES, for Coughs, Epidemics, Catarrh, &c. (For linseed tea, compound infusion of linseed, barley water, &c., see DRINKS, above.)

1. *Simple Emulsion.* Olive oil 2 oz., honey 3 oz., soft water 1 pint, subcarbonate of potash, 2 dr.; mix.—WHITE.

2. Linseed tea 1 pint, honey 2 oz., syrup of poppies 2 oz., linseed oil 4 oz.

3. B. CLARK'S *Cough Drench.* Linseed oil 2 oz., liquor of potash 40 drops, treacle 1 oz., soft water 10 oz; mix.

4. Powdered gum 2 oz., warm water a quart; dissolve, and add honey 4 oz.—MOIROUD.

5. Marshmallow root 2 oz., water 2½ or 3 pints; boil to a quart, and add 4 oz. of treacle.—MOIROUD.

6. Liquorice and marshmallow roots, of each 2 oz., water a quart; boil, strain, and add honey 4 oz.—LEBAS.

7. Marshmallow root 2 oz., poppy heads 4, water a quart; boil for 10 minutes, strain, and add to the liquor before quite cold, 4 oz. olive oil, 6 oz. of honey, and the yolk of 4 eggs, previously well beaten together.—MOIROUD.

8. Compound decoction of linseed (page 77) 1 quart oxymel 3 ounces.

9. Spermaceti ½ oz., olive oil 3 oz.; melt together, and add of honey 4 oz., water (by little at a time) to make up a quart; repeat it twice a day.—LEBAS.

10. *Camphorated Emulsion.* Powder with a few drops of spirit, 1 or 2 dr. of camphor, add 12 drops of oil of aniseed, and 12 oz. of simple emulsion.—WHITE.

11. Oxymel of squills 2 oz., opium ½ dr. to 1 dr., linseed oil 2 oz.; mix the opium with 8 oz. of water, and add the others; for one dose.—WHITE.

12. For chronic coughs: Tar-water ½ pint, lime-water ½ pint, powdered squill 1 dr.; every morning.—BLAINE.

13. In inflammation of the lungs, or catarrhal fever: Tartarized antimony 2 dr., digitalis 1½ dr., nitre 3 dr. simple oxymel 4 oz., compound decoction of linseed 8 oz.—BLAINE.

14. The same, omitting the digitalis, and substituting 6 oz. of warm water for the dec. linseed. In influenza, when soreness of throat prevents swallowing balls.—BLAINE.

15. In inflammation of the lungs: Ipecacuanha 2 dr. laudanum 4 dr., powdered camphor 2 dr., Mindererus' spirit 4 oz., linseed tea ½ pint.—BLAINE.

16. In pleurisy: Boil pearl barley, split figs, and raisins, each 6 oz., and liquorice root 2 oz., in 4 quarts of

water, down to 3; strain, and add honey 1 ℔, vinegar 1 pint; give 1 oz. nitre in a pint of this decoction every 6 hours.—TAPLIN.

17. In epidemic (epizootic) catarrh: Spirit of nitrous ether 1 oz., Mindererus' spirit 6 oz., with linseed tea. —BLAINE.

18. GIBSON'S *Drink for Catarrhal Epidemic.* Coltsfoot, hyssop, chamomile, of each a handful, linseed and garlic each 1 oz., liquorice root sliced 1 oz., saffron ½ oz.; infuse in 2 quarts of boiling water; give half in the morning, the rest in the afternoon.

19. In influenza (after bleeding.) Oil of croton 5 drops, nitre 4 to 6 dr., tartarized antimony 1 dr., spirit of nitric ether ½ oz. to 1 oz., solution of acetate of ammonia 2 to 4 oz., warm water q. s. Once or twice daily. Sometimes ½ oz. of cream of tartar is added.—SPOONER.

20. For malignant epidemic. Oxymel 4 oz., spirit of Mindererus 4 oz., beer yeast 4 oz., sweet spirit of nitre 1 oz.

DIURETIC DRENCHES, for Dropsical Complaints, &c. The use of stimulating diuretics in retention of urine from inflammation of the neck of the bladder, is dangerous.

1. MARKHAM'S *Dropsy Drench.* Decoction of wormwood in ale 2 quarts, soap 1 oz., grains of paradise 6 dr., long pepper 6 dr., treacle 3 oz.; for one dose, fasting.

2. For dropsy of the belly: Castile soap 2 oz., strong beer 1 pint; dissolve, and add cascarilla 2 dr., ginger 3 dr., oil of juniper 2 dr. (or balsam of copaivi 1 oz.;) mix; for 1 dose.—WHITE.

3. White soap 1 oz., spirit of turpentine 1 oz., honey 4 oz.; decoction of linseed 2 quarts; for 2 doses.—MOIROUD.

4. Strained turpentine 2 oz., yolk of 6 eggs; triturate together till incorporated, and add gradually 2 quarts of linseed tea; for 2 doses.—MOIROUD.

5. White wine and water 4 quarts, nitre 3 oz., honey 4 oz.; for 3 doses.—LEBAS.

6. Acetate of potash 2 or 3 oz., honey 6 oz., decoction of hemp or linseed 2 quarts; for one dose.—MOIROUD.

7. Acetate of potash 2 oz., camphor (rubbed with yolks of 2 eggs) 2 dr., decoction of linseed 2 quarts; for 2 doses, at an interval of some hours; in irritation of the urinary passages, especially arising from cantharides or resinous irritants.—MOIROUD.

8. *Squill drench.* Decoction of pellitory of the wall 1 quart, oxymel of squills 4 oz.—MOIROUD.

9. *Colchicum Drench.* Colchicum wine 2 oz., simple oxymel 4 oz., barley water 1 quart.

10. Sweet spirit of nitre 4 oz., white wine 1 quart, water 2 quarts; for 3 doses; in dysuria not arising from mechanical obstruction or inflammation of the neck of the bladder.—LEBAS.

11. *Saline Diuretic Drink.* Glauber salt 2 oz., nitre 6 dr., warm water 1 pint, sweet spirit of nitre 1 dr. —CLARK.

DRENCHES FOR FARCY AND GLANDERS.

1. Expressed juice of cleavers 6 oz., strong decoction of hempseed 6 oz.; essence of spruce 6 oz.; mix; give every evening; and a mercurial or arsenical ball in the morning.—BLAINE. See Farcy Balls.

2. *For Glanders.* Sulphate of copper 3 to 6 dr., gum Arabic 2 or 3 oz., dissolved in 2 or 3 pints of water.—SEWELL.

FEVER DRENCHES.

1. Nitre 2 dr., tartar-emetic ½ dr., warm water or thin gruel 12 oz.; once or twice a day.—B. CLARK.

2. Sweet spirit of nitre 1 oz., spirit of Mindererus 6 oz., water 4 oz.

LAXATIVE AND PURGATIVE DRENCHES.

1. Castor oil 6 oz., linseed oil 8 oz., gruel q. s.—BLAINE.

2. Glauber's or Epsom salts 6 or 8 oz., whey or gruel 1 quart, castor oil 6 or 8 oz.—WHITE.

3. Barbadoes aloes 2 dr. tartarized antimony 1 dr., warm water 4 oz.; mix, and add castor oil 4 oz.—WHITE.

4. *Laxative Febrifuge in Influenza.* Linseed oil 12 oz., nitre 3 dr., camphor powdered 1 dr., sweet spirit of nitre 1 oz., warm water ½ pint.—CLATER.

5. *Laxative Anodyne Drink.* In inflammation of the bowels: Linseed oil 1 pint, opium 2 scruples, sweet spirit of nitre 6 dr., warm water 4 oz.—CLATER.

6. Aloes 2 or 3 dr., salt of tartar 1 dr., water or mint water ½ pint; mix, and add castor oil 4 to 6 oz.—WHITE.

7. *A Cooling Purging Drink.* Infuse 2 oz. senna with 3 dr. salt of tartar in a quart of boiling water for 2 hours; strain, and add 4 oz. Glauber's salts, and 2 or 3 dr. of cream of tartar.—BARTLET.

STRONGER PURGATIVE DRENCHES.

1. B. aloes 2 oz., gum Arabic 1 oz.; powder and mix them, and pour on them a pint of boiling water. Take 10 gr. of farina of croton, and add to it gradually 4 oz. of the above solution. Repeat this dose every 6 hours till it operates; in inflammation of the brain.—CLATER.

2. Aloes 1 oz., soap 2 dr., salt of tartar 1 dr., water 1 pint: in apoplexy or staggers.—WHITE.

3. Infuse 1 oz. of senna in a quart of boiling water, strain, and add 1 oz., of aloes in powder.—BOURGELAT.

4. Aloes 1 oz., sulphate of magnesia 2 oz., aniseed powder ½ oz., water a quart.—LEBAS.

5. Aloes 1 oz., syrup of buckthorn 4 oz., warm water a quart.—LEBAS.

DRENCHES FOR STOMACH STAGGERS, or Staggers from Indigestion.

1. After a ball of aloes and calomel, and clyster of salt water—Spirit of sal volatile ½ oz., cascarilla powder 2 dr., warm water ½ pint; twice a day; and the same without the cascarilla every hour.—WHITE.

2. Aloes 3 dr., pimento 2 dr., ginger 1 dr., infuse in a quart of hot water, and when cold add 2 oz. spirit of turpentine, and 1 oz., of spirit of hartshorn. Repeat in an hour if required.—BLAINE.

3. *Laxative Tonic Drinks.* Linseed oil 1 pint, powdered gentian 2 dr.; every 6 hours till the bowels are properly opened.—CLATER.

4. Common salt 4 oz., ginger 2 dr., magnesia 1 oz., warm water 1 quart.—WHITE.

5. Valerian 1 oz., serpentary ½ oz., saffron 2 dr.; infuse in a pint of boiling water, and when nearly cold, strain off, and add 1 oz. tincture of assafœtida and 2 dr. of laudanum.—TAPLIN.

6. *After a purgative.* Volatile tincture of valerian 1 oz., powdered valerian 1½ oz., peppermint water 8 oz.; mix, for a dose.—WHITE.

TONIC DRENCHES. Tonics are more generally administered in the form of balls.

1. *Mild Tonic in latter stage of epidemic catarrh or distemper.* Gentian 1 dr., powdered ginger ½ dr., cascarilla 1 dr., warm water ½ pint, sweet spirit of nitre ½ oz. to 1 oz.; to be repeated night and morning unless they quicken the pulse.—CLATER.

2. Gentian root 2 oz., smaller centaury 1 oz., wormwood ½ oz.; boil in 3 pints of water to a quart.—M. VATEL.

3. CLARK'S *Bitter Drench.* Quassia chips 2 oz., water 3 pints; boil to 2 pints; for 3 doses.

4. Quassia 1 oz., ginger 2 dr., water 2 pints; boil for 10 minutes; for 2 doses.

5. *Metallic Tonic.* Sulphate of zinc ½ dr., ginger or pimento 1 dr., treacle 1 oz.; mix, and add gradually 12 oz. warm water.—B. CLARK.

6. *Egyptian Tonic Drink.* In farcy and nasal gleet. Ægyptiacum ½ oz., pimento or ginger ½ dr., warm water 12 oz.—CLARK.

7. *Cantharides Tonic Drench* (for the same.) Sulphate of zinc 15 gr., cantharides 7 gr., pimento 15 gr., treacle 1 oz., warm water to form a drench.

DEOBSTRUENT DRENCHES.

1. Guaiacum wood 2 oz., sassafras 1 oz., linseed ½ oz., water q. s. to yield a quart of decoction; boil, strain, and add of corrosive sublimate 10 gr., sal ammoniac 2 dr.—LEBAS.

2. Iodide of potassium 40 gr., iodine 10 gr., water a quart.—MOIROUD.

3. Muriate of lime 2 oz., water a quart.—MOIROUD.

WORM DRENCHES.

1. Common salt 2 oz., infusion of wormwood a quart. Repeat it for some days.—MOIROUD.

2. A quart of linseed oil.—CLATER.

3. Oil of turpentine 4 oz., linseed or castor oil 8 oz., gruel a pint; preceded by a mild dose of aloes, and bran mashes.

4. Fern root 2 oz., valerian 1 oz., DIPPEL'S animal oil (empyreumatic oil of hartshorn) 1 oz., yolks of 2 eggs, honey 2 oz.; boil the roots in 2 pints of water to half, incorporate the oil with the egg, and then the honey, and mix the whole with the decoction.—VATEL.

5. Animal oil 1 oz., yolks of 2 eggs, honey 1 oz., water or some bitter infusion a quart. CHABERT recommends infusion of savory as a vehicle for the oil.—LEBAS.

6. Soot (wood soot?) in fine powder 2 oz., spirit of wine 2 oz.; mix, and add a quart of infusion of rue, or of tansy. Some practitioners prefer milk as a vehicle for worm medicines.—MOIROUD. For other worm remedies, see Worm Balls.

DRENCHES for the MALIGNANT EPIDEMIC, or DISTEMPER—Pestilential or Putrid Fever.

1. Gentian 1 dr., calumba 2 dr., ginger 1 dr., laudanum ½ oz., spirit of nitrous ether ½ oz., peppermint water 3 oz.—CLATER.

2. Gentian 2 oz., willow bark 6 oz., water 3 pints; boil to a quart, and add solution of acetate of ammonia 6 oz.—MOIROUD.

3. Dissolve ½ dr. of chloride of lime in 8 oz. water, and add spirit of nitric ether ½ oz., laudanum ½ oz., tincture of calumba 1 oz.; twice a day.—CLATER.

4. Bruised bark 3 oz., acetate of ammonia 4 oz., camphor 1 dr.; boil the bark in 2 quarts of water in a covered vessel for a quarter of an hour; strain, and when cool, add the camphor (rubbed with yolk of egg or honey,) and the acetate of ammonia.—LEBAS.

5. Spirit of nitric ether 1 oz., Mindererus' spirit 4 oz., infusion of chamomile 6 oz., beer yeast 6 oz., tincture of opium 3 dr.—BLAINE. See also Antiseptic Drenches (below.)

ANTISEPTIC DRENCHES, *to check Mortification.*

1. Peruvian bark 1 oz., ginger 2 dr., opium 1 dr., fresh beer q. s.—WHITE.

2. Opium 1 dr., carbonate of ammonia 1 dr., aromatic powder 2 dr., camphor 1½ dr., good ale or porter a pint.

3. Chloride of lime or soda 2 to 3 dr., serpentary in powder 1 oz., fresh beer or sweet wort 1 quart.—WHITE.

DRENCH FOR POISONING BY YEW. Stronger purgative drink (No. 1) 4 oz., vinegar 4 oz., thick gruel 4 oz.; repeat it every 6 hours, *without the croton*, till purging is produced.—CLATER.

DRENCH FOR PREVENTING HYDROPHOBIA. Box leaves 8 oz., rue 8 oz.; cut them very fine and boil in 3 pints of milk, in a close vessel, for an hour, and strain; boil the ingredients another hour in 3 pints of water, and strain; mix the decoctions: give a third part every morning fasting.—BLAINE.

DRENCHES TO PROMOTE PARTURITION.

1. Ergot of rye in fine powder 2 or 3 dr., pennyroyal water, or infusion of rue, 1 quart.

2. Saffron 6 dr., chamomiles 2 oz., boiling water a quart; make an infusion, to be given warm. 1 oz. of dried savin, with 1 oz., of cassia, may be substituted for the saffron.—MOIROUD.

ANODYNE DRENCHES.

1. Opium 1 dr. dissolved in warm water, ½ pint; add 1 quart of starch gruel.

2. Oil of peppermint 50 drops, dissolved in a pint of warm water, with 2 oz., of gum Arabic; add tincture of opium ½ oz.

3. Mix tincture of opium ½ oz., with sweet spirits of nitre 1½ oz., essence of peppermint 1 dr., and water 1 pint.

IODINE DRENCH. Iodide of potassium 2 scruples, iodine 12 gr.; triturate together, and add gradually a quart of water.—MOIROUD.

MISCELLANEOUS LIQUID MEDICINES.

TINCTURES, SOLUTIONS, &c.

Solution of Aloes. Aloes 1 part, water 7 parts, proof spirit 1 part; dissolve the aloes in water by means of a water bath, and when removed, add the spirit.—MORTON.

Anodyne Carminative Tincture. Opium 1 oz., cloves 1 oz., ginger 1 oz., old brandy (or rum, or gin) 1 quart; digest in a corked bottle, shaking daily.—WHITE.

Ethereal Tincture of Opium. Turkey Opium 1 ℔, spirit of nitric ether 8 ℔; macerate for a month. Dose, ½ oz. to 1 oz., in spasmodic colic.—MR. DICKENS.

Gripe Tincture. Tincture of Pimento. Ground pimento 1 ℔, rectified spirit, and soft water, of each 3 pints; digest for some days and strain: give 4 fluid oz. at once, and repeat every hour till relieved.—MR. B. CLARK.

Tincture of Fox-glove. Digest 3 oz. of dried fox-glove in a quart of any spirit.—YOUATT.

Infusion of Fox-glove. Infuse 1 oz. of powdered fox-glove in a quart of boiling water till cold.—YOUATT.

Tincture of Myrrh. Myrrh 2 oz., sand 2 oz., rectified spirit and soft water, of each ½ pint.—B. CLARK.

Tincture of Aloes and Myrrh. Aloes 12 oz., myrrh 6 oz., rectified spirit 1 gallon, water ½ gallon; digest 14 days, frequently shaking, and filter. For outward use, rectified wood naphtha may be substituted for the spirit.—V. C.

Tincture for Colic. Opium 1 dr., horseradish 2 oz., capsicum 1 oz., spirit of nitric ether 1 ℔; macerate 14 days; dose, 1 oz., with 2 oz. of spirit of nitric ether, every 2 hours as long as necessary.—GREGORY.

Tincture of Croton. Bruised croton seeds 1 oz.; rectified spirit 16 oz. Digest for 7 days, and filter. Dose ½ oz. to 1 oz., in water.

Tincture of Iodine. Iodine 1 part, rectified spirit 8 parts; dose, 1 to 2 dr.—V. C. But the following is preferable:—

Compound Tincture of Iodine. Iodine 1 oz., iodide of potassium 2 oz., spirit of wine 12 oz.

Solution of Chloride of Lime. 1. Chloride of lime, 1 dr., water 8 oz.; mix in a mortar, and filter.—CLATER.

2. Chloride of lime 1 part, water 10 parts.—CHEVALLIER.

Chloride of lime, 1 part, water 48 parts.—LABARRAQUE. See LOTIONS, page 100.

Solution of Nitre. Nitre 1 part, water 7 parts.—V. C.

Solution of Ammonio-Sulphate of Copper.—Dissolve 1 part of sulphate of copper in 4 parts of water, and add ammonia until it begins to precipitate. 4 ounces every 8 hours as a tonic.—Mr. JECKYLL.

Solution of Henbane. Extract of henbane 4 dr., spirit of nitric ether 4 oz. Antispasmodic; dose, 2 oz, with or without solution of Aloes.—WRIGHT.

For SOLUTIONS and TINCTURES *for outward use,* see EXTERNAL APPLICATIONS, further on.

CLYSTERS.

Laxative. 1. Aloes 1 oz., water 2 or 3 quarts.—YOUATT.

2. Water gruel 1 gallon, olive oil a pint.—WHITE.

3. Epsom salts 6 oz. (or common salt 6 oz., or soap 2 oz.,) thin gruel or broth 5 quarts.—BLAINE.

4. Soft soap 2 oz., warm water ¾ of a pailful.—B. CLARK.

5. Infuse 3 oz. senna in 2 quarts of water, and add Epsom salts 4 oz., honey 6 oz.—MOIROUD.

6. Chamomiles, fennel seed, coriander seed, of each 1 oz., caraways, ½ oz.; boil in 2 quarts of water to 3 pints; strain, add 2 oz. Epsom salts, and when nearly cool, ¼ pint of olive oil and ¼ pint of tincture of senna. —TAPLIN.

Purgative. 1. Aloes 8 to 12 dr., salt 8 oz., water 1 gallon; in staggers.—WHITE.

2. Senna 2 oz., tobacco 2 oz.; boil for a quarter of an hour in 2 quarts of water, strain, and add common salt 4 oz., emetic tartar 1 dr.; for 2 doses. *Very irritating.*—LEBAS.

Emollient. Dried mallow leaves, or marshmallow root 1½ oz., linseed ½ oz., water 2 quarts; boil and strain: to be used warm.—MOIROUD.

Emollient and Anodyne. 1. Mix 6 dr. of starch in powder with a little cold water, and add it to a decoction of 6 poppy-heads in 2 quarts of water; boil for an instant and strain; in intestinal irritation.—MOIROUD.

2. Gruel 2 pints, liquid starch or arrowroot 1 pint, powdered opium 1 dr. to 1½ dr.—WHITE.

3. Boil 6 poppy-heads in 4 quarts of water till reduced to 2 quarts; add prepared chalk 2 oz., boiled starch 2 quarts: once or twice a day in diarrhœa.—BLAINE.

4. A double handful of coarse bran, 6 poppy-heads, 2 quarts of water; boil and strain.—MOIROUD.

5. Tripe liquor (or suet boiled in milk) 3 pints, thin starch a quart, laudanum ½ oz.: in diarrhœa.

Cooling. Butter-milk or whey, barley-water, of each a quart.—MOIROUD.

Carminative and Stimulant. 1. Chamomiles 3 oz., aniseed or fennel seed 1½ oz., 4 poppy-heads; boil the poppies in sufficient water, and infuse the flowers and seeds in the hot decoction.—M. VATEL.

2. *To expel wind.* Boil 1 ℔ of figs in 3 quarts of water for half an hour, then add two handfuls of chopped rue; boil a few minutes, strain, and add 8 oz. of olive oil.—SOLLEYSELL.

For Gripes. Mash 2 onions, pour over them 2 oz. of oil of turpentine and 4 quarts of thin gruel.—BLAINE.

Astringent. 1. Alum whey 1 quart, thin starch a quart.

2. Suet milk 3 pints, starch gruel 2 pints, laudanum ½ oz.

Vermifuge. 1. *For thread worms.* Powdered aloes ½ oz., powdered gum Arabic ½ oz.; mix with half pint of boiling water; then mix the white of an egg with a quart of linseed oil, and gradually add the solution of aloes.—CLATER.

2. Infuse 4 oz. of tansy in 2 quarts of water; strain and add 2 oz. of animal oil (empyreumatic oil of hartshorn;) also the worm drenches Nos. 4 and 6 may be used in this method.—MOIROUD.

Uterine Stimulants. 1. Infuse a handful of rue in 2 quarts of water, and add 2 oz. of common salt.

2. Savine 2 oz., sal ammoniac 4 dr.: as the last.

Diuretic. 1. Nitre 1 oz., decoction of linseed 3 pints.

2. *Camphorated.* Incorporate 4 dr. of camphor with the yolks of 2 eggs, and add it to the last.—MOIROUD.

For Irritable Bladder. 1. Belladonna leaves 3 oz., water 3 pints; boil, and administer warm.—MOIROUD.

2. Extract belladonna ½ oz., boiling water 1½ pint.

Nourishing. 1. Thick gruel 3 quarts, ale 1 quart.—BLAINE.

2. Milk 2 quarts, yolks of four eggs; mix, and give warm.—BOURGELAT.

3. Strong broth 2 quarts, thickened milk 2 quarts. —BLAINE.

4. Tripe liquor or broth 3 quarts, flour 4 oz.; mix the flour in the hot broth; repeat frequently.—MOIROUD.

External Applications.

LINIMENTS AND EMBROCATIONS.

BLISTERING LINIMENTS, OR LIQUID BLISTERS, AND SWEATING OILS.

1. Powdered Spanish flies 1 oz., spirit of wine 6 oz., water of ammonia 2 oz.; let it stand for a week, shaking it frequently, and strain. (See No. 11.)—WHITE.

2. Flies 1 oz., euphorbium ½ oz., oil of turpentine 4 oz.; digest for 2 or 3 days, and pour off the liquid; digest the flies, &c. in 4 oz. of spirit of wine and 2 oz. of water of ammonia for 3 or 4 days, shaking frequently; strain off this liquid, and mix it with the former. This is more active than the last.—WHITE.

3. BLAINE'S *Liquid Blister.* Spanish flies, coarsely powdered, 8 oz., oil of turpentine 2 quarts; steep for 3 weeks, strain, and add a quart of olive oil.

4. BLAINE'S *Milder or Sweating Liquid.* Mix 4 oz. of the last with 6 oz. of oil.

5. CLATER'S *Strong Liquid Blister.* Spirits of turpentine, coloured with alkanet, 1 gallon, powdered flies 1 ℔; macerate for a month, shaking daily, then pour off the clear fluid for use.

6. *Common, or Sweating Liquid.* Mix the last with equal parts of spermaceti oil.

7. Powdered flies 2 oz., spirit of turpentine a pint; digest for a few days.—YOUATT.

8. *Blistering Liniment for immediate use.* Spanish flies in fine powder 1 oz., oil of turpentine 6 oz. To be rubbed on the belly in inflammation of the bowels. —WHITE.

9. *Croton Liniment.* A tincture of croton nuts with oil of turpentine is used as a blister, but is not so efficacious as Cantharides.—Mr. YOUATT.

10. WHITE'S *Mustard Blister.* Best flour of mustard 8 oz., water enough to form a paste, oil of turpentine 2 oz., water of ammonia 1 oz.

11. *Blistering Tincture.* Flies 1 oz., proof spirit 8 oz.; macerate 2 or 3 weeks; mix, and filter. To be rubbed in, and repeated next day if necessary.—WHITE.

12. Saturated tincture of cantharides 1 oz., bichloride of mercury 6 grains.—KENT.

13. Powdered cantharides 1 dr., olive oil 2 oz. To be applied every 48 hours for a week, in old spavin.—TAPLIN.

14. *Oil of Cantharides* (by infusion.) Digest 1 part of powdered cantharides in 8 oz. of olive oil, in a water-bath, for two hours, and strain.

15. *Cantharidal Solution* (for setons.) Digest 1 part of p. flies with 8 of oil of turpentine, with a gentle heat, for 14 days; strain and add to the clear liquid an equal weight of Canada balsam. Soak the cotton cord in the solution, draw it between the finger and thumb, and dry it.—MORTON.

STIMULATING LINIMENTS.

1. Soft soap 4 oz., camphor 1 oz., proof spirit 2 pints, water of ammonia ½ pint.—V. C.

2. Sweet oil 2 oz., spirit of hartshorn 1 oz., oil of turpentine ½ oz.—WHITE.

3. Common oil 6 oz., liquid blister 2 or 3 oz.; in chronic sprains.—BLAINE.

4. *Soap Liniment.* Soft soap 4 oz., water 8 oz.; dissolve, and add 1 pint of rectified spirit, in which is dis-

solved 2 oz. camphor, 1 oz. oil of rosemary, and 2 to 4 oz. strong water of ammonia.—WHITE.

5. For splints: Oil of origanum 1 oz., oil of turpentine 1 oz., spirit of wine ½ oz. To be applied night and morning for a few days, discontinuing it as often as any moisture appears.—LANCET.

6. For the same purpose: Oil of origanum ½ oz., oil of turpentine ½ oz., camphorated spirit of wine 2 oz.—TAPLIN.

7. For sprains, old swellings, rheumatism, &c.: Spirit of hartshorn 2 oz., camphorated spirit 2 oz., oil of turpentine 1 oz., laudanum ½ oz., oil of origanum 1 dr.

8. Camphorated oil 4 oz., oil of turpentine 1 oz., oil of origanum 1 dr.

9. For callous swellings after bruises: Soap liniment 4 oz., camphor 2 dr., water of ammonia 1 oz.

10. For indolent tumours: Mercurial ointment 2 oz., olive oil 2 dr., camphor 2 dr.

11. Olive oil 4 oz., water of ammonia 2 oz., oil of turpentine 2 oz.

12. For strains: Barbadoes tar 2 oz., spirit of turpentine 2 oz., opodeldoc 4 oz.—TAPLIN.

13. Oil of turpentine 2 parts, muriatic acid 1 part. —POTT.

14. Camphorated oil 4 parts, oil of turpentine and tincture of cantharides, of each 2 parts, acetic acid 1 oz.—LEBAS.

15. *Turpentine Liniment.* Equal parts of oil of turpentine and olive oil. Digestive and rubefacient.—V. C.

16. *Compound Turpentine Liniment.* Soft soap 4 oz., camphor 1 oz., oil of turpentine 16 oz.; mix.—V. C.

LINIMENT FOR BOG SPAVIN. Mercurial ointment 2 oz., oil of cantharides 4 dr.—MORTON.

LINIMENT FOR SORE BACKS. Extract of lead ½ oz., vinegar 1 oz., olive oil 2 oz.—WHITE.

LINIMENTS FOR ITCHING HUMOURS, MANGE, LICE, &c.

1. Equal parts of oil of tar, oil of turpentine, and

seal oil. Apply every second day for 2 or 3 times, then wash.—V. C.

2. Sulphur 4 oz., turpentine 4 oz., oil of tar and train oil 6 or 8 oz. The parts to be first washed with soft soap and dried.

3. For lice: Sublimate 1 dr., muriatic acid 3 dr., tobacco water 2 pints, oil of turpentine 4 oz.—WHITE.

Liniment for Mange. Goulard's extract of lead 2 oz., olive or rape oil 2 oz., sulphur 1 oz.

LINIMENTS FOR CANKER OF THE FOOT AND BAD THRUSHES. See also CAUSTICS and LOTIONS.

1. Barbadoes tar 1 oz., oil of turpentine 1½ oz.; mix carefully, and add oil of vitriol 1 dr.—WHITE.

2. Butter of antimony alone.

3. Crystallized verdigris in fine powder 1 oz., honey 2 oz., bole and alum, of each ½ oz., vinegar to form a liniment; to be mixed over a gentle fire. Greasy applications are to be avoided.—WHITE.

See also DETERGENT LINIMENTS.

DETERGENT LINIMENTS.

1. Oil of turpentine 1 oz., oil of vitriol 2 dr., by measure; mix in a large gallipot, and when cool, add 2 oz. of linseed oil.—WHITE.

2. *Ægyptiacum.* Bruised sulphate of copper 12 oz., vinegar 4 lb., treacle 3 lb.; place over a clear fire, and let it boil up.—B. CLARK.

3. *Wash for Grease.* Sulphate of copper 2 dr., and alum 2 dr., in water 1 pint.

MISCELLANEOUS LINIMENTS AND MIXED OILS.

(See also EMBROCATIONS.)

Creasote Liniment. Creasote 2 oz., oil of turpentine 4 oz., olive oil 4 oz.; mix: in fistulous sores, unhealthy wounds, &c.—V. C.

Oil of Cantharides. Powdered flies 1 oz., olive oil 8 oz.; digest in a water-bath for 2 or 3 hours, and filter.—V. C.

Goulard Liniment. Extract of lead 1 oz., olive oil 4 oz., —MORTON. For excoriated surfaces, &c.

Saturnine Balsam. Acetate of lead 1 oz., oil of turpentine 2 oz.; digest with a gentle heat.—MOIROUD.

Drying Liniment. Linseed oil and spirit of wine of each equal parts.—SOLLEYSELL.

Marshmallow Liniment. Olive oil and marshmallow ointment, of each 4 oz.; melt the ointment, and add the oil. —BOURGELAT.

Emollient and Anodyne Liniment. Neatsfoot oil 4 oz., poplar ointment, and marshmallow ointment, of each 2 oz.—MOIROUD.

Lime-water Liniment. Lime-water 8 oz., olive or linseed oil 2 oz.

Narcotic Liniment. Olive oil 4 oz., laudanum 2 oz.—MOIROUD.

Liniment for Confirmed Grease.—Verdigris, sugar of lead, of each ¼ oz., honey 1 oz.; mix.—CLATER.

Compound Iodine Liniment. Iodine 1 oz., soap liniment 8 oz.—V. C.

Turpentine Liniment. Equal parts of turpentine and olive oil.—V. C.

Resolvent Liniment. Olive oil 2 oz., strong mercurial ointment 2 dr., water of ammonia 2 dr.

Black Oils. Olive (or rape) oil 1 pint, oil of turpentine 2 oz.; mix, and add gradually 6 dr. of sulphuric acid; leave the bottle open till cold.—PERCIVALL.

Oils for Mange. Oil of turpentine 1 pint; add to it very gradually and cautiously 2 oz. of oil of vitriol, stirring the mixture constantly, then add a quart of linseed oil; from 4 to 8 oz. to be rubbed in with a brush every second day, for 3 or 4 times.—CLATER.

WARD'S *White Oils.* Spirit of wine, oil of turpentine, rape oil, beef brine, camphor, of each equal parts.

White Oils, or Egg Oils. 1. Yolks of 2 eggs, 3 oz. solution of ammonia, 1 oz. oil of origanum, 4 oz. oil of turpentine, a pint of vinegar; mix, s. a.—PHARMACEUTICAL JOURNAL.

2. Distilled vinegar 1½ pint, oil of turpentine 1½ dr., spirit of wine 1½ oz., GOULARD'S extract of lead ½ oz., whites and yolks of 2 eggs; mix the turpentine and

Goulard with the eggs, gradually add the vinegar, and lastly the spirit.—REDWOOD'S GRAY'S SUPPLEMENT.

Liniment of Ammonia. This is sometimes termed *White Oils.* Olive or rape oil 4 oz., water of ammonia 1 oz. Sometimes 1 oz. of oil of turpentine is added, to increase its activity.

Darby's Oils. Equal parts oil of amber, Barbadoes tar, and balsam of sulphur.

MARSHALL'S *Oils.* Linseed oil 1 ℔, olive or rape oil 1 ℔., green oil ½ ℔, oil of turpentine ½ ℔, oil of vitriol 1½ dr.

Newmarket Oils. Linseed oil, oil of turpentine, green oil, of each 3 ℔, oil of vitriol 1 oz.

Nine Oils. Train oil 23 ℔, oil of turpentine 6 ℔, oil of bricks 1 ℔, oil of amber 1 ℔, spirit of camphor 2 ℔, Barbadoes tar 7 ℔, oil of vitriol 2 oz.—GRAY'S SUPPLEMENT.

RADLEY'S *Oils.* Barbadoes tar 8 oz., linseed 4 oz., oil of turpentine 4 oz.

LORD STAMFORD'S *Mixed Oils.* Oil of origanum 6 oz., oil of turpentine 24 oz., spirit of wine 16 oz., green oil 6 ℔., camphor 3 oz.

EMBROCATIONS, VARIOUS.

(See also LINIMENTS & LOTIONS.)

Embrocation for Strains. 1. Soft soap 1 oz., spirit of wine 4 oz., oil of rosemary 2 dr., camphor 2 dr.

2. For strains in the shoulder: oil of turpentine 1 oz., camphorated spirit 2 oz.—BLACKER.

3. Equal quantities of soft soap, oil of turpentine, spirit of wine, and elder ointment.—WHITE.

4. Soft soap 2 oz., oil of bays 1 oz., water of ammonia 1½ oz., oil of origanum ½ oz.

5. Barbadoes tar 2 oz., spirit of turpentine 2 oz., opodeldoc 4 oz. After fomenting with hot vinegar and Goulard.—TAPLIN.

Mustard Embrocations. 1. Mustard flour 4 oz., water of ammonia 1½ oz., oil of turpentine 1 oz., water enough to bring it to the consistence of cream.

2. Camphor 1 oz., oil of turpentine 2 oz., water of ammonia 2 oz., flour of mustard 8 oz., water to form a thin paste.—WHITE.

Embrocation for Poll Evil. Spirit of wine ½ pint, camphor 2 dr., Goulard's extract of lead 1 dr.; mix.—HINDS. See DISCUTIENT LOTIONS.

Embrocation for Saddle Galls, or Warbles. 1. Goulard's extract of lead 2 dr., distilled vinegar 3 oz., spirit of wine 4 oz.—WHITE.

2. Soap liniment and Mindererus' spirit, equal parts.

3. Sal ammoniac ½ oz., muriatic acid 2 dr., water 8 to 12 oz.

4. White vinegar 3 oz., spirit of wine 3 oz., sugar of lead 2 dr., water 6 oz.; mix.—HINDS.

CLARK'S *Embrocatio Frigorifera.* Vinegar 4 oz., camphor (dissolved in spirit) ½ oz., water to fill up a wine bottle.

CLARK'S *Embrocatio Excitans.* Olive oil 3 oz., camphor ½ dr., spirit of turpentine ½ oz., water of ammonia 3 dr.

TAPLIN'S *Embrocation for Windgalls.* Oil of Origanum, spirit of turpentine each ½ oz., camphorated spirit 1 oz. Applied with tow, and covered with a piece of lead bound on.

LOTIONS OR WASHES.

COOLING LOTIONS, for external inflammation.

1. Sal ammoniac 1 oz., nitre 2 oz., water 16 oz. To be used as soon as made.—MORTON.

2. Goulard's extract of lead 1 oz., vinegar 2 oz., camphorated spirit 3 oz., water 16 oz.; for recent spavin.—TAPLIN.

3. V. C. *Goulard Water.* Goulard's extract 2 dr., spirit 2 dr., soft water 1 pint.

4. WHITE'S *Saturnine Lotion.* Sugar of lead 1 oz., vinegar and water 1 pint.

5. B. CLARK'S *Lotio Refrigerans.* Liquor of diacetate of lead 1 dr., spirit of nitric ether 1 dr., water 2 pints. In slight rubs and bruises.

DISCUTIENT LOTIONS, for dispersing indolent tumours and saddle-galls, and for chronic strains, &c.

1. Mindererus' spirit 4 oz., camphorated spirit 4 oz., water 16 oz.—PERCIVALL.

2. Sal ammoniac 1 oz., vinegar 8 oz., camphorated spirit 1 oz.—MORTON.

3. For saddle-galls and warbles: Goulard's extract 2 dr., distilled vinegar 3 oz., spirit of wine 4 oz.—WHITE.

4. Muriate of ammonia ½ oz., muriatic acid 2 dr., water 8 to 12 oz.: for saddle-galls and wind-galls.—WHITE.

5. BLAINE'S *Saline Embrocation.* Sal ammoniac 8 oz., vinegar 3 pints.

6. Mindererus' spirit 2 oz., soap liniment 2 oz.—WHITE.

7. For Warbles: White Vinegar 3 oz., spirit of wine 3 oz., sugar of lead 2 dr., water 6 oz.—HINDS.

8. Strong solution of salt 1 oz., tincture of myrrh ¼ oz.: for saddle-galls.—YOUATT.

9. Common salt 4 oz., vinegar ½ pint, cold water 1 quart, spirit of wine and laudanum, each 1 oz.: in incipient poll-evil.—CLATER.

10. White vinegar 1 pint, extract of lead 2 oz., camphorated spirit 4 oz., soft water 1 pint.—TAPLIN.

11. For strains: Bay salt ½ ℔., sal ammoniac 2 oz., sugar of lead ¼ oz., vinegar 1½ pint, water 1 pint.

ASTRINGENT LOTIONS, for drying up sores or diminishing their discharge, (especially in grease and scratched heel,) after the inflammation has been subdued by linseed or carrot poultices.

1. Alum 4 oz., boiling water 1 pint: for grease and cracked heel. TAPLIN.

2. Alum 2 dr., sulphate of zinc 1 scruple, water 1 pint.—YOUATT.

3. Mild, for cracks: sugar of lead 2 dr., sulphate of zinc 1 dr., infusion of oak bark 1 pint.—BLAINE.

4. For confirmed grease: Nitric Acid 1 oz., water 8 oz.—BLAINE.

5. Strong: Blue vitriol ¼ oz., alum 3 dr., water 1 pint.—SPOONER.

6. Sugar of lead 1 oz., blue vitriol 1 oz., water 1 quart.—WHITE.

7. Lime water 16 oz., spirit of camphor ½ oz., sugar of lead 1 dr.—BOURGELAT.

8. Sulphate of iron 2 oz., alum 2 oz., vinegar 8 oz., water 3½ pints.—MOIROUD.

9. Tincture of myrrh 1 oz., camphorated spirit 1 oz., distilled vinegar and water, each 2 oz.—TAPLIN.

10. For anburies: Alum 2 oz., water 1 pint, sulphuric acid 1 dr.

11. Sulphate of iron 1 oz., water 1 quart; dissolve, and add ¼ oz. (by weight) of oil of vitriol. To wash farcy buds after they have been opened.—CLATER.

DETERGENT LOTIONS, for foul ulcers.

1. Sulphate of copper 1 oz., nitric acid ½ oz., water 6 oz.—WHITE.

2. Sulphate of copper 1 oz., sulphuric acid 12 drops, water 4 oz.

3. Sulphate of copper 2 dr., water 1 pint; for stimulating old ulcers.—YOUATT.

4. Sulphate of copper 1 oz., water 1 pint: to remove fungous granulations.

5. Nitrous acid 1 oz., quicksilver ½ oz., dissolve, and add water 8 oz.

LOTIONS FOR MANGE.

1. White hellebore 2 oz., tobacco 2 oz., water 3 pints; boil, strain, and add, when cold, a pint of fresh lime water.—BLAINE.

2. Boil 4 oz. of white hellebore in 3 pints of water to 2 pints, and add corrosive sublimate 2 dr., previously dissolved in 3 dr. of muriatic acid.—WHITE.

3. Boil 2 oz. of tobacco in a quart of water, strain, and add common salt 3 oz., soap 2 oz.—M. LEBAS.

4. Liver of sulphur 2 oz., water 1 quart.—MOIROUD.

5. Liver of sulphur 4 oz., soft soap 16 oz., water 2 gallons.—LEBAS.

6. Acid nitrate of mercury 2 dr., distilled water 16 oz.—MOIROUD.

7. *Mercurial Wash.* Sublimate 2 dr., spirit of wine 2 oz., water 2 pints.—CLARK.

8. Chloride of lime 1 ℔, water a gallon. Mix.—LUCAS.

VARIOUS LOTIONS.

Conglutinum. Sulphate of zinc 4 oz., water a pint.—BRACY CLARK.

Black Wash. For sluggish ulcers: Calomel 2 dr., lime-water 1 pint.

Yellow Wash. Sublimate 8 gr., lime water 4 oz.

Nitric Acid Lotion. Nitric Acid 2 or 3 dr., water 1 pint; for exciting sluggish ulcers.—MORTON.

Lotion of Nitrate of Silver. For the same: Nitrate of silver 10 gr., distilled water 1 oz.—YOUATT.

Lotion for Farcy. Dissolve 1 oz. of sulphate of iron in a quart of water, and add ½ oz. of oil of vitriol.—CLATER.

Styptic Lotion, for stopping bleeding. Alum 2 oz., sulphate of zinc 2 dr., water 1 quart.

Catechu Lotions, for ulcers of the mouth. Infuse 2 oz. of catechu in a quart of boiling water for an hour; strain, and add 1 oz. of spirit of wine. (For saddle-galls, add 4 oz. of tincture of catechu, and 8 oz. common salt.)—CLATER.

Lotion of Chloride of Lime. To chloride of lime 1 ℔, add gradually 1 gallon of water; mix and filter or decant; for mange, and as a stimulant to unhealthy wounds and fistulous sores. Diluted with 10 or 15 parts of water, it is used as a lotion for grease, exfoliated bones, &c., and as a disinfectant for foul stables. For ulcers of the tongue, mix 1 dr. of chloride of lime with a pint of water; for mange, 4 dr. to a pint.

Wash for destroying Lice about the legs. Corrosive sublimate 1 dr., muriatic acid 3 dr., tobacco water 1 quart, oil of turpentine 4 oz.—WHITE.

Alum Mouth Wash. Alum 2 dr., sage tea a quart.—ECKEL.

For Bruised Gums. Alum 2 dr., tincture of myrrh 1 oz., honey 1 oz., water 2 oz.—SPOONER.

Acid Collutorium. Infusion of sage a quart, muriatic acid 1 oz., flour 3 oz., honey 8 oz. To be applied to the mouth frequently.—ECKEL.

LOUSE WATER.

1. Tobacco 4 oz., boiling water a quart; infuse for 24 hours.—CLARK.

2. *Mercurial.* Sublimate 2 dr., spirit of wine 2 oz., water 1 quart.

LIQUID CAUSTICS, for canker and thrush, for foul, unhealthy wounds, to remove proud flesh, &c. See also LINIMENTS (Detergent.)

MILDER.

1. Tincture of muriate of iron.

2. Sulphate of copper 1 oz., water from 4 oz., (V. C.) to a pint.—CLATER.

3. Saturated solution of sulphate of zinc, in quittors. —WHITE.

4. Alum ½ oz., borax ½ oz., boiling water 4 oz., styptic tincture 1 oz.—TAPLIN.

5. Muriatic acid, alone or diluted.

6. Ægyptiacum 2 oz., nitrous acid 20 drops.

7. Any of the stronger caustics (except butter of antimony) diluted with water.

8. Goulard's extract 4 oz., sulphate of zinc 2 oz., sulphate of copper 2 oz., white vinegar 32 oz.—VILLATE.

9. Aloes 5 oz., weak spirit 10 oz.; dissolve, and add 6 oz. of sulphuric acid.—DUVILLE.

STRONGER.

1. Butter of antimony. This is the safest and most useful caustic in canker.

2. Dissolve 1 oz. of quicksilver, by heat, in 2 oz. of nitric acid, and evaporate till the liquid weighs 2¼ oz.

3. Verdigris 1 oz., nitrous (red nitric) acid 1 oz.; dissolve.—WHITE.

4. Red precipitate 1 oz., nitrous acid 2 oz.—WHITE.

5. Nitrous acid, alone or with a little water.

6. Sulphuric acid, alone or with a little water.

7. Sublimate 1 dr., muriatic acid 2 dr., water q. s.—WHITE.

8. For Canker: Dissolve corrosive sublimate ¼ oz. in

muriatic acid 1 oz., then add spirits of wine 4 oz., and water 4 oz.

9. Chloride of zince with enough water to dissolve it; or SIR WM. BURNETT'S PATENT SOLUTION.

CAUSTICS FOR POLL-EVIL.

1. Lunar caustic 1 dr., distilled water ½ oz.—BLAINE.

2. Corrosive sublimate 2 dr., water 3 oz.

Scalding mixture for Poll-Evil. 1. Sublimate 2 dr., verdigris 2 dr., blue vitriol 2 dr., sulphate of iron 4 dr., honey 2 oz., oil of turpentine 8 oz., spirit of wine 4 oz; to be applied hot, and confined by stitches.—GIBSON.

3. Sublimate 1 dr., finely powdered and mixed with 4 oz. of basilicon, and melted to scalding heat.—BLAINE.

4. Caustic potash 1 dr., rubbed down with 4 oz. oil of turpentine.—BLAINE.

CAUSTIC FOR FARCY BUDS. Sublimate 1 dr., muriatic acid 3 dr., spirit of wine 1 oz., water ½ oz.—WHITE.

SOLID CAUSTICS. Lunar Caustic, Caustic Potash, and Chloride of Zinc. See Argenti nitras, Potassæ hydras, and Zinci chloridum, Pocket Formulary.

Canquoin's Caustic is made by mixing chloride of zinc with twice its weight of flour and a little water into a stiff paste, which is to be rolled out to the required thickness, and cut to the size of the part to be destroyed, the skin being previously removed by a blister. Another caustic is made with 2 parts of chloride of zinc, 1 of butter of antimony, and 5 of flour.

Sulphuric Caustic is made by triturating bay saffron with oil of vitriol, so as to form a ductile mass. BOUCHARDAT recommends solidifying the acid by ivory or lamp black.

Solidified Nitric Acid is merely lint soaked with strong nitric acid, squeezed, and formed to the required shape.

Filho's Caustic is made by melting together in an iron ladle 2 parts of caustic potash and 1 of lime, over a quick fire, and pouring it into leaden tubes of the desired size. The air must be excluded when not in use, by bees'-wax, or other means.

FOMENTATIONS.

These should be applied moderately warm (about 120°) by means of flannel dipped in the liquid, and frequently renewed from time to time, keeping the parts covered.

Emollient. 1. Coarse bran 2 double handfuls, water 6 quarts, boil and strain.

2. Mallow-leaves, 8 oz., water 4 quarts; boil and strain; 6 poppy-heads may be added.

Anodyne. 1. Boil 24 poppy-heads and 2 handfuls of hemlock in 6 quarts of water for 2 hours, and strain.—WHITE.

2. Belladonna 2 handfuls, 6 poppy-heads, water 3 quarts; boil and strain.—MOIROUD.

3. Dried wormwood, and chamomile, of each 4 oz., bay-leaves 2 oz., rue 3 oz.; boil in a gallon of water.

4. Take wormwood, and chamomile, mallow, (or either of them,) cut them to pieces, and put 2 handfuls into a bucket, pour scalding water on them, and cover with a cloth.—B. CLARK.

Discutient and Astringent. Vinegar or verjuice 1 quart; make it hot, and add 2 oz. of Goulard's extract of lead; apply warm, in strains of the sinews of the legs.—TAPLIN.

COLLYRIA OR EYE-WATERS.

1. Acetate of lead, and sulphate of zinc, each ½ dr. to 1 dr. dissolve them separately in ½ pint of water; mix, and filter.

2. Sugar of lead 10 to 20 grains, water 8 oz.—MORTON.

3. Extract of lead 1 dr., spirit 2 dr., water 8 oz.—WHITE.

4. Acetate of ammonia 3 oz., rose water 6 oz.—BLAINE.

5. Sugar of lead 2 dr., vinegar ½ oz., soft water 16 oz., rose water 4 oz.—BLAINE.

6. Infuse 1 oz. of foxglove in 2 pints of boiling water, and strain.—YOUATT.

7. Tincture of opium 2 dr., water 8 oz., extract of lead 1 dr.—WHITE.

8. Brandy 1 oz., vinegar 1 oz., tincture of opium 2 dr., rose-water 8 oz.—BLAINE.

9. Extract of henbane 1 dr., water 8 oz.—WHITE.

10. Decoction of poppies 8 oz., saffron ½ dr.; infuse the saffron in the hot decoction.—LEBAS.

11. Lapis divinus 3 dr., soft water ½ pint.—CLATER.

12. Common salt ½ dr., water 6 oz.—YOUATT.

13. *For Watery Bloodshot Eyes.* Burnt alum 1 oz., calcined white vitriol 1 oz., boiling water 3 pints.—BRACKEN.

14. *Emollient.* Infusion of marshmallow leaves or flowers 1 quart, starch (rubbed smooth with a little water) ½ oz.; mix, and boil. To be used warm.—MOIROUD.

15. *Astringent.* Alum 2 dr., whites of 2 eggs, water ¼ pint; mix in a mortar.—BOURGELAT.

16. Tincture of digitalis ½ oz., soft water 8 oz.—CLATER.

17. *To remove Opacity of the Cornea.* Nitrate of silver 10 gr., distilled water 1 oz. 1 or 2 drops to be dropped in the eye.—Mr. YOUATT.

18. *For Cloudiness of the Eye.* Sublimate 4 gr., spirit of wine 20 drops; rub together, and add soft water 4 oz. A few drops to be introduced into the eye 3 or 4 times a day.—CLATER.

19. Tincture of aloes 1 oz., rose water 8 oz.—LEBAS.

20. *Stimulating.* Infusion of elder flowers 16 oz., brandy 2 oz.—MOIROUD.

21. Lapis mirabilis ½ oz., water 4 to 8 oz. The *Lapis mirabilis* is thus made—White vitriol 2 ℔, rock alum 3 ℔, fine bole ½ ℔, litharge 2 oz., water 3 quarts; boil together to dryness.—SOLLEYSELL.

22. *Alum Collyrium.* Decoction of marshmallow 16 oz., alum 2 dr., camphorated spirit 1 dr. Mix. To be used towards the decline of inflammation.—STRAUSS.

23. *Tannin Collyrium.* Dissolve 1 dr. of tannin in 13 oz. of water, and add 3 oz. of cherry-laurel water.

24. Sulphate of zinc 8 grains, water 4 ounces. In chronic inflammation.—CLATER.

25. In *Specific Ophthalmia.* Tincture of opium 2 dr., extract of belladonna 1 dr., with distilled water 1 pint.

SUNDRY SOLUTIONS, &c.

Styptic Stone. Sulphate of iron 8 oz.; sal ammoniac, sulphate of zinc, and oxide of copper, each 1 oz.; mix, and melt together with a gentle heat. About the size of a nut of this compound to be dissolved in a quart of warm water, and applied with compresses renewed every 3 or 4 hours: for saddle-galls, kicks, sprains, bruises, ulcers, and a collyrium.—KNAUP.

Lapis Divinus. Sulphate of copper, alum, nitre, of each 3 oz.; melt together, and stir in one dr. of camphor: used in eye-waters and lotions.

Wound Stone. Alum, sulphate of zinc, of each 3 oz., verdigris and sal ammoniac, of each 1 dr.; melt together, and add ½ dr. of powdered saffron: detergent and drying.

Clark's Conglutinum. Sulphate of zinc 4 oz., water a pint.

Solution of Alum. Alum 1 oz., water 16 oz. Dissolve. V. C.

Solution of Sulphate of Zinc. Sulphate of zinc 1 oz., water 3 oz.—V. C. *In quittors* it is usually diluted.

Solution of Sulphate of Copper. Sulphate of copper 1 oz., water 4 oz.—V. C.

Compound Solution of the same. Sulphate of copper 3 oz., alum 3 oz., water 2 ℔, sulphuric acid 1½ oz.

Solution of Bichloride of Mercury. Sublimate, hydrochloric acid, each 1 part; spirit, *or* water, 7 parts.—V. C.

Goulard Water. Extract of lead 1 oz., camphorated spirit 2 oz., rain water a quart.—TAPLIN. V. C. use extract of lead and rectified spirit each 2 dr., soft water 1 pint.

Tincture of Catechu. See P. F. Used externally for wounds.

Tincture of Euphorbium. Euphorbium 1 oz., rectified spirit 6 oz.

Alkaline Tincture of Euphorbium. Euphorbium 8 oz., solution of subcarbonate of potash 3 pints: used as caustics and stimulants, particularly in *curbs* after the inflammation has been subdued.

Compound Tincture of Cantharides. Powdered flies 4, euphorbium 1, proof spirit 24.—LEBAS.

Styptic Tincture. Tincture of myrrh, spirit of camphor, and Friar's balsam, equal parts.—TAPLIN.

Ægyptiacum. (Veterinary.) Sulphate of copper in powder 12 oz., vinegar 4 oz., treacle 48 oz.; boil together to a proper consistence.—B. CLARK.

Ægyptiacum with Turpentine. Honey 28 oz., pyroligneous acid 14 oz., powdered verdigris 10 oz., boil together in a copper vessel till the mixture has a reddish purple colour and the consistence of thin honey; add Venice turpentine 28 oz., and keep it on a slow fire, stirring constantly for a quarter of an hour.—LELOUP.

Liniment of Verdigris. V. C. Verdigris in fine powder 9 oz., alum 6 oz., treacle 1½ ℔. Boil until the compound assumes a brown colour.

Liniment of Sulphate of Copper. Powdered sulphate of copper 1 part, treacle 4 parts. Simmer in a pipkin over a slow fire until the whole assumes a reddish-brown colour. *In canker, severe thrush, &c.*—MORTON.

POULTICES OR CATAPLASMS.

These are useful in reducing inflammation and relieving pain. They should not be used too hot, nor applied too tightly, especially to the feet.

COMMON POULTICES.

1. Bran moistened with hot water, and as much linseed meal added as will give it tenacity.—V. C.

2. Boil a quart of bran for 10 minutes with enough water to make a thin mash, then add to it 4 oz. of linseed meal; apply it in a flannel bag.—BLAINE.

3. Fine bran 3 parts, linseed meal 1 part, hot water q. s.

CHARCOAL POULTICES.

1. Oatmeal ½ pint, linseed meal ½ pint, charcoal 4 oz., beer grounds q. s.

2. Carrots scraped, or carrots boiled, with charcoal powder q. s. *Antiseptic.*—BLAINE.

YEAST POULTICES.

1. Linseed meal, oatmeal, boiling water, q. s.; mix, and ferment with a tablespoonful of yeast: in old grease with an offensive smell.—BLAINE.

2. In Gangrene: Add 2 oz. of turpentine to the last. —BLAINE.

ANODYNE POULTICES.

1. Boil poppy heads in water, strain, and add linseed meal to stiffen it.—YOUATT.

2. Sprinkle the surface of a simple poultice with laudanum.

CLEANSING POULTICES. Mashed turnips, not pressed, with enough linseed meal, or oatmeal, to give them consistence; or, the charcoal poultice above.

DRAWING POULTICES.

1. Boil 2 ℔ of chopped onions in water, and add to it the crumb of a 4 ℔ loaf.—HINDS.

2. Sorrel boiled and squeezed 4 parts, onions baked in ashes 1 part, basilicon ointment 1 part; mix, and apply warm.—M. VATEL.

RESOLVENT POULTICES.

1. Rye meal 8 oz., prepared chalk 2 oz., vinegar 10 oz., mix, warm, and stir, till no more gas is disengaged; apply cold.—SOLLEYSELL.

2. Linseed meal 12 oz., powdered hemlock 4 oz., muriate of ammonia 4 oz., vinegar q. s.: to indolent glandular tumours.—LEBAS.

GOULARD POUTICES.

1. To a linseed meal poultice add 1 or 2 dr. of Goulard's extract of lead.—YOUATT.

2. Bread and barley-meal equal parts, Goulard water q. s., lard 4 or 6 oz.—TAPLIN.

CHLORINE POULTICE. Chloride of lime ½ oz., water 1 pint, linseed meal, q. s.: to grease, when offensive.—YOUATT.

POULTICES FOR GREASE.

1. The herb cleavers (or goose grass beaten to a paste.)

2. Mash bread and boiled turnips with stale beer, and stir in 1 oz. flour of mustard, turpentine 2 oz., linseed meal 2 oz., lard 6 oz.; night and morning.—TAPLIN.

MUSTARD POULTICE.

1. Mustard flour and linseed meal, equal parts; mix with sufficient hot vinegar to give a proper consistence.

2. Flour of black mustard 3 ℔, hot vinegar, or water, q. s.—MOIROUD.

RUBEFACIENT POULTICE.

1. Fresh horse-radish root, grated and immediately applied.—MOIROUD.

2. *Stronger.* Old yeast 2 ℔, flour of black mustard 1 ℔, euphorbium powder 4 oz., vinegar q. s.; mix, and apply cold.

OINTMENTS, CERATES, CHARGES, &c.

SIMPLE EMOLLIENT OINTMENTS.

1. *Simple Cerate.* Olive oil a pint, beeswax 4 oz.

2. *Spermaceti Ointment.* Lard 12 oz., white wax 2 oz., spermaceti 1 oz.

BLISTERING OINTMENTS. The Spanish flies should be finely powdered and the heat moderate.

1. Lard 4 oz., common turpentine 1 oz., p. flies 1 oz.; melt the lard and turpentine, and stir in the powdered flies.—V. C. Mr. YOUATT subsitutes resin for the turpentine.

2. Venice turpentine and resin, of each 1 ℔, palm oil or lard 2 ℔; melt together, and gradually stir in 1 ℔ of powdered flies.—BLAINE.

3. Palm oil 4 ℔. resin 1 ℔; melt together, and stir in 1 ℔ of powdered flies.—CLATER.

4. *Mild.* Lard 4 oz., Venice turpentine 1 oz., p. flies 6 dr.—WHITE.

5. *Stronger.* Mercurial ointment 2 oz., oil of bays 2

oz., Barbadoes tar 1 oz., oil of rosemary 2 dr., p. flies 1 oz.—WHITE.

6. *Strong.* Oil of turpentine 1 oz., oil of vitriol 2 fluid dr.; mix in a basin, and add melted lard 6 oz., oil of origanum 1 oz., powdered flies 1 to 2 oz.—WHITE.

7. *Strongest.* Strong mercurial ointment 4 oz., oil of origanum ½ oz., finely powdered euphorbium 3 dr., p. flies ½ oz.—WHITE.

8. BLAINE'S *Mercurial.* Common blister (No. 2, above) 4 oz., sublimate in fine powder ½ dr.: for splints, spavins, &c.

9. *For common purposes.* Lard 6 oz., Venice turpentine 4 oz., bees' wax 2 oz., yellow resin 1 oz., oil of origanum ½ oz., powdered cantharides 3 oz. It may be softened in winter by rubbing it with a little turpentine.—WHITE.

10. Powdered flies 5 dr., lard 4 oz., oil of turpentine 1 oz.—HINDS.

11. *Mustard Blister.* Best flour of mustard 8 oz., water to form a paste.—MR. YOUATT. Others add 2 oz. of oil of turpentine, and 1 oz. pure water of ammonia.

Note.—The hair should be clipped closely, or shaved off, the part fomented with warm water, and the blistering ointment well rubbed in. In inflammation of the lungs, &c., blistering is more successful after bleeding. In 24 hours a little olive or neatsfoot oil should be applied, and repeated night and morning. The head should be tied up for the first 2 days, and the litter removed from the stable. If strangury is produced, give plenty of linseed tea. The simplest blisters are perhaps the best for common purposes. Sublimate blemishes. *Sweating down* is effected by milder stimulants; for this purpose, the liquid blister (see p. 91) is lowered by some mild oil, &c.

DETERGENT OINTMENTS, for cleansing foul and indolent ulcers.

1. Suet 4 oz., Venice turpentine 6 oz., red precipitate, finely powdered 2 oz.—WHITE.

2. Citrine ointment, alone or with ¼ its weight of Venice turpentine.

3. Sulphate of zinc 1 dr., sulphate of copper 1 dr., oil of turpentine 2 dr.; grind smooth, and mix it with 4 oz. of melted tallow. See also DIGESTIVE OINTMENTS, No. 4.

4. Yellow basilicon 2 oz., black basilicon 1 oz.; melt together, remove from the fire, and add 1 oz. of turpentine, ½ oz. finely powdered red precipitate.—TAPLIN.

5. *Verdigris Ointment.* Verdigris in fine powder 1 part, common turpentine 1 part, lard 12 parts. Mix. —MORTON.

DIGESTIVE OINTMENTS, to promote a discharge from unhealthy and indolent ulcers.

1. Resin 16 oz., linseed oil 12 oz.; melt together with a gentle heat.—CLARK.

2. Strained turpentine, honey, of each 2 oz.; yolks of 4 eggs, myrrh ½ oz., aloes 1 oz.; mix.—SOLLEYSELL.

3. Equal parts of common turpentine and lard melted together.—WHITE.

4. To 1 ℔. of the last add 1 oz. of finely powdered verdigris.—WHITE.

5. Yellow wax 3 oz., common turpentine 3 oz., black pitch 1 oz., resin 6 oz., linseed oil 16 oz.: melt together with a gentle heat, then add oil of turpentine 4 oz., and stir till cold.

6. Olive oil 1 pint, yellow wax and black resin, of each 4 oz., Burgundy pitch and turpentine, of each 2 oz.; melt the other ingredients and add the turpentine when it is removed from the fire.—TAPLIN.

7. Common turpentine 1 part, lard 3 parts; melt together.—V. C.

8. (Basilicon.) Resin 5 oz., yellow wax 2 oz., lard 8 oz. melt together.

9. (Black Basilicon.) Pitch, wax, resin, of each 11 oz.; olive (or rape or linseed) oil, a pint.

EYE OINTMENTS. The powder should be very fine, and the whole rubbed smooth.

1. Nitrate of silver 5 to 10 gr., lard 1 oz.; rub till perfectly smooth. The size of a pea to be introduced between the lids, in chronic ophthalmia.—MORTON.

2. Calamine ½ oz., tutty ½ oz., sulphate of copper ½ dr.,

sulphate of zinc ½ oz., alum ½ oz., camphor 2 dr., fresh butter 3 oz.; mix, and apply warm, with a feather, to watery, inflamed eyes.—BRACKEN.

3. Ointment of nitrated quicksilver 1 dr., zinc ointment 1 oz., camphor 1 dr.

4. In inflammation of the eyelids: Verdigris 1 part, Venice turpentine 1, lard 12.—MORTON.

5. For wounds in the eye: Tutty ointment 1 oz., honey of roses 2 dr., calcined white vitriol 20 gr.; apply with a feather night and morning, and sponge daily with warm milk and water.—BRACKEN.

6. For removing opacity of the cornea: Iodine 2 gr., iodide of potassium 20 gr., lard or butter ½ oz.

EUPHORBIUM OINTMENT. Euphorbium 1, lard 8 parts; mix.—DELAFOSSE.

OINTMENTS FOR SCURVY AND CRACKED HEELS. AND CONFIRMED GREASE. The inflammation should be first subdued by poultices. The milder preparations (which are here placed first) should be employed in the first instance, and afterwards those for confirmed grease.

1. For scurvy heels: Goulard's extract ½ dr., lard 1 oz., mix. The heel should first be gently rubbed with soap and water.—CLATER.

2. For scurvy or cracked heels: Sugar of lead ¼ oz., oxide of zinc ¼ oz., lard or palm oil 4 oz.

3. Melt together 3 oz. white diachylon, 4 oz. olive oil; mix, and when nearly cold, add 3 dr. of sugar of lead in fine powder. First wash the heel, then apply the Astringent Lotion No. 9, and afterwards this ointment; or, elder ointment 4 oz., camphor 6 dr., laudanum 2 dr., extract of lead 2 dr.; mix.—TAPLIN.

4. Melt yellow wax 2 oz., with sweet oil 8 oz., and sugar of lead ¼ oz.

5. Healing ointment for cracked heel: lard 4 ℔, resin 1 ℔; melt together, and stir in 1 ℔ true calamine.—CLATER. See also SOFTENING and COOLING OINTMENTS, below.

6. For cracked heels and grease: Alum 1 oz., turpentine 1 oz., lard 3 oz. Melt the turpentine and lard, and stir in the powdered alum.—V. C.

7. For grease: Venice turpentine 4 oz., wax 1 oz., lard 4 oz.; melt together, and add sugar of lead 1 oz., (or alum 2 oz.) in fine powder.—WHITE.

8. Lard, honey, common turpentine, each 8 oz.; melt together, and add powdered alum 6 oz., white vitriol 2 oz.

9. Common turpentine 1 ℔; melt, and add powdered alum 1½ ℔, bole 2 ℔; stir till cold; spread on brown paper, and tie over with list.

10. Lard ½ ℔, honey ½ ℔, common turpentine ½ ℔; melt, and add p. alum 1 ℔, white vitriol 2 oz., stir till cold.

11. For confirmed grease: Common verdigris ½ oz., alum, sulphate of zinc, sugar of lead, of each ½ oz.; tar 6 oz.—BLAINE.

12. Citrine ointment 3 oz., lard 2 oz., turpentine 2 dr., saturated solution of nitrate of copper 2 dr.—BLAINE.

13. Ægyptiacum 8 oz., lard 4 oz., sulphate of zinc in powder 1 oz.; rub together till perfectly mixed.—LASSAIGNE.

14. Prepared verdigris 1 oz., lard 4 oz., honey a sufficient quantity.—DELAFOSSE.

15. Chloride of lime 1 to 2 parts; lard 8 parts. Mix. *To remove the fœtor, in grease.*—MORTON.

OINTMENTS TO PROMOTE THE GROWTH OF THE HAIR, and remove the blemish from broken knees.

1. Camphor ½ dr., oil of rosemary 1 dr., weak mercurial ointment 1 oz., ivory black and bole to colour.—WHITE.

2. Poplar-bud ointment and honey, applied twice a day for 15 or 20 days.—PYE.

3. Calamine 2 dr., prepared charcoal 1 dr., oil of turpentine 1 dr., lard 4 dr.; rub well together with 1 dr. of blister ointment.—CLATER.

4. Liquid blister (No. 3, 6, or 7) 1 dr., ivory black 1 dr., camphor 1 dr., palm oil 1 oz.

5. Citrine ointment 1 oz., camphor 1 dr., colour as above.

HELLEBORE OINTMENT. Powdered white hellebore 1 part, lard 8 parts: an irritating dressing for rowels and setons.—V. C.

HOOF OINTMENT. Tar and tallow equal parts, melted together.—WHITE.

IODINE OINTMENT, Simple. Iodine 1 part, lard 8 parts. Mix.—V. C.

FARCY OINTMENT. Iodine 1 dr., lard 1 oz., mercurial ointment 1 oz. Mix. Useful when the complaint is confined to one leg; from 5 to 10 grains of iodide of potassium being given daily, with a mineral tonic.

IODINE OINTMENT, Compound. Iodine 1 dr., iodide of potassium 2 dr., lard 2 oz.—V. C.

IODIDE OF MERCURY OINTMENT. Red iodide of mercury 1 part, lard or palm oil 7 parts; mix; the size of a nut to be rubbed on daily: in thoroughpin.

OINTMENTS FOR MANGE AND LICE.

1. Sulphur 4 oz., soft soap 4 oz., oil of bays 4 oz., train oil q. s.

2. Sulphur 1 oz., train oil 1 oz., Venice turpentine, 2 oz.—YOUATT.

3. Train oil 3 oz., sulphur 1 oz., oil of turpentine 6 oz.—WHITE.

4. Sulphur 8 oz., common turpentine 2 oz., strong mercurial ointment 2 oz., linseed oil 1 pint; rub the flowers of sulphur with a fourth part of the oil, then rub in the turpentine and ointment, and gradually add the rest of the oil; half to be rubbed in daily for 3 days; on the sixth day, wash off with soft soap and warm water.—CLATER.

5. Oil of turpentine 3 oz., oil of vitriol 1 oz.; mix cautiously, avoiding the fumes, and add melted lard 8 oz., train oil 4 oz., oil of turpentine 2 oz., flowers of

sulphur, or sulphur vivum 4 oz.; stir till cold; apply daily for 3 or 4 times, and give an alterative powder twice a day.—WHITE.

6. Oil of bays 16 oz., strong mercurial ointment 6 oz., oil of turpentine 2 oz., soft soap 4 oz.; mix, and apply in the sun; but it is not quite safe.—BRACKEN.

7. Oil of turpentine 4 oz., oil of tar 4 oz., train oil 8 oz., sulphur 4 oz.

8. Sulphur vivum 8 oz., powdered stavesacre 1 oz., mercurial ointment 2 oz., turpentine 2 oz., lard or train oil 8 oz.—BLAINE.

9. Soft soap and tar equal parts.

10. Weak mercurial ointment ½ ℔, sulphur vivum 4 oz., white hellebore 3 oz., black pepper 3 oz., oil of tartar 1 oz., olive oil enough to make it soft: use daily for 7, 10, or 14 days.—TAPLIN.

OINTMENTS FOR MALLENDERS AND SALLENDERS. (Scurvy eruptions.)

1. Citrine ointment 2 oz., tar ointment 1 oz. Mix.

2. Lard 2 oz., finely powdered red precipitate 2 dr.—WHITE.

3. Sugar of lead 1 part, tar 2, lard 6; mix; give a diuretic ball occasionally.—YOUATT.

4. Lard 4 oz.; melt, and stir in Goulard's extract 1 oz.—WHITE.

5. Quicksilver 1 oz., common turpentine 3 oz.; mix. —BRACKEN.

6. Sublimate 10 gr., mercurial ointment 1 oz.; mix.

7. Iodide of potassium 1 dr., lard 2 oz., Goulard's extract 4 dr.; mix.

8. Camphor 1 dr., sugar of lead ½ dr., mercurial ointment 1 oz.; mix, and apply after washing with soap and water.—BLAINE.

9. Naphthaline 1 dr., cod-liver oil 1 oz., zinc ointment 1 oz.

MARSHMALLOW OINTMENT. The following is often substituted for the pharmacopœia preparation: Rape oil 1 ℔, yellow wax 6 oz., palm oil ½ ℔, common turpentine 1 oz.

MERCURIAL OINTMENT. This is prepared in the usual way; but Venice turpentine is often used to kill the quicksilver more speedily, as it does not interfere with its veterinary uses.

Strong Mercurial Ointment. Quicksilver 16 oz., Venice turpentine 2 oz.; rub together till the metal is killed, then add 16 oz. of lard.

2. Quicksilver 16 oz., liquid styrax 5 dr., lard 3 oz.; triturate until the metal disappears, and add 12 oz. more lard.—CRESSENT.

Weaker Mercurial Ointment. Strong mercurial ointment 1 part, lard 2 parts.

2. Quicksilver 2 oz., balsam of sulphur ½ oz.; rub together till the globules disappear, and add 6 oz. of lard.—TAPLIN.

Compound Mercurial Ointment. Mercurial ointment 1 part, soft soap 2 parts.—V. C.

RESOLVENT OINTMENTS, for indolent tumours of the withers, spavins, wind-galls, farcy buttons, splints, &c.

1. Strong mercurial ointment 4 oz., cantharides in powder ½ oz., oil of rosemary 2 dr.—WHITE.

2. Biniodide of mercury 1 part, lard or palm oil 7 parts; rub together in a mortar; the quantity of a nut to be rubbed on daily till a scurf is produced: for spavin and thoroughpin.—SPOONER.

3. Blister ointment 2 oz., strong mercurial ointment 1 oz., soft soap ½ oz., oil of bays 3 dr., yellow wax 3 dr., melt the wax by a gentle heat, add the other ingredients, mix by stirring, remove, and stir till cold.—LEBAS.

4. Common turpentine 12 parts, corrosive sublimate 1 part; mix.—GIRARD.

OINTMENT OF NITRATE OF SILVER. Nitrate of silver 5 to 10 gr., lard 1 oz.—MORTON.

CREASOTE OINTMENT. Creasote 2 parts, lard 8 parts. —V. C.

MILD CITRINE OINTMENT. Ointment of nitrate of quicksilver 1 part, lard and oil 2 parts. *In tarsal ophthalmia.*

SOFTENING AND COOLING OINTMENTS, for cracks and ulcers on the heel, &c.:

1. Spermaceti ointment 4 oz., olive oil 1 oz., sugar of lead 2 dr., oxide of zinc 1 oz.—WHITE.

2. Extract of lead ½ dr., lard 1 oz.; mix.—CLATER.

3. Marshmallow ointment 4 oz., extract of lead 3 dr., elder ointment ½ oz., calamine 1 oz.

OINTMENT FOR SIT-FASTS, and all hard tumours. Strained ammoniacum 4 oz., mercurial ointment 8 oz., oil of turpentine 10 oz.—HINDS.

OINTMENTS FOR SORE BACKS AND SADDLE-GALLS. (See LOTIONS.)

1. Camphor 2 dr., oil of rosemary 1 dr., elder ointment or lard 3 oz.

2. Marshmallow ointment 4 oz., extract of lead 1 oz. —WHITE.

SULPHURIC ACID OINTMENT.

1. Sulphuric acid 1 dr., lard 1 oz.; mix.

2. Sulphuric acid 1 fluid oz., lard 8 oz., oil of turpentine 1 oz.

OINTMENTS FOR SPAVINS AND WIND-GALLS. See RESOLVENT OINTMENTS, above.

TAR OINTMENT. Equal parts of tallow and tar melted together.

OINTMENTS FOR THRUSH AND CANKER.

1. Common verdigris ½ oz., calamine ½ oz., sulphate of zinc 1 dr., tar 3 oz.—BLAINE.

2. Blue vitriol 2 oz., white vitriol 1 oz., rubbed down and mixed with lard 2 ℔, tar 1 ℔; a pledget of tow covered with it to be introduced into the cleft of the frog every night, and renewed in the morning.—YOUATT.

3. *Thrush Paste.* Alum, blue vitriol, white vitriol, of each 1 oz.; rub them into a fine powder; melt 2 ℔ of tar with 1 ℔ of lard, and when getting cool, stir in the powder.—CLATER.

4. Verdigris 1½ oz., (or burnt alum 8 oz.,) red lead

8 oz., treacle 4 lb; boil to a proper consistence, and add 1 oz. of nitrous acid.—FERON.

5. *In Canker.* Tar 4 parts, nitric acid 1 part; mix. —MORTON.

OINTMENTS FOR FARCY-BUDS. 1. Sublimate 1 oz., white arsenic ½ oz., yellow arsenic ½ oz., euphorbium ½ oz., oil of bays 4 oz.; mix.—M. LAMOTTE.

2. (*Topique Terrat.*) Corrosive sublimate 1 oz., white and yellow arsenic each ½ oz., oil of bays 4 oz. Mix with a gentle heat.

TURPENTINE OINTMENT. Common turpentine 1 part, lard 3 parts; melt together.—V. C.

VERDIGRIS OINTMENT. Verdigris in powder 1 part, common turpentine 1 part, lard 12 parts: for foul ulcers and tarsal ophthalmia.—MORTON.

OINTMENT FOR WARTS AND ANBURIES. Muriate of ammonia 2 dr., powdered savin 1 oz., lard 1½ oz.; to be applied daily.—BLAINE.

OINTMENTS FOR CHRONIC VIVES.

1. Emetic tartar 2 dr., olive oil 1 dr.; rub together till smooth, and add lard 1 oz.

2. Iodide of potassium 1 dr., palm oil 1 oz.; rub together till quite smooth.—CLATER.

ASTRINGENT PASTE, for broken knees, and for wounds after the inflammation has subsided.

1. Powdered alum and pipe clay, mixed with water to the consistence of cream. For broken knees it may be coloured with bole and lamp-black.—WHITE.

2. *Paste for Open Knee-joint.* Flour and stale beer, boiled to the consistence of paste, and coloured as above. To be spread thick all round the joint, and covered with a pledget of tow, and ½ sheet of brown paper; and the leg of a cotton stocking drawn over the whole. The stocking to be covered with the paste, and enveloped with 2 calico bandages regularly applied.—TURNER.

STOPPING FOR THE FEET.

1. Cow-dung beaten with a fourth part of clay.—Youatt.

2. Soft soap 4 oz., Barbadoes tar 16 oz., linseed meal 2½ ℔.—White.

3. Tallow and tar, equal parts, melted together.

4. Common tar 2 parts, soft soap 1 part, linseed meal q. s. To be spread over the sole of the foot ¼ of an inch thick, covered with a layer of tow, and a leather sole over all.—V. C.

HOOF OINTMENTS.

1. Equal parts of wax, olive oil, lard, veal suet, turpentine, and honey; melt the wax and lard with the oil by a gentle heat, remove from the fire, and add the honey and turpentine, stirring till cold; when intended to embellish the hoof as well as to soften it, it may be coloured with lamp black, or ivory black.—Bourgelat.

2. Tallow 4 ℔, bees'-wax 4 oz., tar ½ ℔; melt slowly, remove from the fire, and when they begin to cool, stir together. A portion of pitch may be added when intended to fill fissures, &c.—Bracy Clark.

COMPOSITION FOR SAND CRACKS. Bees'-wax 4 oz., yellow resin 2 oz., common turpentine 1 oz., tallow ½ oz., melt together; fill the cracks with the composition, and turn the horse out to grass.

SUPPLING LINIMENT FOR BRITTLE HOOF. Oil of tar 1 pint, fish oil 2 pints.—Clater.

CHARGES.

The usual means of applying charges is to soften the compound by heat, and apply it with a large spatula to the part, as warm as the animal can comfortably bear it, and while warm to cover it with cut tow. They are used for old sprains of the loins, strains of the back sinews, wind-galls, &c. Cold charges are spread on cloth or leather, and renewed as they become dry.

1. *Simple Charge.* Pitch 4 oz., turpentine 1 oz.—Gasparin.

2. *For Strains of the Loins.* Pitch 4 ℔, turpentine 6 oz., olive oil 4 oz.; melt together.—B. CLARK.

3. Burgundy pitch 4 oz., wax 4 oz., yellow resin 4 oz., common turpentine 1 oz.; melt together, and when it begins to thicken, stir in 1 oz. of bole.—WHITE.

4. Burgundy or common pitch 5 oz., tar 6 oz., wax 1 oz.; melt together, and when they are becoming cool, stir in ½ dr. of powdered cantharides.—YOUATT.

5. Pitch 3 ℔, tar 1 ℔, bees'-wax ½ ℔; melt together. —CLATER.

6. Resin 2 oz., Burgundy pitch 4 oz., Barbadoes tar 2 oz., wax 3 oz., red lead 4 oz.—WHITE.

7. Pitch 8 oz., suet 4 oz., oil of turpentine 3 oz., tincture of cantharides 3 oz.—DELAFOSSE AND LASSAIGNE.

8. *Cold Charge.* Bole ½ ℔, white of egg and vinegar, to form soft paste, to be applied on double cloth or leather, and renewed as it dries: for sprains in the back sinews.—BRACKEN.

9. Bruised leaves of elder, or cabbage, or mallow.—B. CLARK.

10. *Mercurial Charge.* B. pitch 1½ ℔, wax 1½ ℔; melt, and add, while cooling, 6 oz. of mercurial ointment previously mixed with 6 dr. of iodine.—Mr. S. FISHER.

11. *Soot Charge.* Common turpentine 4½ oz., soot 3 oz.: mix.—DELAFOND.

POWDERS FOR OUTWARD USE.

ASTRINGENT POWDERS; chiefly used for sprinkling greasy or ulcerated heels, after the inflammation has been subdued by poultices, and in joint wounds.

1. Calamine (true) 4 parts, alum 1 part; mix.—MORTON.

2. Burnt alum, dried sulphate of iron, and myrrh, equal parts.—V. C. (Comp. powder of alum.)

3. Alum 1 dr., charcoal ½ oz., chalk 2 oz.—BLAINE.

4. Sulphate of zinc, chalk lightly calcined, white pepper, in equal parts.—B. CLARK.

5. Alum 4 oz., bole 1 oz.—WHITE.

6. Oak-bark 1 oz., verdigris 2 dr.—BLAINE.

7. White vitriol 2 oz., oxide of zinc 1 oz.—WHITE.

8. Prepared chalk 4 oz., sulphate of zinc 1 oz., charcoal 1 oz., Armenian bole 2 oz.—SPOONER.

DETERGENT AND ESCHAROTIC POWDERS; for cleansing foul ulcers and repressing fungous or proud flesh. They should all be very finely powdered and well mixed.

1. Equal parts of calcined white vitriol and alum.—BRACKEN.

2. Bole 2 dr., blue vitriol or verdigris 1 oz.—WHITE.

3. Red precipitate ½ oz., acetate of copper ½ oz., calamine ½ oz.—BLAINE.

4. Red precipitate ½ oz., burnt alum 2 dr.

5. Blue vitriol 1 oz., alum 1 oz., white lead 1 oz.

6. Equal parts of verdigris and sugar of lead—CLATER.

7. Alum, dried sulphate of iron, and myrrh, equal parts: in joint wounds.

8. Alum, sulphate of iron, of zinc, and of copper, of each 1 oz., muriate of ammonia ½ oz., camphor and saffron, of each 1½ dr.—BOUCHARDAT.

STYPTIC POWDER. Alum, with an equal or double weight of flour.—WHITE.

STYPTIC STONE. See SOLUTIONS, page 105.

SNEEZING POWDERS. The ingredients to be very finely powdered and mixed.

1. Asarabacca 4 dr., white hellebore 1 dr.; mix, and keep it in a bottle for use.—BRACKEN.

2. Snuff 1 oz., hellebore 1 dr., euphorbium 10 to 20 gr.—PECK.

3. *In Incipient Cataract.* Turpeth mineral 2 dr., asarabacca 4 dr.; mix, and apply as much as will lie upon a sixpence, daily.—BRACKEN.

MEDICINES FOR NEAT CATTLE.

DRINKS OR DRENCHES.

Note.—The peculiar structure of the digestive organs in cattle renders it proper to give their medicines in a liquid form. For the same reason, drenches should be given very slowly, so as to enter at once the third or fourth stomach. It is only in cases of hoven or *blown*, that it is desirable to introduce medicine into the first stomach or *rumen*.

PURGING and LAXATIVE DRENCHES. These are given when fever exists, or is threatened; to prevent downfalls of the udder; after calving, to prevent milk-fever; to remove undue accumulations in costiveness; in the first stage of red-water, and jaundice; and in all inflammatory complaints.

1. Epsom salts 8 oz., sulphur 4 oz., ginger 2 dr., warm water a pint, linseed oil 12 oz,—SPOONER.

2. Epsom salts 6 or 8 oz., castor oil 8 oz., gruel 1½ pint, ginger ½ oz.

3. Glauber or Epsom salts 16 oz., (or in bad cases with fever 24 oz.) caraways 1 oz., warm gruel a quart. —CLATER.

4. Castor oil from 16 to 24 oz., with gruel; but it is not to be depended on.

5. To No. 3, add 2 or 3 dr. of gamboge, or 4 dr. of aloes.

6. Sulphur 8 oz., ginger ½ oz., warm gruel a quart: in rheumatism, or joint-felon.—CLATER.

7. Common salt 6 oz., flour of mustard a tablespoon-

ful, grated ginger or ground pepper, of either a teaspoonful, gin ¼ pint, water 2 pints.

8. Common salt 1 ℔, warm water, or gruel, q. s. The last three are only proper where there is not much fever.

9. *In Red-water.* Sulphate of magnesia 8 to 16 oz., sulphur 2 to 6 oz., carbonate of ammonia ½ oz., ginger ½ oz., warm water q. s.; a fourth of this every 6 hours till the bowels are sufficiently acted on.—SPOONER.

10. *When the last does not operate.* Calomel 20 gr., yeast ½ pint.—HARRIS.

11. Aloes 4 to 6 dr., common salt 4 to 6 oz., ginger 1 to 3 dr., water a quart, anodyne tincture 2 oz.: in red-water.—WHITE.

12. *Cordial Purgative.* Aloes 4 dr., Epsom salts 4 oz., ginger 1 dr., carminative tincture 2 oz., water 1 quart.—WHITE.

13. In the commencement of puerperal or milk fever: Epsom salts 6 or 8 oz., powdered croton seeds 20 to 30 gr., ginger 4 dr.; in 3 or 4 pints of gruel: repeat in 6 hours, if required, without the croton seeds.—BLAINE.

14. In locked jaw: Barbadoes aloes 1½ oz., powdered croton kernel 10 gr., boiling water q. s.; given when cool.—CLATER.

15. *Mild laxative and tonic.* Epsom salts ½ ℔, sulphur 4 to 6 oz., ginger ½ oz., gentian ½ oz., warm water q. s.—EVESON.

16. In flatulent colic with costiveness: Aloes 1½ oz., carbonate of potash 3 dr., ginger ½ oz., warm water 1 pint, linseed oil 8 oz.—WHITE.

17. Palm oil 16 oz., Glauber's salts 12 oz., boiling water q. s.—PECK.

18. *Laxative drink for cows that are kept on hay.* Aloes 4 dr., ginger 1½ dr., water a quart, Epsom salts 6 oz., carbonate of soda ½ oz.; for one dose.—YOUATT.

FEVER DRENCHES, for fevers, colds, influenza, &c.

1. Tartar emetic 1 dr., digitalis ½ dr., nitre 3 dr.; mix, and give in a quart of gruel: in simple colds or catarrh.—CLATER.

2. Antimonial powder 2 dr., opium a scruple; rub together, and mix with thick gruel: after bleeding, in inflammation of the bladder.—WHITE.

3. In influenza, or epidemic (epizootic) colds: Nitre ½ oz., salt of tartar 1 oz., camphor 2 dr., valerian, liquorice, turmeric, of each 1 oz., mustard 2 oz., juniper berries 1 oz., gruel a quart.—SKERRET.

4. For the same: After bleeding and a laxative, give antimonial powder 2 dr., camphor 1½ dr., ginger 3 dr., laudanum ½ oz., in gruel.—WHITE.

5. In bad colds attended with fever: Nitre 1 oz., camphor ½ dr., tartar-emetic ½ dr., in gruel.—PECK.

FEBRIFUGE TONIC DRENCHES.

1. Antimonial powder ½ dr., camphor 1 dr., Peruvian bark 1 oz., gruel, or decoction of arrowroot or starch q. s., for 2 doses.—PECK.

2. In the decline of fevers and influenza: Emetic tartar ½ dr., nitre 2 dr., gentian 3 dr., chamomile 1 dr., ginger ½ dr.; pour on them a pint of boiling ale, and give when cool.—CLATER.

3. Emetic tartar ½ dr., gentian 2 dr., digitalis ½ dr., nitre ½ oz., spirit of nitric ether 4 dr., gruel q. s.

TONIC DRENCHES.

1. Cascarilla 3 dr., ginger 3 dr., carbonate of soda 2 dr., in gruel.—WHITE.

2. Gentian ½ oz., ginger 1 dr., Epsom salts 2 oz., warm gruel a pint.—CLATER.

3. Tartarized iron 1 dr., gentian 2 dr., ginger 1 dr., gruel 1 pint: after laxatives, in indigestion.

DRENCHES FOR INFLAMMATION OF THE LIVER.

After bleeding give—

1. Calomel 1½ dr., opium ½ dr., ginger 2 dr., thick gruel q. s. Six hours afterwards, give Epsom salts 1 ℔, sulphur 6 oz., linseed oil ½ pint, gruel q. s.—SPOONER.

2. Epsom salts 1 ℔, caraway ½ oz., Barbadoes aloes ¼ oz.; in a quart of warm gruel.—CLATER. After the yellowness appears give

3. Half of No. 2, with 20 gr. of calomel morning and night.—CLATER.

DRENCHES FOR JAUNDICE OR YELLOWS.

1. Opium 10 gr., calomel 10 gr., thick gruel q. s., at night, and the tonic drink (No. 2) in the morning.—CLATER.

2. Mr. SPOONER says salts in ½ lb doses, with a little ginger, are generally sufficient.

3. Muriate of soda ½ oz., carbonate of soda ½ oz., turmeric 2 oz., Glauber's salts 6 oz., powdered gentian and chamomile 2 dr., gruel q. s.

4. Castile soap ½ oz., Venice turpentine ½ oz., ginger 3 dr., gentian 1 oz.; rub the soap and turpentine in a mortar, and gradually add a pint of water, and afterwards the ginger and gentian.—WHITE.

5. Castile soap 1 oz., salt 1 oz., Venice turpentine 1 oz., yolks of 2 eggs; mix together, and gradually add a strong decoction of barberry-bark.

6. Powdered cummin seed, aniseed, and turmeric, each 2 oz., grains of Paradise and salt of tartar, each 1 oz.; mix. Slice 1 oz. of Castile soap, to mix with 2 oz. of treacle. Pour a quart of boiling ale upon all the ingredients, and administer when lukewarm. To be repeated 2 or 3 times a day.

CLEANSING DRINKS, for cows after calving. These are often applied for, but are condemned as useless or hurtful by veterinarians of the new school. The following are some of the forms in use; probably a gentle laxative would be in most cases preferable.

1. Spermaceti, Irish slate, and birthwort, in powder, of each 1 oz., powdered aniseed 2 oz., liquorice powder 2 oz.; in linseed tea.

2. Aniseed, myrrh, birthwort, allspice, cummin seed, of each 1 oz., in a quart of gruel.—MCEWEN.

3. Juniper-berries 3 oz., birthwort 2 oz., fenugreek 1 oz., spermaceti 2 oz., antimony 1 oz., saffron ½ oz., in a quart of warm ale.—DOWNING.

4. Resin, soap, of each ½ oz., spermaceti ½ oz., aniseed, caraway-seed, of each 1 oz., ginger ½ oz., treacle 4 oz., warm gruel a quart.

5. 1 oz. spermaceti, 1 oz. birthwort, 2 oz. powdered bay-berries, 1 oz. myrrh; in juniper-berry tea.

LAXATIVE DRINK AFTER CALVING. Epsom salts 12 oz., aniseed 1 oz., olive oil 6 oz., gruel a pint, or q. s.

DRENCH FOR STRANGURY. After laxatives and a clyster, give, Camphor 2 dr., spirit of nitrous ether ½ oz., tincture of opium ½ oz., nitre 1 oz., gruel a pint.—WHITE.

DRENCHES FOR HOVEN OR BLOWN, (flatulent distention of the paunch.) It appears doubtful whether any liquid enters the paunch in these cases. More dependence is now placed on the introduction of a tube constructed for the purpose.

1. Ginger ½ oz., spirit of nitric ether 2 oz., oil of peppermint 30 drops, warm water a pint.—WHITE.

2. Liquid ammonia, or spirit of hartshorn ½ oz. to 1 oz., (1½ oz.—WHITE) cold water 3 pints.—MOIROUD.

3. Chloride of potash 4 dr., water 4 oz., ether 3 dr. The solution of chlorinated soda may be substituted for chloride of potash (Eau de Javelle.)—CHARLOT.

4. Aloes 3 dr., pimento 2 dr., oil of turpentine 2 oz., spirit of hartshorn 1 oz., in gruel or warm water.—BLAINE.

5. Chloride of lime 2 dr., water a quart. Administer it by means of a stomach-pump, and repeat in an hour if required.—MR. YOUATT.

RHEUMATIC DRENCH.

1. Sulphur 8 oz., ginger ½ oz.; in gruel, every third day, if necessary.—CLATER.

2. Antimonial powder 2 dr., Dover's powder ½ dr., aniseed 1 oz., thick gruel a pint; night and morning, the bowels having been opened by No. 1.—CLATER.

3. Rhododendron leaves 4 dr., water a quart; boil to a pint, strain, and add powdered gum guaiacum 2 dr., caraway-seeds and aniseed, each 2 dr., warm ale ½ pint.

ANTISPASMODIC DRENCH FOR LOCKED-JAW. Camphor 1 dr. (rubbed with spirit,) powdered opium 1 dr., thick gruel ½ pint.

CORDIAL CARMINATIVE DRENCHES. Drenches for indigestion, and colic without inflammation.

1. In Indigestion: Salt 3 or 4 oz., carbonate of soda 2 dr., ginger ½ dr., anodyne tincture (below) 2 oz., water 10 or 12 oz.—WHITE.

2. The same: Aloes 4 dr., common salt 4 oz., ginger 2 dr., anodyne tincture 2 oz., water q. s.

3. In Colic: Salt 4 oz., aloes 3 dr., ginger 1 dr., opium ½ oz., water 1 pint, peppermint water 1 pint.

4. *Carminative.* Oil of turpentine 1 oz., tincture of opium 6 dr., spirit of nitric ether 2 oz., water 1 pint.—WHITE.

5. *Warm Cordial.* A bottle of red wine, extract of juniper 1 oz., powdered cinnamon ½ oz.—LEBAS.

6. *Mild.* Peppermint 2 oz., chamomiles ½ oz., hot water 5 pints; infuse, and give while warm.

7. Chamomile 2 oz., aniseed 1½ oz.; infuse in hot water, and strain; when cold add ether 2 oz.—VATEL.

DRENCHES FOR BLOODY URINE.

Bloody Urine (Hæmaturia) and Red-water are often confounded, but are different diseases, and require a different treatment. Hæmaturia is distinguished by the presence of actual blood in the urine, in a state of coagulation, and by great tenderness across the loins. It generally occurs in oxen of good condition. It is to be treated by bleeding, purgatives, stimulating applications to the loins, emollient drinks and opiates. [SPOONER.] After bleeding, give one of the following drenches:—

1. Epsom salts 6 to 8 oz., water a quart, castor oil 4 to 6 oz.—WHITE. Or,

2. Linseed oil 1 pint, gruel 1 pint, caraways 2 dr., Epsom salts 8 oz. (in warm water ½ pint,) tincture of opium 2 dr. Or either of the laxative drenches for red-water, below.

3. After the above, when the pain and difficulty have abated, but the water continues bloody, give—Catechu 2 dr., opium ½ dr., alum 3 dr., gum Arabic ½ oz., water ½ pint; simmer for a few minutes, and add ½ pint of ale. Repeat, if required.

4. In obstinate cases: Oil of juniper ½ oz., oil of tur-

pentine 1 oz., laudanum 1 oz., in a pint of linseed tea; at first twice, and afterwards once a day.—RUSH.

5. Three-quarters of a pint of black beer, and 2 oz. Irish slate.—KNOWLSON.

DRENCHES FOR RED-WATER.

This commonly attacks milch cows, and appears generally to arise from the nature of the pasture. Moderate bleeding is recommended, but is less necessary than in hæmaturia. Laxatives should then be given.

1. Epsom salts 8 to 12 oz., sulphur 2 to 4 oz., carbonate of ammonia ½ oz., ginger ½ oz., warm water 4 pints; give a fourth part every 6 hours till the bowels are acted on.—SPOONER. Or,

2. Glauber's salts 12 oz., carbonate of soda ½ oz., nitre ¼ oz., sugar 1 oz., powdered caraways ½ oz., in a quart of gruel. Or the Purging Drenches, No. 1, 2, or 3. After the bowels are well opened, give astringents, or mild stimulants.

3. The laxative drench, No. 11, page 122.—WHITE. This is WHITE's drench for red-water, No. 1. To be followed by drenches of whey.

4. *Astringent.* Powdered oak-bark ½ oz., catechu 2 dr., opium 10 gr., gruel 1 pint.—CLATER.

5. Catechu 2 dr., mucilage 4 oz., lime water 6 oz.—BLAINE.

6. Laudanum ½ oz., sugar of lead ½ dr., catechu 4 dr., gruel 1 quart.—WHITE.

7. After laxatives: Ginger, gentian, each 1 dr., spirit of nitrous ether 1 oz., gruel q. s.; twice a day.—SPOONER.

8. Powdered oak-bark 1 oz., charcoal 1 oz., bole 2 oz., in a quart of new milk.—PYE.

9. Catechu 1½ oz., alum 1½ oz., diapente 2 oz., Locatelli balsam 2 oz., warm gruel 3 pints.—MCEWEN.

10. Dragon's blood 2 oz., rust of iron 1 oz., nitre 3 oz., oil of turpentine 2 oz.; mix; for 2 doses, in gruel. DOWNING.

11. Sulphuric acid 1 dr., tincture of opium ½ oz., treacle 4 oz., warm gruel 4 quarts; daily, for a week.—BLAINE.

DRINK FOR ACUTE DIARRHŒA. Sulphate of soda, sulphate of magnesia, of each 2 oz., ipecacuanha ½ dr., sulphate of iron 6 gr.—BLAINE.

FOR CHRONIC DIARRHŒA. Calomel ½ dr., aloes 1 dr., gentian 2 dr., opium 5 gr., decoction of chamomiles 1 pint.—BLAINE.

ASTRINGENT DRENCHES, for dysentery (scouring rot) or lax.

1. After purging drenches: Prepared chalk 2 oz., oak bark 1 oz., catechu ½ oz., opium 2 scruples, ginger 2 dr., warm gruel 1 quart.—CLATER.

2. Two quarts of alum whey.

3. First give blue pill 2 or 3 dr., rhubarb 3 dr., castor oil 4 oz., gruel 1 pint, well stirred before giving it; repeat this 3 or 4 mornings; then give—thick starch (made with 4 oz. of starch) 3 or 4 pints, tincture of opium 2 dr., ginger 3 dr., catechu ½ oz.—WHITE.

4. Mutton suet 1 ℔, new milk 2 quarts; boil, and add opium ½ dr., ginger 1 dr.—CLATER.

5. *Cordial Astringent Drench.* (After the laxative drench No. 2.) Catechu ¼ oz., allspice ¼ oz., caraways ½ oz., ale ½ pint, water ½ pint.—WHITE.

6. Decoction of sloes, with prepared chalk.—TUSSER.

7. Decoction of wormwood a quart, gum Arabic 2 oz., aromatic confection 1 oz., catechu 2 dr.; with linseed tea, repeated every 6 days for 3 times.—MR. RAWLINGS.

8. Sheep's heart, liver, and lights, all chopped up together.—MR. SUMNER.

EXPECTORANT & COUGH DRENCHES, IN HOOSE or CATARRH. [For Hoose, in Calves, see page 134.]

1. Bruised liquorice 2 oz.; boil in a quart of water to a pint, strain, and add powdered squill 2 dr., gum guaiacum 1 dr., tincture of tolu 4 dr., honey 2 oz.—CLATER.

2. Balsam of sulphur 2 oz., Barbadoes tar 1 oz., yolks of 2 eggs, honey 4 oz., salt of tartar ½ oz., oil of aniseed 1 dr., elecampane 1 oz., gruel 1 quart: in chronic coughs.

3. Fresh squill 2 oz., garlic, 2 oz., vinegar 24 oz.; di-

gest for a day with a gentle heat; strain, and press, and boil the liquor with 24 oz. of treacle: for 6 doses, in chronic cough.

4. For recent coughs: Digitalis 20 gr., emetic tartar ½ dr., nitre, 3 dr., squill 1 dr., opium 20 gr., gruel 1 pint.

5. Boil 4 oz. Iceland moss and 1 oz. liquorice root in 4 quarts of water, for a quarter of an hour, and strain; add to the liquor 1 oz. nitre, cream of tartar 2 oz. In hoose from cold, if inflammation of the lungs and fever be present, bleed before giving the drink. See also Fever Drenches.

If the disease be connected with worms in the air passages, give the following:—

Worm Drench.—For cough from worms: Oil of turpentine 2 oz., sweet spirit of nitre 1 oz., laudanum ½ oz.; mix, and give in a pint of gruel.—Clater.

DRENCHES FOR THE RECENT EPIDEMIC, affecting the feet and mouth, and attended with a low fever.

1. Glauber's salts 1 ℔., treacle 4 oz., sulphur 4 oz., aniseed ½ oz., cream of tartar 2 oz., warm water 3 pints; give it new milk warm. The above is for a full-grown beast. The mouth to be washed with a strong solution of blue vitriol, burnt alum and vinegar. If the feet crack, apply a mixture of equal parts of muriatic acid and water.

2. Some cattle-masters give common salt in gruel with great success.—Blaine.

3. After a mild dose of salts—sweet spirit of nitre 1 oz., ale yeast 6 or 8 oz.—Blaine.

4. Epsom salts 8 oz., sulphur 2 oz., nitre ½ oz., ginger ¼ oz.; half of this to be given in warm water, with 1 oz. of sweet spirit of nitre. Repeat daily. When the bowels are properly relaxed, and the fever reduced, but much weakness remains, give the following:—

5. *Tonic Drench.* Gentian 4 dr., ginger 2 dr., sulphate of iron 2 dr., sweet spirits of nitre 1 oz., warm water q. s.; wash the mouth with the *lotion*, page 135; dress the feet, after paring and poulticing, with equal parts of tincture of myrrh and butter of antimony; and afterwards apply the *astringent powder*, page 140.—Spooner.

6. Linseed oil a pint, oil of turpentine 8 oz., aloes ½ oz., ginger ¼ oz., laudanum 1 oz.; mix. For 2 doses, to be given with gruel.

REMEDIES FOR THE EPIZOOTIC PNEUMONIA.

In the fatal form of this disease lately prevailing, the following treatment is said to have proved effectual:—Bleed freely; then administer ½ pint of brandy every 2 hours. Mr. Jeckyll gives, in pleuro-pneumonia, when a tonic is indicated, ½ oz. of the following solution every 8 hours:—Sulphate of copper 1 part, water 4 parts; dissolve, and add ammonia until it begins to precipitate.

MURRAIN DRENCHES.

1. Sweet spirit of nitre ½ oz., laudanum ½ oz., solution of chloride of lime 2 dr., prepared chalk 1 oz.; mix, and give in a pint of warm gruel.—CLATER.

2. Cascarilla powder 2 oz., spirit of nitrous ether ½ oz., liquid acetate of ammonia 4 oz., beer yeast 8 oz.; every four hours.—BLAINE.

3. Opiate confection 1 oz., liquid acetate of ammonia 2 oz., water 1 quart: for one dose.—VATEL.

4. *Tonic.* Calumba 2 dr., canella 3 dr., ginger 1 dr., sweet spirit of nitre ½ oz., thick gruel 1 pint.—SPOONER.

5. *Ceylon Remedy.* A small piece of lard the size of a walnut. Said to be used with perfect success.

6. *To prevent Murrain.* Myrrh 1 oz., Epsom salts 2 oz., sulphur 1 oz., liver of antimony ½ oz., diapente 1 oz.: in rue tea after bleeding.—DOWNING.

FOR THE DISTEMPER.

Warm tar-water is much recommended by some. It should be given in doses of 3 quarts 3 or 4 times a day, gradually diminishing the quantity.

DIURETIC DRINKS.

1. Common turpentine ½ oz., ginger 2 dr.; mix with a little treacle, and add gradually spirit of nitrous ether 1 oz., gruel a pint.—CLATER.

2. *Tonic Diuretic.* Common turpentine 4 dr., ginger 2 dr., gentian 2 dr., tartrate of iron 1 dr.; rub together with a little treacle, and add gradually 1 oz. of sweet spirit of nitre.

BULLING DRENCHES. These are strongly condemned by modern veterinary writers; those drenches, at least which contain cantharides.

1. Aniseed, grains of paradise, bay berries, of each 1 oz.; cantharides in fine powder 20 to 30 gr.; to be given in a quart of milk.

2. Black hellebore ½ oz., capsicum 2 dr., birthwort ½ oz., bay berries 1 oz., cantharides 20 gr.; in a quart of warm ale.—DOWNING.

3. A quart of milk from a cow in season.—CLATER.

4. Powdered cantharides 20 gr., aniseed 2 oz., black hellebore ½ oz.; in ale, gruel, or milk.—PECK.

DRYING DRENCHES; for drying a cow's milk. Bleed the night before, and give the drink, warm, in the morning.

1. Boil 6 dr. of alum in milk, and strain.—WHITE.

2. Alum 6 ℔, bole 2 ℔, cream of tartar or red tartar 1 ℔; mix. Give from 6 to 9 oz. in stale beer; or in gruel with ½ pint of vinegar.

3. Roche or common alum 4 oz., dragon's blood ½ oz., turmeric 1 oz., in a pint of rennet water, and a pint of vinegar.—DOWNING. [These large doses of alum, though often given, are not regarded as necessary or proper by modern veterinary writers.]

DRENCH FOR THE BITES OF VIPERS. Olive oil 2 pints, spirits of hartshorn 1 oz.; mix.

ALUM WHEY. Boil ½ oz. of alum in 2 quarts of milk for 10 minutes, and strain.

ANODYNE CARMINATIVE TINCTURE; and Tincture of Pimento. See MEDICINES FOR HORSES.

ALTERATIVE POWDERS.

1. Sulphur 4 oz., black antimony 1 oz., Æthiop's

mineral ½ oz., nitre 2 oz.; mix, for 4 doses: to be given daily in gruel.

2. *Alterative Tonic.* Add to the last 2 oz. gentian and 1 oz. ginger; and make 6 doses.

FEVER POWDERS, IN INFLAMMATION, &c.

1. Antimonial powder a scruple, camphor ½ dr., nitre 1 oz.; mix: give twice a day in gruel.—PECK.

2. Peruvian bark 16 oz., nitre 24 oz.; for 16 doses.

CORDIAL POWDERS.

1. Black mustard ½ oz., flowers of sulphur 1 oz., aromatic powder (see HORSE POWDERS) 1 oz., fenugreek 4 oz., common salt 16 oz.; a large pinch on a slice of bread.—MATTHIEU.

2. *Cow Spice.* As Horse Spice, No. 2, page 73. Or,

3. Powdered turmeric, liquorice, aniseed, and diapente, each 1 oz.

CLYSTERS.

1. Salt 1 ℔, warm water a gallon.

2. Linseed oil 8 oz., Epsom salts 8 oz., gruel 3 quarts.

MASTICATORIES.

1. Bruised garlic 4 cloves, salt a tablespoonful, ground pepper 1 oz., honey 4 oz. Boil for a short time in a glass of vinegar, immerse it in a piece of linen, and roll it up. Keep it in the animal's mouth for an hour night and morning. *Antiputrescent;* in epizootic maladies, and in ulcers of the mouth.—J. ROBINETT.

2. Bruised mustard and pepper, each ½ oz., rolled up in linen, and sprinkled with vinegar: to be kept in the mouth not more than half an hour, morning and evening, in epizootic diseases.

MEDICINES FOR CALVES.

PURGATIVE DRENCHES.

1. Epsom salt 1 oz. to 2 oz., according to the age and size of the calf; dissolve in ½ pint of gruel, and add 20 gr. of ginger, and 3 drops of essence of peppermint.—CLATER.

2. Salts 1½ oz., castor oil 2 oz., ginger 10 gr., caraway 2 dr., gruel ½ pint.

3. In costiveness, and accumulation in the paunch and stomach: dissolve 2 oz. of Epsom salts in 2 or 3 quarts of water, or 4 oz. in a gallon, according to the age of the calf, and throw it gently by means of a stomach pump.

4. *Laxative.* Epsom salts 2 or 3 oz., carbonate of soda 2 dr., water 6 or 8 oz., ginger 1 dr.; mix. After it has operated, give the cordial, No. 3, below.—WHITE.

DRENCHES FOR DIARRHŒA, OR CALVES' CORDIAL.

1. YOUATT'S *Cordial.* Prepared chalk 2 oz., catechu 1 oz., ginger ½ oz., opium 1 dr., peppermint water 1 pint; dose for a calf, from 2 to 4 tablespoonfuls.

2. Prepared chalk 2 dr., opium 10 gr., catechu ½ dr., ginger ½ dr., essence of peppermint 5 drops; mix, and give twice a day in ½ pint of gruel.—CLATER.

3. Caraway ½ oz., ginger ½ dr., subcarbonate of soda 1 dr., brandy or gin 1 oz., water 8 oz.—[WHITE'S *Cordial.*]

4. Half a bottle of Dalby's carminative.

5. Suet boiled in milk ½ pint, opium 5 gr., alum 5 gr., prepared chalk ½ oz.; mix.

6. If No. 2 fails: Dover's powder 2 scruples, aromatic powder 1 dr., kino ½ dr.; give it night and morning, with 1 oz., of arrowroot boiled in a pint of water.—CLATER.

INFLAMMATORY DISORDERS. Bleed; give 2 to 6 oz. Epsom salts. [Give to a calf of six months old ¼ the dose for cattle; at a year and a half, ½ the dose.—SPOONER.]

MEDICINE FOR PILES IN CALVES.

Oil of vitriol 15 drops, tincture of opium ½ oz.—PECK.

SOLUTION OF POTASH, FOR CORDS, &c. Subcarbonate of potash 2 oz., fresh lime water 8 oz. To correct acidity in the stomach, give 1 or 2 teaspoonfuls in gruel; the first dose to be given with an ounce or two of Epsom salts in ½ a pint of thin gruel. If the disorder is attended with griping pains, add a tablespoonful of anodyne carminative tincture.—WHITE.

ALUM WHEY. See page 131.

TO PROMOTE THE FATTENING OF CALVES.

Aniseed ¼ ℔, fenugreek ¼ ℔, linseed meal 1℔; make it into a paste with milk, and cram them with it.

Fattening Powder. Common salt with a little carbonate of soda; a small quantity added to the food promotes fattening, and prevents scouring, &c.

HOOSE, OR COUGH FROM WORMS IN AIR PASSAGES.

1. ½ pint lime water every morning, and a tablespoonful of salt every afternoon, to each calf.—MR. MAYER.

2. Linseed oil 4 oz., oil of turpentine 1 oz., oil of caraways 20 drops; repeated once or twice at intervals of 10 days. This dose for calves of 6 to 10 months old.—MR. DICKENS.

3. A tablespoonful of oil of turpentine, a little sweet oil, and 6 or 8 oz. of warm water.—WHITE.

External Applications for Neat Cattle.

LOTIONS OR WASHES. (See also EMBROCATIONS.)

LOTIONS FOR CANKER IN CALVES.

1. Alum 1 oz., water 8 oz., tincture of myrrh 1 oz., honey of roses 1 oz.

2. Equal parts of tincture of myrrh and water.—CLATER.

3. Alum ½ oz., water 1 pint, tincture of myrrh 1 oz.

LOTION FOR COW-POCK. Sal ammoniac ¼ oz., white vinegar ½ pint, camphorated spirit 2 oz., Goulard's extract 1 oz.; mix.—CLATER.

LOTIONS FOR SLIGHT BRUISES.

1. Extract of lead ½ oz., vinegar 4 oz., soft water 1 pint.—WHITE.

2. Acetate of ammonia 4 oz., water ½ pint, spirit of camphor ½ oz.

DISCUTIENT LOTION, for dispersing tumours. Bay salt 4 oz., vinegar 1 pint, water 1 quart, oil of origanum 1 dr.; rub the oil with the salt, and gradually add the others.

LOTIONS FOR STRAINS.

1. Bay salt 4 oz., oil of origanum 1 dr.; rub together, and add vinegar ½ pint, spirit of wine 2 oz., water 1 quart.

2. Common salt 1 oz., sal ammoniac 1 oz., water 1 pint.

LOTIONS FOR FOUL IN THE FOOT. After poulticing and removing loose horn, apply—

1. Butter of Antimony, or
2. Strong solution of alum.
3. Solution of sulphate of copper.
4. (When the above are not sufficient.) Dissolve 2 dr. of corrosive sublimate in 12 ounces of water.—WHITE.

LOTIONS FOR WOUNDS.

1. Tincture of myrrh and aloes.
2. For proud flesh: strong solution of sulphate of copper.
3. For offensive wounds: chloride of lime 1 oz., water 1 pint; mix well, and strain.

LOTION FOR BULL-BURNT. Goulard's extract 1 oz., spirit of wine 2 oz., water ½ pint.

LOTION FOR BLAIN IN THE MOUTH. After lancing the bladder, apply a saturated solution of salt in water. YOUATT.

LOTION FOR THE MOUTH, in the lately prevailing epidemic. Alum 1 oz., sulphate of zinc ½ oz., warm water 1 pint, treacle ¼ lb.—SPOONER.

WASHES FOR DESTROYING VERMIN. They are all poisonous.

1. Stavesacre seeds 4 oz., water 4 pints; boil to 2 pints, and apply it daily.—PECK.

2. Sublimate 2 dr., spirit of wine 2 oz., water 1 pint. —CLATER.

3. Stavesacre 4 oz., white hellebore root 2 oz., water 1 gallon; boil to half; apply with a sponge.

LOTION FOR MANGE. Corrosive sublimate 2 dr., muriatic acid ½ oz., water 12 to 16 oz.; mix. In obstinate cases only.—WHITE. See Liniments.

EYE WATERS, OR COLLYRIA,

1. White vitriol a scruple, spirit of wine 1 dr., water a pint.—CLATER.

2. Sugar of lead 10 to 20 gr., soft water 8 oz.—V. C.

3. *Sedative Eye Drops.* Powdered digitalis 1½ oz.; infuse in a pint of Cape wine for a fortnight, and filter: a few drops to be introduced into the eye twice or thrice a day.—SPOONER.

4. Extract of lead 2 dr., wine of digitalis (No. 3) 2 dr., tincture of opium 2 dr., water a pint.

EMBROCATIONS AND LINIMENTS.

STRONG EMBROCATION, for deep-seated strains, &c.

1. Oil of origanum ½ oz., oil of turpentine ½ pint, sweet oil 1½ pint, powdered cantharides 1 oz.—CLATER.

2. Olive oil 4 oz., oil of turpentine 1 oz., water of ammonia 1 oz. (For strains and bruises, after the inflammation has subsided.)—WHITE.

CROTON LINIMENT. Bruised croton seeds 1 part, oil of turpentine 8 parts. Macerate for 14 days, and strain. It irritates the skin powerfully: for general purposes it requires to be diluted with olive oil.—MORTON.

MUSTARD EMBROCATION. Flour of mustard 4 oz., oil of turpentine 2 oz., water of ammonia 2 oz.—WHITE.

RHEUMATIC EMBROCATIONS.

1. Olive oil 2 oz., strong water of ammonia 1 oz., marshmallow ointment 1 oz.

2. Neatsfoot oil 4 oz., camphorated oil 1 oz., oil of turpentine 1 oz., laudanum 1 oz., oil of origanum 1 dr. —CLATER.

3. Sweet oil 4 oz., oil of turpentine 2 oz. Mix.—WHITE.

EMBROCATIONS FOR GARGET, or Downfall of the Udder.

1. Oil of elder 4 oz., water of ammonia ½ oz., Mindererus' spirit 1 oz., camphorated oil 2 oz.

2. Olive oil 3 oz., oil of turpentine 1 oz., camphor 2 dr.—WHITE.

3. Soft soap 8 oz., oil of bays 8 oz., oil of turpentine 8 oz., spirit of camphor 4 oz. See also OINTMENTS, below.

DRIFFIELD OILS. Barbadoes tar 1 oz., linseed oil 1 ℔, oil of turpentine 3 oz., oil of vitriol 1 oz. or 1½ oz. (by weight.)

LINIMENT FOR MANGE. Sulphur vivum, or flower of sulphur 4 oz., train oil 12 oz., oil of turpentine 4 oz.; mix.

LINIMENT FOR SORE THROATS. Oil of turpentine 1 oz., sweet oil 1 oz., water of ammonia 2 oz.—WHITE.

BLISTERING LINIMENTS. Cantharides bruised 1 oz., oil of turpentine 8 oz.; digest 14 days, and strain. To be applied by friction on the skin.—YOUATT.

LIQUID CAUSTIC. Butter of antimony alone, or mixed with an equal quantity of tincture of myrrh.

LIQUID SNUFF. Alum, sulphate of zinc, capsicum, of each 1 oz.; camphor 2 dr.; pulverize, and macerate in 32 oz. of strong vinegar, and 1 oz. of turpentine; shake up when used, and introduce a teaspoonful into the nostrils, to promote a discharge for the relief of inflammation of the chest.—MATTHIEU.

OINTMENTS.

BLISTERING OINTMENTS.

1. Resin cerate 1 oz., cantharides finely powdered 3 dr., oil of turpentine 2 dr.; for setons.—CLATER.

2. Lard 12 oz., resin 4 oz.; melt together, and when sufficiently cool, add oil of turpentine 4 oz., powdered cantharides 5 oz.; stir till cold: to be rubbed in after removing the hair.—CLATER.

OINTMENT FOR MANGE, LICE, &c. (See also LOTIONS, above.)

1. Sulphur 1 ℔, common turpentine 4 oz., mercurial ointment 2 oz., linseed oil a pint. Melt the turpentine with the oil, and when nearly cold, stir in the sulphur, and afterwards the mercurial ointment.—YOUATT. *Note.* —Cattle are easily salivated, and greatly weakened by it. Mercurials should therefore be used with great caution.

2. Sulphur 1 ℔, strong mercurial ointment 2 oz., common turpentine ½ ℔, lard 1½ ℔.—CLATER.

3. *French Liniment.* Olive oil a pint, sulphur 4 oz., heat till the oil becomes coloured by the sulphur; remove from the fire, and when nearly cold, add 4 oz. of oil of turpentine; apply with a feather.

4. Lard 2 ℔; melt and add oil of turpentine 8 oz., sulphuric acid 2 oz., sulphur vivum 8 oz.; stir till cold.

5. *Mange Liniment.* Sulphur vivum finely powdered 4 oz., train oil 12 oz., oil of turpentine 4 oz.; mix.—WHITE.

IODINE OINTMENT, for Empyema. Rub together 1½ dr. of iodine, and 1 dr. iodide of potassium, with a few drops of water, then add 3 oz. of strong mercurial ointment, and ½ oz. of powdered camphor. To be rubbed over the chest every night till it causes an exudation, then occasionally keep it up.

GARGET OINTMENT, for Downfall of the Udder.

1. Soft soap 1 ℔, mercurial ointment 2 oz., camphor (powdered with spirit) 1 oz.; mix: give first as a laxative, then a fever or diuretic drink.

2. Green elder ointment 2 oz., water of ammonia ¼ oz.

3. Beat fox-glove leaves with twice their weight of whey butter; to every pound add 1 oz. of sal ammoniac, 1 oz. of turpentine, and ½ oz. of bole; mix and apply 2 or 3 times a day.—DOWNING.

4. Spirit of Camphor 1 oz., mercurial ointment 1 oz., elder ointment 8 oz.—YOUATT.

5. In obstinate cases. Iodide of potassium 1 part, lard 7 parts. To be rubbed in once daily.—MR. SPOONER.

FOOT OINTMENT (for all domestic animals.) Equal parts of tar, lard, and resin, melted together.

OINTMENT FOR ULCERS ABOUT THE JOINTS. Equal parts of basilicon and citrine ointments.—CLATER.

HEALING AND CLEANSING OINTMENT. Lard 2 ℔, yellow resin ½ ℔; melt together, and when it begins to cool, add calamine in powder ½ ℔.

APPLICATION TO WOUNDS. Mix the whites of eggs with flour to a proper consistence. Applied over the part, it soon dries, and shields it from the air.

DIGESTIVE OINTMENT. Lard, common turpentine, of each 4 oz.; melt, and add 1 oz. powdered verdigris. —WHITE.

2. Boil leaves of black hellebore with an equal weight of lard, until the leaves are crisp; strain, and add an equal weight of common turpentine. [A similar ointment made with ivy leaves is likewise very stimulating.]

OINTMENT FOR FOUL IN THE FOOT, OR LOW.

1. Melt 4 oz. of lard with 4 oz. of common turpentine, and add 1 oz. of finely-powdered sulphate of copper, stirring until cold.—WHITE.

2. Melt together equal weights of soft soap and common turpentine.—SKERRET.

OINTMENT FOR CANCEROUS TUMOURS. Hydriodate of potash ¼ oz., hot water ¼ oz.; dissolve, and mix with 2 oz. of lard.

CHARGE FOR OLD STRAINS. Burgundy pitch 4 oz., common pitch 4 oz., wax 2 oz., tar 6 oz.; apply hot, and cover with cut tow.

SETONS.

1. *Common.* A piece of cord, or coarse tape; or horse-hair and tow platted together.

2. *Irritating.* Root of common dock; or of black hellebore.

3. Cotton cord soaked in Morton's cantharidal solution, (page 92.)

PASTE FOR STOPPING BLEEDING. Equal quantities of white, green, and blue vitriol, flour, and bole; beaten up with fresh nettles and a little vinegar.

ASTRINGENT POWDER FOR SORE FEET, &c. Sulphate of copper ½ oz., prepared chalk 2 oz., powdered alum ½ oz., bole 1 oz.; rub together.—SPOONER.

MEDICINES FOR SHEEP AND LAMBS.

THESE are best given in a liquid form, and should be carefully and slowly administered. Sheep generally require one-sixth (or from one-eighth to one-sixth) of the doses given to cattle.

PURGING DRENCHES.

1. Epsom salt 2 oz., powdered caraway ¼ oz., warm thin gruel, sufficient to dissolve the salts. The editor of CLATER says that this is the best purging drink that can be used. For *Lambs* give a fourth of this, and repeat in 6 hours if necessary.

2. Epsom salt 1½ oz. or 2 oz., ginger 1 dr., treacle 1 oz., hot water 4 oz.

3. Castor oil 2 oz., ginger and salt of tartar, of each 2 scruples, moist sugar a spoonful, gruel q. s.—M'EWEN.

4. Epsom or Glauber's salt from 1 to 2 oz., common salt a teaspoonful, boiling water sufficient to dissolve the salts, and a little gruel. A teaspoonful of tincture of ginger or of pimento, or of anodyne carminative tincture (see p. 88,) may be added.

5. Sulphur ¼ oz., Epsom salt 1 oz., common salt a teaspoonful, thin gruel ¼ pint.

6. Linseed oil 2 or 3 oz., croton oil 2 or 3 drops, warm gruel q. s.

7. *For Lambs.* Epsom salt 2 to 4 dr., ginger ½ dr., in gruel.—SPOONER.

8. *For Sheep on the first attack of Small-Pox.* Epsom salt 2 oz., ginger ½ dr., in chamomile tea or an infusion of gentian, (or with 1 dr. of powdered gentian or chamomile.)—WARNECKE.

FEVER DRENCH. Powdered digitalis 20 gr., emetic tartar 10 gr., nitre 2 dr. Twice a day, mixed with gruel. —CLATER.

TONIC DRENCHES.

1. *General Tonic.* Gentian 2 dr., calumba 1 dr., ginger ½ dr., all in powder; tincture of orange peel 1 dr., gruel 4 oz.; for one dose.—CLATER.

2. *In the last stage of Fever.* Gentian 1 dr., ginger 20 gr., spirit of nitrous ether 1 dr., tincture of cardamom 20 drops, in gruel.

3. *For Debility and Indigestion, after a purgative.* Gentian, caraway, each 1 oz., calumba and ginger, of each ½ oz. (all sliced or bruised,) boiling water a quart; infuse till cool, and strain. Give a tablespoonful daily, with the same quantity of gruel.—CLATER.

DRENCHES FOR RED WATER. The pasture should be changed for shorter, the animal bled, and the bowels kept open with the above purging drinks. If these means do not remove the disease, give one of the following:—

1. Epsom salts 6 oz., nitre 2 oz., bole ½ oz., hot water 3 pints, oil of turpentine 4 oz.; mix, and give 3 or 4 tablespoonfuls, (from a horn that will measure that quantity,) shaking the bottle well before each dose is poured out.

2. Powdered catechu 30 gr., alum 20 gr., ginger 20 gr., decotion of oak-bark 4 oz., for a dose.

3. Olive oil 1 oz., oil of turpentine 1 oz., thick gruel ¼ pint.

FOR EXTERNAL RED WATER. (Vesicles on the skin, containing a reddish fluid.)

1. Sulphur 2 to 3 dr., in gruel, once or twice a day. If it continues, give

2. Epsom salts 1 oz., gruel sufficient to dissolve it.—Sir JAMES MACKENZIE.

DRENCHES FOR DIARRHŒA (SCOUR) &c. IN LAMBS. [The Purging Drink, No. 6, or a fourth of No. 1, should be given before the Astringent Drinks.]

1. Prepared chalk 2 oz., catechu 1 oz., ginger ½ oz., opium 1 dr., peppermint water a pint. Dose, for lambs, a tablespoonful night and morning.—YOUATT.

2. Prepared chalk ¼ oz., ginger ½ dr., catechu ½ dr., opium 2 gr., in gruel; once or twice daily.

3. A tablespoonful of Calves' Cordial, p. 133.

4. Compound powder of chalk with opium 2 dr., gentian 1 dr., essence of peppermint 3 drops; in a little thin starch, morning and night.—CLATER.

5. Ginger 2 dr., caraway 4 dr., prepared chalk 4 dr.; mix; give a teaspoonful in gruel.—WHITE.

6. In white skit: a teaspoonful of WHITE'S alkaline solution (p. 133) in a little gruel; and afterwards No. 7.

7. Epsom salt 3 dr., common salt a scruple, powdered ginger a scruple, thin gruel 4 oz. Repeat if necessary.

DRENCH FOR THE LATE PREVAILING EPIDEMIC. Epsom salt 1 oz., sulphur 2 dr., nitre ½ dr., ginger 15 gr., in warm water. Repeat half this, with a teaspoonful of sweet spirit of nitre, daily.—SPOONER.

DRENCH FOR COW-POX. Mix 3 parts of flowers of sulphur, 1 of common salt, and 1 of honey, into an electuary; give ½ oz., of this daily, in gruel. Keep the mouth and nose clean with vinegar-and-water. See also Purging Drench No. 7, above.

DRENCH FOR INFLUENZA. Epsom salt ½ oz., chamomile tea 4 oz. Afterwards give half doses of the Fever Drench, above.—DARBY.

DRENCHES FOR BLOWN OR BLAST.

1. Glauber's salt 1 oz., hot water 1 oz., peppermint water 4 oz., tincture of ginger 1 dr., tincture of gentian 1 dr.; every six hours till the bowels are opened, and half the quantity the next 4 mornings.—CLATER.

2. Common salt 1 oz., solution of potash (WHITE'S) 1½ dr., castor or olive oil, 2 tablespoonfuls, water 8 oz., (After letting out the air by a tube or probang.)—WHITE.

DRINK TO PREVENT RESP OR MEADOW SICKNESS. Pearlash 1½ dr., hot water 8 oz. To be given from a flat bottle the second and fourth morning after putting them to keep.—HOLDITCH.

DRENCH FOR STURDY AND APOPLEXY. After bleeding, 2 oz. of Epsom or Glauber's salts, in warm water or thin gruel.

DRENCHES FOR FLUX, OR SCOURING, OR DYSENTERY.

1. Epsom salt 1 oz., hot water or thin gruel to dissolve it; add castor oil 2 oz., laudanum 30 drops. When it has operated, give No. 2.—BLAINE.

2. Ipecacuanha 15 gr., prepared chalk 1 dr., opium 2 gr., boiled starch or arrow-root 4 oz. Night and morning.

3. Linseed oil 2 oz., powdered opium 2 gr., linseed tea q. s. Afterwards give No. 4.—SAYER.

4. Opium 2 gr., ginger ½ dr., gentian ½ dr., linseed tea or gruel q. s.

5. Epsom salt 1½ oz., hot water 4 oz.; dissolve, and add castor or olive oil 1½ oz.—WHITE. Afterwards give No. 6.

6. Catechu ½ dr., allspice ½ dr., caraway 1 dr., water or beer 4 oz.; simmer together.

DRENCHES FOR DRY BRAXY, OR INFLAMMATION OF THE BOWELS.

1. After bleeding: Epsom salt 1½ oz., warm water a pint.—Mr. STEVENSON.

2. After bleeding: Common salt 1 oz., water ½ pint, laudanum a teaspoonful.—WHITE.

DRENCH FOR BITES OF VENOMOUS REPTILES. Olive oil 4 oz., spirit of hartshorn ¼ oz., gruel or arrowroot ¼ pint.—WHITE.

DRENCHES TO PROMOTE PARTURITION IN THE EWE.

1. A decoction of horsemint, or any other kind of mint.

2. Bruised ergot of rye 1 dr., boiling water a pint; infuse for a ¼ of an hour, and give a third part. Repeat if necessary.

DRENCHES AND POWDERS FOR THE ROT.

1. Juniper berries 6 oz., gentian 1 oz.; boil in 3 gal-

lons of water for a quarter of an hour, strain, and add common salt 4 ℔, powdered ginger 4 oz., tartarized iron 2 oz.; stir; and let it stand till cool. Put it into wine bottles filled two-thirds full, and add to each 1½ oz. oil of turpentine and ½ oz. sweet spirit of nitre. Give a tablespoonful night and morning, shaking the bottle before pouring it out.

2. Common salt 8 oz., gentian powder 8 oz., ginger 1 oz., tincture of calumba 4 oz., water to make up a quart.—CLATER. See the next.

3. To a quart of No. 2, add spirit of turpentine 3 oz.; shake well together, and give 2 tablespoonfuls at night, before the night's food is given, and a tablespoonful of No. 2 every morning.

Powders for the same.—A French recipe. 1. Dry bran 10 ℔, salt ½ ℔, aromatic herbs (as thyme, sage, juniper, rosemary, &c.) cut small, 6 oz., green anise and coriander of each 5 oz.; mix, and give morning and night every third day. The above quantity is for 30 sheep.

2. Juniper-berries 4 oz., bay-berries 1 oz., grains of paradise ¼ oz., bay salt 1½ ℔, loaf sugar ½ ℔; powder all together, and keep the powder in a bottle for use. Give the sheep dry and sweet hay, sprinkled with the powder.—LAWRENCE.

DRENCHES FOR INFLAMMATION OF THE LUNGS; CATARRH, HOOSE, AND COUGH. After bleeding from the neck, give Epsom salt 2 oz., gruel or linseed tea q. s.

DRENCH FOR INFLUENZA. Epsom salt ½ oz., chamomile tea 4 oz. Afterwards small doses of digitalis, opium, tartarized antimony, and vegetable tonics.—DARBY.

External Applications for Sheep.

EYE WATERS.

1. *Strong.* For cloudiness of the eye: corrosive sublimate 4 gr., spirit of wine ½ oz.; dissolve, and add water a pint.—CLATER.

2. Tincture or wine of opium a teaspoonful, water ½ pint.

WASHES FOR THE SCAB, LICE, AND TICKS. (The scab ointments will also destroy them, and are less hazardous, and less injurious to the wool.)

1. *Arsenical Wash.* White arsenic ½ ℔, salt of tartar ½ ℔, water 12 gallons; boil for half an hour.—YOUATT.

2. Arsenic 2 ℔, soft soap 4 ℔, water 30 gallons; dissolve. The sheep to be immersed in this liquid, (the head only being kept out,) and while in it the fleece to be well rubbed. When taken out the fluid should be well pressed out of the fleece, and the sheep kept from cold and wet for a few days.—CLATER. MR. SPOONER says 2 ℔ of arsenic should make 48 gallons of the liquid.

3. Arsenic 1 ℔, yellow soap 6 ℔, pearlash 12 oz., water 30 gallons.—MATTHEWS.

4. *Mercurial.* Corrosive sublimate 1 oz., spirit of wine 2 oz.; rub together till dissolved, then add cream of tartar 1 oz., bay salt 4 oz., dissolve the whole in 2 quarts of water, and apply it with a sponge wherever lice appear.—CLATER.

5. Tobacco 4 oz., water 1 gallon; boil, and add soft soap 1 ℔, sulphur vivum 1 ℔, when cold add a pint of oil of turpentine.

6. Equal parts of decoction of tobacco and lime water.—YOUATT.

WASH TO KILL MAGGOTS. Shake up in a bottle together 1 quart of water, spirits of turpentine 1 oz., and corrosive sublimate 10 grains. Stop with a cork in which a quill is inserted. When the maggots are observed, a small quantity of the mixture is to be shaken on the spot through the quill, and they will shortly creep out and die.

SMEARING MIXTURE.

1. One gallon of common tar, and 12 ℔ of any sweet grease, melted together.

2. Oil of tar is used as a preventive of the *fly;* but fish oil is equally so, according to Mr. HOGG; and is less

injurious to the wool. Oil of tar has sometimes destroyed sheep.

FLY POWDER, FOR SHEEP.

1. White lead 2 ℔, red lead ½ ℔, sulphur 1½ ℔, oil of wormwood, animal oil (empyreumatic,) or creasote ¼ oz.; mix.

2. White lead 2 ℔, red lead 1 ℔; mix, and apply by sprinkling from a dredger, following a stick drawn through the wool.—Clater.

3. Powdered colocynth 3 dr., black brimstone 1 ℔, tincture of assafœtida ½ oz.; mix.

4. White lead 4 parts, arsenic 1 part, sulphur 6, vermilion 2.—Spooner.

POWDER FOR THE EYES. Equal parts of sal ammoniac, white sugar, and oxide of zinc, triturated together. It may be mixed either with rose water or honey.—Spooner.

ASTRINGENT POWDER FOR THE FEET, in the recent epidemic. The same as for cattle. See above, page 140.

OINTMENTS FOR THE SCAB OR SHAB.

1. Quicksilver 1 ℔, Venice turpentine ½ ℔; rub them together until the globules are no longer visible; then add ½ pint of oil of turpentine, and 4 ℔ of lard. The mode of applying this ointment is as follows:—Begin at the head of the sheep, and proceeding from between the ears along the back to the end of the tail, divide the wool in a furrow till the skin can be touched; and let a finger slightly dipped in the ointment be drawn along the bottom of the furrow. From this furrow similar ones must be drawn along the shoulders and thighs to the legs, as far as the wool extends. And if much infected, 2 or more should also be drawn along each side, parallel with that on the back; and one down each side before the hind and fore legs. It kills the sheep-fag, and probably the tick and other vermin. It should not be used in very cold or wet weather.—Sir Joseph Banks.

2. Strong mercurial ointment 1 part, lard 5 parts; mix.—YOUATT.

3. Quicksilver 1 ℔, Venice turpentine ½ ℔, spirit of turpentine 2 oz., lard 4½ ℔; to be made and used as No. 1. In summer 1 ℔ of rosin may be substituted for a like quantity of lard.—CLATER.

4. Strong mercurial ointment 1 ℔, lard 4 ℔, oil of turpentine 8 oz., sulphur 12 oz.—WHITE.

5. *Mild.* Flowers of sulphur 1 ℔, Venice turpentine 4 oz., rancid lard 2 ℔, strong mercurial ointment 4 oz.; mix well.—CLATER.

6. Lard or other fat, with an equal quantity of oil of turpentine.—DAUBENTON.

7. *Without Mercury.* Lard 1 ℔, oil of turpentine 4 oz., flowers of sulphur 6 oz.—WHITE.

8. Strong mercurial ointment 1 ℔, lard 4 ℔, Venice turpentine 8 oz., oil of turpentine 2 oz. If mixed by heat, care must be taken to use no more heat than is necessary; and to add the oil of turpentine when the other ingredients begin to cool, and to stir till cold.—M'EWEN.

9. Corrosive sublimate 2 oz., white hellebore 3 oz., fish oil 6 quarts, rosin ½ ℔, tallow ½ ℔. The sublimate and then the hellebore to be rubbed with a portion of the oil till perfectly smooth, and then mixed with the other ingredients melted together.—STEVENSON.

10. The following once had considerable local celebrity; but it obviously requires to be used with caution. Dissolve 2¼ oz. of corrosive sublimate in the same quantity of muriatic acid, and beat up the solution with 6 ℔ of strong mercurial ointment; put it in a large pan, and pour on it 19½ ℔ of lard, and 1½ ℔ of common turpentine, melted together and still hot, and stir the whole continually until it becomes solid.

OINTMENT FOR DEEP WOUNDS OR ULCERS FROM FLIES. The fly powder No. 2, mixed with tar.—CLATER.

OINTMENT FOR SORE HEADS. Black pitch 2 ℔, tar 1 ℔, flowers of sulphur 1 ℔; melt together, taking care that it does not boil. To be spread thickly on leather while warm, and fitted to the head.

CAUSTIC ASTRINGENTS FOR FOOT ROT.

1. Blue vitriol 1 oz., white vitriol 1 oz., burnt alum 2 oz., bole ½ oz., honey to form a stiff paste.—M'Ewen.

2. Sulphate of copper 2 oz., water 12 oz., dilute sulphuric acid 2 dr.—White.

3. Butter of antimony, alone, or mixed with tincture of myrrh.

4. Verdigris, bole, and sugar of lead, in equal parts, rubbed together into a fine powder. Sprinkle on the sore, cover with tow, and bind down with tape for 24 hours, using afterwards No. 3, or No. 2.—Clater.

5. *Strong*. Verdigris 1 oz., nitrous acid 2 oz., water 4 oz.—White.

6. *Strongest*. Red precipitate 1 oz., nitrous acid 2 oz.; dissolve, and add water 2 oz., spirit of wine 1 oz. —White.

7. Aloes 16 oz., weak spirit 32 oz., sulphuric acid 17 oz.; mix.—Duville.

8. Dissolve sulphate of copper 2½ oz. in 1½ pint of water, and add a solution of 3½ dr. of sulphate of iron previously calcined. Diffuse ¾ oz. slaked lime in water, and add the mixed solution; then add 7 oz. common salt, 1 oz. wood vinegar, and water to make up a quart. [Nearly the composition of a celebrated French nostrum.]

9. Leloup's Terebinthinated Oxymel of Copper. Honey 14 oz., pyroligneous acid 7 oz., powdered verdigris 5 oz., boil it in a large copper pan until it assumes a reddish purple colour; then add, keeping the mixture on a slow fire, 14 oz. Venice turpentine; stir with a wooden spatula for ¼ of an hour, and pour it into jars. To be applied twice, at 12 hours' interval, by means of a small piece of wood, after cleaning the part with an iron blade.

10. White vinegar 78 parts, powdered sulphate of copper 10 parts; dissolve, and add 12 parts of sulphuric acid. Apply it with a feather. (A French remedy.)

11. *Detersive Ointment*. Burnt alum 4 parts, verdigris 1 part, camphor 1 part, green ointment of elder or poplar 16 parts.—Lebas.

12. Honey 4 oz., burnt alum 2 oz., Armenian bole ½ lb; mix with as much train oil as will convert these ingredients into a salve. The honey must first be completely dissolved in the oil made hot, then the bole stirred in, and lastly the alum.

BLACKLOCK condemns all caustic applications, using only mild poultices and emollient ointments.

MEDICINES FOR SWINE.

ALTERATIVE MEDICINES, in mange and other skin diseases, and obstinate costiveness.

1. Sulphur ¼ oz., Ethiop's mineral 3 gr., nitre ½ dr., cream of tartar ½ dr.; daily, in thick gruel or wash.—CLATER.

2. Black antimony ½ oz., sulphur 2 oz., nitre ½ oz.; mix; for 8 doses.

FEVER MEDICINE. Digitalis 3 gr., antimonial powder 6 gr., nitre ½ dr.; after bleeding, in a little warm swill milk, or mash, morning, noon, and night.—CLATER.

PURGING MEDICINES.

1. Epsom salts 1, 2, or 3 oz., in broth or swill.

2. Sulphur 2 dr., daily; full dose ½ oz., with milk or other food. This may be repeated for 2 or 3 days, in surfeit from overfeeding.

3. Jalap 1 dr.; if insufficient, add 10 or 12 gr. of scammony, or 10 gr. of calomel.—WHITE.

4. Jalap ½ dr., sulphur 2 dr., antimony ½ dr.

5. Jalap ½ dr., Epsom salts 1 ounce.

6. Castor oil 1 oz. to 2 oz., with gruel.

7. Castor oil 1 oz., gruel q. s., Epsom salts 2 oz., salt ¼ oz.; mix.

8. Calomel 5 gr.; but this must not be repeated more than twice.

CARMINATIVE DRENCH, for flatulent distention, from sour whey, &c. After using the probang, or where it cannot be had, give—

1. WHITE'S solution of potash (see p. 133) 2 oz., anodyne carminative tincture 1 tablespoonful, water 8 oz.

2. A tablespoonful of common salt in warm water, a teaspoonful of mustard or powdered ginger, and a glass of gin.

THRIVING POWDER, to promote fattening. Powdered fenugreek, alone, or mixed with a fourth of liquorice powder; an ounce daily with the food. Cleanliness greatly conduces to the same end.

REMEDIES FOR MEASLES. After bleeding by tail, ear, palate, or vein inside the forearm, an inch above the knee, give one of the purging drinks, and turn it into the open air.

REMEDIES FOR THE LATE PREVAILING DISTEMPER, affecting the Mouth and Feet. The same drink, and astringent powder, as for SHEEP.

DRENCH FOR INFLAMMATION OF THE BRAIN. Castor oil 2 oz., with gruel: afterwards 2 gr. white hellebore powder twice or thrice a day.—Mr. CUPISS.

HEALING OINTMENT FOR SORE EARS.

1. Lard 1 ℔, resin 4 ℔; melt together, and stir in ½ ℔ lapis calaminaris.—CLATER.

2. Zinc ointment 1 oz., yellow basilicon 3 oz.

3. Tar ointment mixed with a little soap.

MANGE OINTMENT.

1. Sulphur 4 oz., Venice turpentine 1 oz., old lard 8 oz., mercurial ointment 1 oz.; the animal to be previously scrubbed all over with a good soap lather. [The above alterative powders should be given at the same time.]

OINTMENT FOR SORE TEATS. Soft soap 4 oz. camphor (powdered with spirit) ¼ oz., mercurial ointment ½ oz. It must be carefully washed off.

MEDICINES FOR DOGS.

N. B.—The doses required vary considerably, according to the strength and size of the dog, which should always be duly considered.

PHYSIC BALLS AND OTHER PURGATIVE MEDICINES.

1. Barbadoes aloes 8 oz., antimonial powder 1 oz., ginger 1 oz., palm oil 5 oz.; beat together into a mass. Dose from ½ dr. to 2 dr., every 4 or 6 hours, till the bowels are relieved.—YOUATT.

2. The same, with the addition of 1 oz. of calomel. He directs from 45 grains to 2 dr. for a dose.—CLATER.

3. Aloes ½ dr. to 2 dr. made into a ball with syrup of ginger.

4. Aloes ½ dr. to 1½ dr., calomel 2 to 5 gr., syrup to form a ball: in inflammation of the bowels, and in worms. —BLAINE.

5. Cape aloes ½ dr. to 1 dr., calomel 2 to 3 gr., oil of caraway 6 drops, syrup to form a ball.—M'EWEN.

6. Calomel 12 gr., aloes 3 dr., opium 1 gr., syrup q. s. to form a mass, for 4, 6, or 8 balls; one every 4 or 5 hours till the bowels are relieved.—BLAINE.

7. Croton oil 1 drop, Castile soap 20 gr., conserve to form a ball.

8. Castor oil 3 parts, syrup of buckthorn 2 parts, syrup of poppies 1 part; dose from 1 to 2 tablespoonfuls.—Mr. YOUATT's purge. [Mr. Clark says syrup of buckthorn for dogs should be made with treacle, and the spices omitted.]

9. Epsom salts, from 1 to 4 dr., wrapped in tissue paper, dividing the doses into convenient sized packets.

10. In costiveness with inflammation: ½ oz. to 2 oz. castor oil.—Mr. SPOONER.

11. Jalap, powdered, 30 gr., calomel 8 gr.; make into

a pill with gum water, and administer every morning. In distemper.

ALTERATIVE BALLS AND POWDERS.

1. Sulphur 2½ ℔, nitre ½ ℔, Æthiop's mineral 4 oz., linseed meal ½ ℔, palm oil 1 ℔, or as much as may be required; beat together, and keep in a jar for use: dose, from 2 scruples to 1½ or 2 dr.—CLATER.

2. Æthiop's mineral 20 to 40 gr., cream of tartar 20 to 40 gr., nitre 5 to 10 gr.: night and morning, made into a ball with butter.—SPOONER.

3. *Tonic Alterative.* Mercurial pill 1 dr., aloes 2 dr., myrrh, benzoin, balsam of Peru, of each 1½ dr.; to be divided into 10, 15, or 20 pills: one every evening, for the yellows, after aloes and calomel.—BLAINE.

4. *Alterative Powder.* Æthiop's mineral 2 to 5 gr. cream of tartar 4 to 10 gr., tartarized iron 1 to 3 gr.: once a day.—CLATER.

5. *To give a fine skin.* Give a tablespoonful of tar, made up with oatmeal.—MAYER.

ASTRINGENT BALLS, &c.

1. Catechu 1½ dr., sulphate of quinine 20 gr., opium 3 gr., ginger 1 dr., conserve of roses q. s. to form a mass, to be divided into 8, 6, or 4 balls.—BLAINE.

2. Prepared chalk 2 oz., powdered gum Arabic ½ oz., powdered catechu ½ oz., powdered oak bark ½ oz., powdered ginger ¼ oz., opium 15 gr., palm oil 1 oz.; beat well together: dose, ½ dr. to 2 dr., morning, noon, and night, in the advanced stage of distemper.—CLATER.

3. Opium 5 gr., catechu 2 dr., gum Arabic 2 dr., ginger ½ dr., syrup of poppies q. s.; divide into 12, 9, or 6 balls: in diarrhœa.—BLAINE.

4. Myrrh 1 dr., ipecacuanha 1 scruple, opium 3 gr., chalk 2 dr., carbonate of iron 1 dr.: as No. 3.—BLAINE.

5. In obstinate cases: Alum 1 dr., chalk 2 dr., opium 6 gr., resin 3 dr.: into 4, 6, or 8 balls.

6. In diarrhœa, after 1 to 4 dr. of Epsom salts: Prepared chalk 1 to 3 scruples, catechu 5 to 10 gr., opium ¼ to 2 gr.; twice a day.—SPOONER.

7. *Astringent Drink.* Boil 1 oz. of logwood in a

quart of milk to ½ a pint. A teacupful every morning, *in prolapsus.*

COUGH BALLS, IN ASTHMA, &c.

1. *After a few emetics:* Calomel 3 gr., fox-glove 3 gr., cream of tartar 1 dr., antimonial powder 12 gr., honey to form 6 boluses. One twice a-day.—BLAINE.

2. Digitalis 20 gr., antimonial powder 40 gr., nitre 2 dr., sulphur 3 dr., palm oil 3 dr. or q. s. Divide into 10, 15, or 20 balls, according to the size of dog, morning and night, interposing an emetic every third or fourth day.—CLATER.

3. *In old cases.* P. squill ½ gr. to 1 gr., gum ammoniac 5 gr., balsam of Peru 8 gr., benzoic acid 1 gr., balsam of sulphur to form a ball.

4. Extract of hemlock ½ dr., extract of henbane 10 gr., p. digitalis 20 gr., conserve of roses to form a mass. Divide into 10, 8, or 6 balls. One night and morning. —BLAINE.

DISTEMPER MEDICINES.

1. Turpeth mineral 1 to 3 gr., assafœtida ½ dr., aloes 20 gr., soap 10 gr., syrup of poppies to form a ball. To be preceded by an emetic, and given every third day.

2. After bleeding (if required) and an emetic, give a physic ball; and afterwards the following 2 or 3 times a day: Antimonial powder 2, 3, or 4 gr.; nitre, 5, 10, or 15 gr.; ipecacuanha 2, 3, or 4 gr.; form a ball. If the disease proceed to the debilitating stage, give the *Tonic Ball* No. 2; in the putrid or malignant stage, give the *Astringent Ball* No. 1.—BLAINE.

3. After the emetic powder No. 1 (which should be repeated every 3rd or 4th day) give the *Cough Ball* No. 2, from ½ dr. to 2 dr. in weight. And if the dog loses flesh, give equal parts of the cough ball and the tonic ball (No. 1.) In the more advanced stages give the tonic alone; or the *astringent ball* if diarrhœa comes on.—CLATER.

4. Give a third of a paper of James's powder, mixed with butter, and afterwards warm broth or milk. In 2 hours another third; and if this neither vomit nor purge, give the other third at the end of 4 hours.—Mr. DANIEL.

5. BLAINE'S *Distemper Powders,* which are sold in packets, with directions for use.

6. Camphor 3 to 5 gr., charcoal 10 gr., opium 1 gr., aromatic infection q. s. to form a ball.—In the malignant stage, with diarrhœa.

7. Antimonial powder 2 to 4 gr., nitre 5 to 10 gr., digitalis 1 to 2 gr. Afterwards the tonic pills No. 4.—SPOONER.

Poudre Kusique; a French nostrum. Mix 45 gr. of nitre, 45 of sulphur, and 1 of charcoal. Divide into 3 doses. Give 1 for 2 successive mornings, and the third on the 4th morning, mixed with lard or butter, or in milk. For a large dog a second packet (of 3 powders) may be required.—HABERT.

Another French nostrum, Hemel's powder, is of a similar kind.

8. A strong solution of salt, to the amount of ½ pint daily.

9. Powdered tin, sulphur, gunpowder, of each 1 oz., lard sufficient to form a mass. The size of a nutmeg to be given twice or thrice a week.

10. Physic ball No. 11.

REMEDIES FOR SPASMODIC COLIC.

1. Castor oil ½ oz., oil of peppermint 1 drop, laudanum 20 drops. If it does not open the bowels, give ½ dr. to 1½ dr. of aloes.—BLAINE.

2. Castor oil 3 oz., syrup of buckthorn 2 oz., syrup of poppies 1 oz. Give from a teaspoonful to a tablespoonful. —YOUATT.

3. Ether ½ dr., laudanum ½ dr., camphor 3 to 6 gr., castor oil (unless he is purged) 3 to 5 dr.—BLAINE.

CONVULSIONS.

Give Colic mixture No. 3, and apply warm bath and flannel.

FOR FITS OR EPILEPSY.

1. Calomel 8 gr., carbonate of iron ½ dr., extract of hemlock 20 gr., conserve of roses, or plain oil, to form a mass for 12, 9, or 6 balls.—BLAINE.

2. Give the Alterative Balls No. 1, or the pills of nitrate of silver, as for St. Vitus' Dance.—CLATER.

3. For epilepsy of suckling bitches: Ether 1 dr., laudanum ½ dr., strong ale 2 oz.; give from a dessert spoonful to 1 or 2 table spoonfuls every 2 or 3 hours.—BLAINE.

4. For epilepsy attending distemper: The tonic balls, or the pills for chorea.—CLATER.

5. After an emetic: Gentian 10 to 20 gr., ginger 3 to 6 gr., carbonate of iron 2 to 4 gr., or from an eighth to a fourth of a gr. of nitrate of silver, and ½ gr. of spider's web once a day.—SPOONER.

6. Ether 1 dr., laudanum ½ dr., camphor 6 gr., spirit of hartshorn 1 dr.; in a spoonful of ale: for small dogs give ½ the quantity.—BLAINE.

EMETIC POWDERS.

1. Calomel, emetic tartar, of each 1 oz.; vermilion 10 gr.; rub together: dose, from 1 to 3 gr., dropped on the tongue, or mixed with a teaspoonful of milk.—CLATER.

2. Emetic tartar, from 1 to 3 gr.

3. Turpeth mineral, from 1 to 3 gr.

4. A teaspoonful of common salt.

MEDICINES FOR INFLAMMATORY DISORDERS.

1. In inflammation of the lungs: After bleeding and purging, digitalis 12 gr., emetic tartar 3 gr., nitre 1 dr.; mix, and divide into 6, 9, or 12 powders.—BLAINE.

2. Ditto, with much cough: Tincture of digitalis 1 dr., emetic tartar 3 gr., nitre 1 dr., simple oxymel 2 oz.; dose, 1 or 2 dr. every 3 hours.—BLAINE.

3. In pleurisy, with incipient water in the chest: Digitalis 6 gr., calomel 6 gr., tartarized iron 18 gr.; into 6, 9, or 12 doses.—YOUATT.

4. In inflammation of the liver: Digitalis 8 gr., antimonial powder 16 gr., nitre 1 dr.; divide into 7, 9, or 12 powders, or boluses.—BLAINE.

5. In chronic inflammation of the liver: Calomel 20 gr., antimonial powder ½ dr., myrrh, gentian, aloes, of each 2 dr.; mix, and divide into 15, 20, or 25 balls.

6. In inflammation of the bowels: After bleeding and a warm bath, give the castor oil mixture (Purgatives No. 8.)—CLATER.

7. Bilious inflammation (with offensive, often black, vomiting and purging:) Calomel 10 gr., opium 4 gr.; in 4 or 8 pills—one 3 times a day; afterwards the astringent remedies for diarrhœa.—SPOONER.

MEDICINES FOR RHEUMATISM.

1. After warm bath, and friction, give, tincture of opium 20 drops, ether 30 drops, castor oil ½ oz. to 1 oz. —BLAINE.

2. Calomel 2 to 4 gr., opium ¼ gr., oil of peppermint 1 drop, aloes 1 dr.; form a ball with butter or lard: repeat it every 4 hours till the bowels are well opened; and use the embrocation No. 3.—CLATER.

3. After warm bath, &c., give 40 drops of laudanum, and a teaspoonful of hartshorn, in warm beer; and rub with the Embrocation No. 1.—MAYER.

TONIC MEDICINES.

1. Gentian 1 oz., chamomile ½ oz., oak-bark ½ oz., ginger ¼ oz., carbonate of iron ¼ oz., palm oil 1 oz.; beat them together to form a mass; dose, 2 to 6 scruples.—CLATER.

2. Sulphate of quinine ½ dr., powdered chamomile 3 dr., balsam of Peru 1½ dr., camphor 1 scruple; form a mass with conserve of roses, and divide into 12, 9, or 6 balls; one every 6 hours, in the debilitating stage of distemper.—BLAINE.

3. Chamomile 1 oz., rue ½ oz., ginger ¼ oz., (all in powder;) beat them into a mass with 7 dr. of palm oil, and divide into 12, 16, or 20 balls; one night and morning in gutta serena.—CLATER.

4. Gentian powder 10 to 20 gr., ginger 5 gr., cascarilla 10 to 20 gr.; conserve of roses, or syrup, to form a ball. Once or twice a day.

WORM MEDICINES.

1. Carbonate of iron ½ oz., Æthiop's mineral 1 dr.,

gentian 1 oz., ginger ½ oz., levigated glass 1 oz., palm oil 9 dr.; beat well together; dose, from ¾ to 2 dr.—CLATER.

2. As much finely-powdered glass as will lie on a sixpence, mixed with butter.—BLAINE. Mr. YOUATT says from ½ dr. to 1 dr. powdered glass, with a little ginger, made into a ball with lard.

3. Aloes, sulphur, prepared hartshorn, and juice of wormwood, made into a mass; the size of a hazel nut to be given 3 times a week, fasting, wrapped in butter.—DANIEL.

4. Tin filings, or pewter filings, ½ dr., to 1 dr., with butter or lard.

5. Jalap 10 to 15 gr., calomel 2 to 3 gr., mixed with butter; no cold liquid should be allowed.—WHITE.

6. Cowhage ½ dr., iron filings 4 dr., conserve q. s. to form a mass, to be divided into 4, 6, or 8 balls; one every night and morning; and afterwards the purgative No. 4.—BLAINE.

5. Epsom salts 1 oz., common salt 1 drachm; give a small or large teaspoonful daily.

8. Give green walnut leaves boiled in milk.—MAYER.

9. *For Tape Worm.* Oil of turpentine ½ dr., mixed with yolk of egg; for very large dogs 2 scruples. Some writers prescribe larger doses (1 or 2 dr.) but these sometimes prove fatal.—BLAINE.

10. *For Tape Worm.* Oil of turpentine and olive oil, of each ½ oz.; mix, and give carefully; 3 or 4 hours after give 1 oz. castor oil. But see No. 9.—WHITE.

11. *For Stomach Worms.* Give the emetic powder (above) and afterwards a physic ball.

12. *Thread Worms.* These are destroyed by an aloetic clyster.

MEDICINES FOR THE YELLOWS.

1. After bleeding—Calomel 2 to 3 gr., jalap 10 gr., scammony 4 gr.—WHITE.

2. Aloes 20 to 40 gr., calomel 2 to 4 gr.; afterwards the tonic alterative balls.—BLAINE. See ALTERATIVES.

MEDICINES FOR ST. VITUS'S DANCE, OR CHOREA.

1. Nitrate of silver 8 gr., ginger 10 gr., syrup to form a mass; divide into 64 pills, and give one or two morning and night.—CLATER.

2. Strychnia 1 gr., oxide of zinc 24 gr., assafœtida 24 gr., conserve of roses q. s.; mix very accurately, and divide into 12, 9, or 6 balls.

3. Nitrate of silver 3 gr., carbonate of iron 2 dr., gentian 3 dr., conserve of roses to form a mass, for 12, 9, or 6 balls.—BLAINE.

MEDICINES FOR DROPSICAL COMPLAINTS.

1. Digitalis 9 gr., squill 12 gr., cream of tartar 2 dr., mix and divide into 9, 12, or 15 powders; one night and morning.

2. Fox-glove 12 gr., antimonial powder 15 gr., nitre 1 dr.; as the last.—BLAINE.

3. Fox-glove 1 gr., nitre 10 gr., ginger 8 gr.; night and morning; then iodide of potassium ½ gr. to 1 gr.—YOUATT.

BALLS FOR ENLARGED GLANDS AND CANCEROUS DISEASES.

1. Extract of hemlock 1 to 3 gr., burnt sponge 10 to 20 gr.; make a ball, to be given once or twice a day.

2. Iodine 12 gr., powdered gum 40 gr., syrup to form a stiff mass; divide into 48 pills, and give one or two night and morning.—CLATER.

BALLS TO PROMOTE PARTURITION. Ergot of rye 20 gr.; pulverize, and add ginger 16 gr., syrup q. s.: beat into a mass, and divide into 5 pills; give one every hour, or to a small bitch, half of one.—CLATER.

TO PREVENT RABIES, OR CANINE MADNESS.

1. Powdered leaves of the scutellaria lateriflora 40 gr., powdered belladonna 2½ gr.; to be given night and morning for 6 weeks, gradually increasing the dose.—YOUATT.

2. Infuse a teaspoonful and a half of powdered scutellaria in a quart of hot water; give half a pint morning

and night, omitting the dose every third day, when a mild dose of sulphur must be given.—Dr. SPALDING.

3. Fresh leaves of the tree box 2 oz., rue 2 oz., sage ½ oz., chop them fine, and boil them in a pint of water till reduced to half a pint; strain and press out the liquid; beat the herbs, and boil them in a pint of new milk to half; strain, press the herbs, and mix the liquids. For a man, give a third of this quantity every other morning fasting; double the above quantity makes 3 doses for a horse or cow; two-thirds will suffice for a middle-sized dog, and a third for smaller dogs. It produces extreme nausea and distress, and has occasionally proved fatal to dogs.—BLAINE.

External Applications.

ASTRINGENT & DETERGENT LOTIONS, for wounds, &c.

1. Bruised oak-bark 2 oz., catechu 1 oz., water 3 pints; boil to a pint, and strain.—CLATER.

2. Tincture of myrrh and aloes 1 oz., alum ½ oz., water 1 pint.

3. For sore feet: The Lotion No. 1, 4 oz., tincture of aloes ½ oz., water 1 pint.

4. Nitrate of silver 10 gr., water 1 oz.: to excite sluggish wounds.

LOTIONS FOR CANKER IN THE EAR. See OINTMENTS.

1. Sulphate of zinc 20 gr., sugar of lead ½ dr., water 4 oz.—WHITE.

2. Sulphate of zinc 20 gr., decoction of oak-bark 4 oz. —BLAINE.

3. Nitrate of silver 1 gr., rain water 2 oz.

4. Sugar of lead ½ dr., rose water 4 oz. A teaspoonful to be introduced blood-warm into the ear.

5. *Mild Canker Lotion.* Infusion of fox-glove leaves

½ pint, Goulard's extract of lead ½ oz. Mix. To be used as the last.—CLATER.

6. *Strong Canker Lotion.* Goulard's extract 2 dr., white vitriol 1 dr., alum 2 dr., water ½ pint.

7. Chloride of lime 20 to 30 gr., water ½ pint.

LOTION TO ALLAY ITCHING. Dilute hydrocyanic acid 1 dr., water a pint.—YOUATT.

OINTMENTS FOR CANKER OF THE EAR.

1. Equal parts of zinc ointment, and ointment of nitrate of quicksilver.—BLAINE.

2. Sublimate 3 gr., Turner's cerate 1 dr., sulphur a scruple.

3. White vitriol, alum, each in fine powder, a drachm; lard 4 oz. To be rubbed gently into the crack.—CLATER.

4. *Stronger.* Nitrate of silver 20 gr., lard 1 oz. Rub them well together.—CLATER.

5. Levigated red precipitate ½ oz., lard 2 oz.—MAYER.

EYE WATERS.

1. *Astringent Wash for Weak Eyes.*—White vitriol 4 gr., spirit of wine ½ dr., water 4 oz.—CLATER.

2. Sugar of lead 30 gr., rose water 6 oz.—BLAINE.

3. Laudanum ½ dr., infusion of green tea 4 oz.—M'EWEN.

4. For naturally weak eyes: Laudanum 2 dr., water 8 oz. To be used every morning.—CLATER.

5. Sugar of lead ½ dr., distilled water 6 oz., tincture of opium ½ drachm. In inflammation, after bleeding, physic, and warm fomentations.—SPOONER.

OINTMENTS FOR ULCERATED EYE-LIDS.

1. Red precipitate, levigated, 10 grains, zinc ointment ½ oz.

2. Ointment of nitrate of quicksilver 1 dr., sugar of lead 20 gr., spermaceti ointment 3 dr.—BLAINE.

3. Dissolve a drachm of quicksilver in a drachm and half of strong nitric acid, and mix the warm solution well with 6 oz. of melted lard.—CLATER.

OINTMENTS AND LOTIONS FOR THE MANGE.

N. B.—An alterative ball should be given daily, and a physic ball occasionally. Bleeding is sometimes prescribed.

1. For Scabby Mange: Sulphur 4 oz., sal ammoniac ½ oz., aloes 1 dr., Venice Turpentine ½ oz., lard 6 oz. Mix. After four applications wash well with soap and water.—Blaine.

2. Horse turpentine and palm oil, of each ½ ℔, train oil ½ pint. Melt together, and while cooling stir in 3 ℔ of flowers of sulphur.—Clater.

3. Aloes 2 dr., hellebore ½ oz., sulphur 4 oz., lard or train oil 6 oz.—M'Ewen.

4. Sulphate of zinc 1 dr., snuff ½ oz., white hellebore ½ oz., sulphur 4 oz., aloes ¼ oz., soft soap, 6 oz.—Blaine.

5. Charcoal powder 2 oz., sulphur 4 oz., salt of tartar 1 dr., Venice turpentine ½ oz., lard 6 oz.

6. For Red Mange: Add 1 oz. of strong mercurial ointment to 6 oz. of either of the above.

7. Charcoal 1 oz., chalk 1 oz., sugar of lead 1 dr., white precipitate 2 dr., sulphur 2 oz., lard 5 oz.—Blaine.

8. *Wash for Red Mange.* Sublimate 20 gr., spirit of wine 2 dr.; dissolve, and add milk of sulphur ½ oz., lime water ½ pint. Apply by means of a sponge.—Clater.

9. For Ulcerated Mange: Ointment of nitrated quicksilver 2 dr., sugar of lead 20 gr., flowers of sulphur ½ oz., lard 1 oz.; mix.—Blaine.

ARSENICAL OINTMENT. Yellow sulphuret of arsenic 1½ gr., cerate or lard ½ oz.: in mange and other skin diseases.—Delafond.

SURFEIT OINTMENT. After bleeding and purging, apply sugar of lead 1 dr., spermaceti ointment 2 oz.

OINTMENT AND POWDERS FOR PILES.

Ointment.—Sugar of lead 6 gr., tartar ½ dr., elder ointment 3 dr.—Blaine.

Powders.—Nitre ½ dr., milk of sulphur 3 dr.; mix, and divide into 9, 12, or 15 doses.—BLAINE.

HEALING OINTMENTS.

1. Palm oil 3 ℔, resin 1 ℔; melt together, and when they begin to cool, add 1 ℔ of powdered calamine.—CLATER.

2. Oxide of zinc ¼ oz., lard, 1½ oz., balsam of Peru 1 dr.

OINTMENT FOR SCIRRHOUS TUMOURS. Hydriodate of potash 1 dr., lard 7 dr.; rub together till perfectly smooth.

STIMULATING MERCURIAL OINTMENT. Mercurial ointment 1 oz., simple cerate 1 oz. A small quantity to be rubbed over the region of the liver once a day till the mouth is sore.—BLAINE.

EMBROCATIONS FOR PALSY, RHEUMATISM, &c.

1. Oil of turpentine 2 oz., spirit of hartshorn 2 oz., tincture of opium ¼ oz., olive oil 2 oz.—BLAINE.

2. Cajeput oil 1 oz., soap liniment 2 oz.

3. Spirit of turpentine, spirit of hartshorn, cam[illegible]ted spirit, of each 1 oz., laudanum ½ oz.—CLATER.

LOTIONS FOR STRAINS AND BRUISES.

1. Common salt and cold vinegar.

2. Sal ammoniac ½ oz., vinegar a pint.

3. Oil of turpentine 1 oz., old beer ½ pint, brine ½ pint. For strains.—MAYER.

4. Spirit of Mindererus 4 oz., Goulard water 8 oz.

ASTRINGENT LOTION for WOUNDS, SORE FEET, &c.—Bruised oak bark 2 oz., catechu 1 oz., water 3 pints; boil to 1 pint and strain.—CLATER.

POWDER AND LIQUID CAUSTIC FOR WARTS.

1. Equal parts of sal ammoniac and savine, powdered together.

2. Sublimate 1 dr., muriatic acid 1 dr., spirit of wine 3 dr., water 2 dr. The warts to be touched with the liquid twice a day.—YOUATT.

FLEAS.

1. Rub the skin with powdered rosin and bran.
2. Let the dog sleep on deal shavings.
3. Scotch snuff steeped in gin.—MAYER. (This requires caution.)

CLYSTERS.

Astringent. Alum whey.

Purgative. The purgative medicine No. 8, with gruel.

For Worms. Solution of aloes 2 oz., linseed oil 1 oz. Mix.

Anodyne. Boiled starch ¼ pint, laudanum 5 to 10 drops. —CLATER.

MEDICINES FOR POULTRY, RABBITS,

ETC.

FOR ROUP, POULTRY GLANDERS, AND GARGLE IN GEESE.

1. A saturated solution of common salt. Medium dose half a teaspoonful.

2. Antimonial powder 1 gr., with sopped bread, twice a day.—CLATER.

3. Garlic, rue, brick dust, and butter, beaten together, and a little crammed down the throat.

4. For wet roup in pigeons: Give 3 or 4 pepper corns in 3 or 4 days.—MOORE.

5.—For dry roup: Give 2 or 3 pills of garlic every day. [Some recommend assafœtida to be mixed with the food of Poultry, whenever they manifest disease by drooping their wings.]

FOR RUMP ROUP, OR INFLAMMATION OF THE OIL VESSEL.—Open the tumour and squeeze out the collected oil.

GAPES (OR PIP,) FROM WORMS IN THE AIR PASSAGES.

1. Pills of sulphur, turpentine, and wheat flour.—(Veterinarian, Oct., 1840.)

2. Oil of turpentine 2 dr., linseed oil 1 oz.; or oil of turpentine 2 dr., flour enough to make it into 20 pills. For 20 doses, one every other day for 3 or 4 times.

3. Tobacco smoke.

INFLAMMATION OF THE LUNGS AND ASTHMA.

Give a grain each of calomel and antimonial powder, daily.

PURGING FLUX, OR DIARRHŒA.

1. Change the diet and give whole wheat or rice; and

if obstinate, cram down small pieces of the following mass:—Chalk, p. caraway, and syrup of poppies.—CLATER.

2. Put chalk in their water, or give forge-water.

CROPSICK, OR CONSTIPATION.

If the obstruction is in the crop, endeavour to force the contents into the gullet and mouth by gentle pressure. When partially emptied give rue and butter.

When the obstruction is in the bowels, give bran and pollard, mixed with a little greasy hot liquor, to which, if necessary, a little sulphur may be added; or give a tea-spoonful of the castor oil mixture.—See CHIPPING.

PIP, OR BLAIN IN THE TONGUE.

1. Wash the mouth two or three times a day with a mixture of equal parts of tincture of myrrh and water.

2. Rub the sore with common salt.

3. Solution of chloride of soda 1 dr., water 1 oz., honey of roses 3 dr.

CANKER IN PIGEONS. Apply burnt alum, mixed with honey.

SCABS IN BREAST AND BACK OF PIGEONS. Dill seed, cummin seed, fennel seed, of each 1 ℔, assafœtida 1½ oz., bay-salt ¼ ℔, common salt ¼ ℔; knead them with fine clay and flour. Bake it in earthen pots, and set it for the birds to peck.—MOORE.

Genuine Salt-Cat.—Sifted gravel, brickmakers' earth, rubbish of old walls, of each a peck, cummin seed 1½ ℔, bay-salt ¼ ℔; mix.

FOR FILANDER WORMS IN HAWKS. Aloes, iron filings, nutmeg, and honey; mix, and give a small piece as often as necessary.

CHIPPING, IN CHICKENS. Remove the chickens to a warm place. Mix 1 oz. of castor oil with ¼ oz. syrup of ginger; mix a teaspoonful of this with a little thick gruel, and force a little down several times a day, so that it shall get ½ a teaspoonful of the mixture in the course of the day.

FOR CHILL, IN TURKEY CHICKS. Give ground malt

and barley-meal in equal quantities, adding a little powdered caraway or coriander seed.

PASTE FOR WEAK TURKEY CHICKS. Eggs boiled hard, nettles, and parsley, all chopped up, and moistened with wine or water.

MEGRIMS, OR GIDDINESS. Castor oil 1 oz., syrup of ginger $\frac{1}{4}$ oz., syrup of poppies $\frac{1}{4}$ oz.; mix with gruel, and force a little down occasionally.—CLATER.

CONVULSIONS OF DUCKS. Give to grown-up ducks 4 grains of pepper, mixed with fresh butter.

FOR BLINDNESS. Foment with warm water, then drop a few drops of the following solution into the eyes:—laudanum 1 teaspoonful, water a teacupful.

LOTION FOR WOUNDS.

1. Laudanum a few drops, added to a teacupful of water.

2. Tincture of myrrh and paregoric, each a teaspoonful, water $\frac{1}{2}$ a pint.

TO PROMOTE THE LAYING OF EGGS. A little sulphate of soda, placed within reach of the hens, is said to be useful. Warmth, good feeding, with a little chopped meat in winter, are also recommended. To prevent their laying soft eggs, supply them with old mortar, bruised egg-shells, or chalk.

FUNGUS, OR PROUD FLESH, FROM WOUNDS IN THE HEAD. Burnt alum 2 dr., honey 1 oz.; mix, and apply twice a day.

VERMIN, TO DESTROY. Tobacco smoke, with good food and cleanliness.

MOULTING. It is usual to put saffron into the water of cage birds when moulting; others recommend a rusty nail.

FOR SNIFFLES IN RABBITS. Sulphate of copper 1 to 2 gr., morning and evening, in bran.—CLATER.

FOR ROT, OR POT BELLY. Give them young green broom and bread well toasted.—MAYER.

Patent and Proprietary Medicines,

DRUGGISTS' NOSTRUMS,

ETC.

THIS division consists of those *medicinal compounds* which are excluded from the Pocket Formulary, as belonging rather to empirical than regular practice. It includes, in addition to those secret and patent remedies which are usually termed QUACK MEDICINES, preparations of various drugs made according to private formulæ; some favourite domestic remedies; and a few compounds, which, though not empirical, are better known by the names of individual practitioners than by any other title. The supposed composition of some of the secret remedies is given on the authority of Dr. PARIS, the Philadelphia College of Pharmacy, and others; but without vouching for their correctness.

ABERNETHY'S PILLS. The nostrum to which this distinguished surgeon's name has been applied is said to consist of 2 gr. of blue pill, and 3 of compound extract of colocynth.

AGUE DROPS (tasteless.) A solution of arsenic, probably similar to the *liquor potassæ arsenitis* of the Pharmacopœia.

ANDERSON'S PILLS. See Pilulæ Andersonis, P. F. Other published formulæ are—

1. Barbadoes aloes 1 oz., jalap ¼ oz., soap 1 dr., oil of aniseed ½ dr., tincture of aloes q. s.; mix, and divide into 4-grain pills.

2. Barbadoes aloes 5 oz., water 1 oz.; soften by the heat of a water-bath, and add powdered jalap, powdered aniseed, and ivory black, of each 1 oz., oil of aniseed 1 dr.

3. Barbadoes aloes 16 oz., black hellebore, jalap, subcarbonate of potash, of each 1 oz., oil of aniseed ½ oz., syrup of buckthorn q. s. to form a mass. To be divided into 4-grain pills.

4. Barbadoes aloes 24 oz., soap 4 oz., colocynth 1 oz., gamboge 1 oz., oil of aniseed ½ fluid oz.,; mix, and divide into pills of 3 gr. each. Phila. Coll. of Pharmacy.

ANODYNE NECKLACES. Beads formed of the root of henbane, and used as necklaces, to allay the pain of teething.

ANTIPERTUSSIS. Dr. PARIS states that the basis of this nostrum is a salt of zinc.

ARQUEBUSADE (acid.) 1. Sulphuric acid ½ ℔, vinegar and spirit of wine, of each 3 ℔, clarified honey 1 ℔.—SWEDIAUR.

2. Distilled vinegar, and rectified spirit, of each 10 oz., sulphuric acid, (by weight,) 1½ oz., sugar 2½ oz; mix. For the aromatic spirituous arquebusade water, see Arquebusade Water, under PERFUMERY; also Spiritus Vulnerarius, P. F.

AROMATIC VINEGAR. Strongest acetic acid 1 ℔, camphor 1 oz.; dissolve, and add 1 oz. each of oil of lavender, oil of cloves, and oil of lemon.

APERIENT AND ANTIBILIOUS PILLS. See ANDERSON'S, BAILLIE'S, BARCLAY'S, DIXON'S, &c. Pills. The following are useful forms—

1. Compound extract of colocynth 60 gr., comp. rhubarb pill 30 gr., soap 10 gr. In 24 pills.

2. Compound extract of colocynth 2 dr., extract of rhubarb ½ dr., compound soap pill 10 gr.; mix, and divide into 40 pills; 1, 2, or 3 for a dose.

3. Compound extract of colocynth 8 oz., soap 1 oz., scammony 2 oz., extract of rhubarb 2 oz., oil of cassia 5 dr., spirit q. s. to form a mass. Divide into 4-grain pills.

4. Blue pill, compound extract of colocynth, of each a scruple; scammony, and Castile soap, of each 10 gr., oil of caraway 4 drops. Mix, and divide into 15 pills—3 at bed-time.—Sir B. BRODIE.

5. Compound extract of colocynth 4 scruples, scam-

mony a scruple, extract of rhubarb 12 gr., soap 6 gr., oil of cinnamon 4 drops. Mix, and divide into 24 pills. —Mr. VANCE.

6. Mr. VANCE'S *Stronger Pills, with Calomel.* Compound extract of colocynth 4 scruples, scammony 2 scruples, calomel 24 gr., oil of cinnamon 6 drops, in 24 pills. —1 or 2 at bed-time.

7. Compound extract of colocynth 1 dr., calomel 15 gr., emetic tartar 1 gr., oil of cassia 5 drops. In 24 pills.—Dr. J. JOHNSON.

8. Scammony 10 to 15 gr., compound extract of colocynth 2 scruples, extract of rhubarb ½ dr., soap 10 gr., oil of caraway 5 drops. In 20 pills. One or two when required.—Sir C. SCUDAMORE.

9. Compound rhubarb pill ½ dr., ipecacuanha 6 gr., compound extract of colocynth 20 gr. In 12 pills. One or more at bed-time occasionally.—Dr. BARON.

10. The same as Pil. Coloc. et Hyoscyami, Ed. Ph. —Dr. HAMILTON.

11. (Strong.) Compound extract of colocynth 2 dr., aloes and myrrh pill 2 dr., calomel 1 dr.; mix, and divide into 40 pills. Two for a dose.—Dr. LYNN.

12. Compound extract of colocynth 2 scruples, ipecacuanha 6 gr., soap 10 gr., extract of henbane 30 gr. In 18 pills. Two at bed-time.—Dr. COPLAND.

13. Dr. NELIGAN'S *Purgative Pills for general use.* Comp. colocynth pill, and soap of jalap, of each 1 dr. In 24 pills. Two when required.

14. (Without aloes.) Simple extract of colocynth 24 gr., extract of jalap 12 gr., blue pill 12 gr., ipecacuanha 4 gr., oil of peppermint 3 drops. In 12 pills.

Other formulæ will be found in the P. F. See Pilulæ Colocynthidis; Pil. Coloc. c. Oleo Crotonis; Pil. Catharticæ; Pil. Jalapæ; Pil. Purgantes; &c. Those which do not contain calomel should be preferred for general and repeated use.

ATKINSON'S INFANT PRESERVATIVE. Carbonate of magnesia 6 dr., white sugar 2 oz., oil of aniseed 20 drops, spirit of sal volatile 2½ dr., laudanum 1 dr., syrup of saffron 1 oz., caraway water to make a pint.

Bacher's Tonic Pills. Alkaline extract of black hellebore 2 dr., extract of myrrh 2 dr., powder of holy thistle 1 dr.; mix, and divide into 4-grain pills.

Dr. Baillie's Pills. Compound extract of colocynth 1½ dr., extract of aloes 1½ dr., Castile soap ½ dr., oil of cloves 15 drops: in 38 pills.—3 at bed-time occasionally.

Dr. Baillie's Dinner Pills. Aloes 20 gr., ginger ½ dr., ipecacuanha 8 gr., syrup q. s. Mix, and divide into 16 pills. One daily, before dinner.

Bailey's Itch Ointment. Olive oil 1 ℔, suet 1 ℔, alkanet root 2 oz. Melt, and macerate until coloured; then strain, and add 3 oz. each of alum, nitre, and sulphate of zinc, in very fine powder; adding vermilion to colour it, and oil of aniseed, lavender, and thyme to perfume.

Baking Powder. Tartaric acid 8 oz., bicarbonate of soda 9 oz., arrow root, or rice flour, 10 oz. Mix. Delfort's is said to consist of alum 5 oz., bicarbonate of soda 2¾ oz., bicarbonate of ammonia ½ oz., arrow root 4 oz.

Balm of Gilead (factitious.) 4 oz. of gum benzoin may be dissolved by heat in 1 ℔ of Canada balsam, and to the mixture, when cold, ¼ oz. each of the oils of rosemary, lemons, and cassia, added.

Balm of Rakasiri. Oil of Rosemary dissolved in common gin.

Balsam. See Ford's, Hill's, Friar's, &c.

Barclay's (Rev. D.) Antibilious Pills. Extract of colocynth 2 dr., soap of jalap 2½ dr., extract of guaiacum wood 3 dr., emetic tartar 8 gr., oils of juniper, caraway and rosemary, each 4 drops; into 4-grain pills.

Baregian Balls. Extract of soap-wort (or of artichoke leaves) 3 oz., gelatine 1½ oz., water 3 oz.; heat together till dissolved, pour the solution into a warm iron mortar; add 6 oz. of sulphuret of lime, and 1 oz. of salt, previously powdered and mixed. Stir constantly till a mass is obtained, and divide it into balls of 2¼ oz. each. Use one for a general bath, half of one for a foot bath.

Bark, Essential Salt of. See Extractum Cinchonæ Siccum, P. F.

Barker's Tooth Tincture. An alcoholic solution of pyrethrum, coloured with tincture of red cabbage.

BATEMAN'S PECTORAL DROPS. 1. Compound spirit of aniseed 16 fluid ounces, opium 1 dr., camphor 1 dr., oil of fennel 20 drops, cochineal 2 dr.

2. Proof spirit 4 gal., red sanders 2 oz., digest 24 hours, filter, and add powdered opium 2 oz., camphor 2 oz., catechu 2 oz., oil of aniseed 4 fluid drachms; digest for 10 days. *Philadelphia College of Pharmacy.* The old wine gallon is here intended.

BATEMAN'S ITCH OINTMENT. Carbonate of potash ½ oz., rose-water 1 oz., vermilion 1 dr., sulphur 11 oz., oil of bergamot ½ dr., lard 11 oz.; mix.

BATES' ANODYNE BALSAM. Soap liniment 2 parts, tincture of opium 1 part.

BATES' CAMPHORATED EYE-WATER. Sulphate of copper 15 gr., French bole 15 gr., camphor 4 gr., boiling water 4 oz.; infuse, strain, and dilute with 4 pints of cold water.

BATES' STYPTIC WASH. See Liquor Aluminis Co., P. F.

BATHING SPIRITS. These resemble liquid opodeldoc (soap liniment,) and are usually coloured by the addition of some dark tincture. See FREEMAN'S Bathing Spirits.

BATH DIGESTIVE PILLS. Rhubarb 2 oz., ipecacuanha ½ oz., cayenne pepper ¼ oz., soap ½ oz., ginger ¼ oz., gamboge ¼ oz.; mix, and divide into 4-grain pills.

BATH LOZENGES (in imitation of Dawson's.) Pure extract of liquorice 1 oz., powdered gum Arabic 1 oz., white sugar 1 ℔, hot water q. s. to form a mass; to be rolled into pipes.

BATTLEY'S LIQUOR CINCHONÆ and LIQUOR OPII. See Pocket Formulary.

BATTLEY'S SENNA POWDER. Senna leaves heated until they become light in colour, reduced to powder, and mixed with some finely powdered charcoal.

BAUME DE VIE. Socotrine aloes 2 dr., rhubarb 6 dr., saffron 2 dr., liquorice-root 1 oz., proof spirit 8 oz.; digest for 8 days, and filter. The original Swedish form is this:—aloes 9 dr., rhubarb, gentian, zedoary, saffron, theriaca, agaric, of each a drachm, proof spirit 2 pints.

BAYNTON'S PLASTER. Simple litharge plaster 16 oz., yellow resin 6 dr.; melt together, and spread on linen or calico.

BEDDOE'S PILLS; for Gravel, &c. Carbonate of soda, dried without heat, 1 dr., soap 4 scruples, oil of juniper 10 drops, syrup of ginger q. s. for 30 pills.

BEETLE WAFERS. Red lead, sugar, and flour; made in wafer-irons.

BELLOSTE'S PILLS. Quicksilver, scammony, and jalap, of each 1 ℔, sugar 4 oz., mixed and made up into a mass with sherry wine.

BESTUCHEFF'S NERVOUS TINCTURE. A mixture of a strong solution of perchloride of iron with sulphuric ether and spirit, exposed in long bottles to the rays of the sun until it has quite lost its brown colour.

BETTON'S BRITISH OIL. Oil of turpentine 8 oz., Barbadoes tar 4 oz., oil of rosemary 4 dr.; mix. See British Oils.

BEWLEY & EVANS' CHALYBEATE WATER. Citrate of iron 13 grains; carbonated water 6 oz., syrup of orange-peel 1 oz.

BISCUITS, APERIENT. An ounce of powdered jalap, mixed with 16 ounces of the materials for gingerbread, or other kind of cake. See Gingerbread, purgative.

BLACK DROP (Lancashire.) Fine opium, cut small, 8 oz., verjuice 48 fluid oz., nutmegs grated 1½ oz., saffron ¼ oz., boil together until the opium is dissolved; add sugar 4 oz., yeast 2 tablespoonfuls. Keep it near the fire for 6 or 8 weeks, then place it in the open air till it becomes a syrup; decant and filter.

BLACK DRAUGHT. 1. Infusion of senna 10 dr., sulphate of magnesia 3 dr., syrup of ginger 1 dr., aromatic spirit of ammonia 20 drops.

2. Tartrate of potash 1½ dr., manna ½ dr., tincture of jalap ½ dr., aromatic spirit of ammonia 20 drops, extract of liquorice 4 gr., infusion of senna 11 dr. See Mistura Sennæ Comp., Haustus Sennæ, and Mistura Aperiens, in Pocket Formulary, for other formulæ.

BLAINE'S DISTEMPER POWDERS. The basis of these is said to be aurum musivum (sulphuret of tin.)

BLISTERING TISSUE. *Taffetas Vesicant.* Powdered cantharides is exhausted by ether, the tincture distilled to recover the principal part of the ether for the same use, and the residue heated in a water-bath till it ceases to boil. The green butyraceous oil which remains is to be melted with twice its weight of wax, and spread on waxed silk, or any convenient or adhesive material. An extract prepared by evaporating a tincture made with 4 parts of flies, one of strong acetic acid, and 16 of rectified spirit, is used for the same purpose.

BOCHET'S SYRUP, *for scrofulous affections.* Compound syrup of sarsaparilla, with senna, and 1 per cent. of iodide of potassium.

BRANDISH'S ALKALINE SOLUTION, OR CAUSTIC ALKALI. American pearl ashes 6 ℔, quick lime 2 ℔, wood ashes prepared by burning the branches of the ash 2 ℔, boiling water 6 old gallons (5 imp.;) slake the lime, add the rest of the water and the pearl ashes, and lastly stir in the wood ashes; let it stand in a covered vessel for 24 hours, and decant. To each pint add one drop of true oil of juniper berries. Keep it in stoppered bottles of green glass.

BRANDISH'S ALKALINE TINCTURE OF RHUBARB. Coarsely powdered rhubarb 1 oz., alkaline solution (BRANDISH'S) 32 fluid ounces. The original formula directs only ½ oz. rhubarb, but as smaller doses than were given by Mr. B. are now usually prescribed, the quantity of rhubarb is here increased. Or an alkaline infusion of rhubarb may be made by pouring boiling water 48 parts on rhubarb 3 parts, and carbonate of potash 1 part.

BRITISH HERB TOBACCO. The principal ingredient in this compound is dried coltsfoot leaves, to which a smaller portion of thyme, wood-betony, eye-bright, and rosemary, are added.

BRITISH OILS. Oil of turpentine, and linseed oil, of each 8 oz.; oil of amber, and oil of juniper, of each 4 oz.; true Barbadoes tar 3 oz.; American petroleum (seneca oil) 1 oz.; mix. See BETTON'S BRITISH OILS, above.

BRODUM'S NERVOUS CORDIAL. Iron wine, compound spirits of lavender, tinctures of calumba, gentian, cinchona, and cardamoms,—equal parts of each.

BROCCHIERI'S STYPTIC WATER. Pieces of fresh pine, bruised in a mortar, are distilled with twice their weight of water, till half the water has come over. After standing in a wide vessel, any floating oil is to be removed from the surface, and the water kept for use.

BURNETT'S (SIR WILLIAM) DISINFECTING FLUID. A neutral solution of zinc in commercial muriatic acid.

CACHOU AROMATISE. See PERFUMERY.

CAJEPUT LINIMENT. Soap liniment 7 oz., camphor ½ oz., oil of cajeput 1 oz.

CAMPHOR LINIMENT, EXTEMPORANEOUS. Rectified spirit 17 fluid ounces, strong water of ammonia 2½ oz., camphor 2 oz., oil of lavender 50 minims.

CARRON OIL. Lime water, and linseed oil, equal quantities.

CASTILLON'S POWDERS. Sago meal, salep, tragacanth, each 1 dr.; prepared oyster-shells a scruple; coloured with cochineal. A drachm to be boiled with milk, in bowel complaints.

CEPHALIC SNUFF. Dried asarabacca leaves 3 parts, marjoram 1 part, lavender flowers 1 part; rub together to a powder. BOELI'S consists of 2 dr. valerian, 2 dr. of snuff, 3 drops of oil of lavender, 3 drops of oil of marjoram; mix. This is said to relieve the eyes as well as the head.

CHAMBERLAINE'S PILLS. Common milk of sulphur, and vermilion. Dr. PARIS' statement that they contain sulphate of lime would probably surprise the proprietor, if not aware that a great part of the commercial milk of sulphur contains half its weight of that substance.

CHAMOMILE DROPS. Dr. PARIS states that the nostrum sold under this name is merely spirit flavoured with essential oil of chamomile. A strong tincture of the flowers would probably be more efficacious.

CHAMOMILE PILLS. We are not aware of the composition of NORTON'S chamomile pills. The following is a good form: watery extract of aloes 12 gr., extract of chamomile 36 gr., oil of chamomile 3 drops; make 12 pills. Two every night, or twice a day.

CHELSEA PENSIONER. Powdered rhubarb 2 dr., cream of tartar 1 oz., guaiacum 1 dr., sulphur 2 oz., 1 nutmeg grated fine, clarified honey 16 oz.; mix: take 2 spoonfuls night and morning: for chronic rheumatism, &c.

CHELTENHAM SALTS (factitious.) Sulphate of soda 16 oz.,

sulphate of magnesia 8 oz., muriate of soda 1 oz., sulphate of iron 8 gr.; dissolve in the smallest quantity of hot water, strain, and evaporate to dryness by a gentle heat; or dry the salts separately, and mix.

CHILBLAINS, Popular Remedies for. 1. Soap liniment 1 oz., cajeput oil ¼ oz., tincture of cantharides ¼ oz.; mix.

2. Sal ammoniac ½ oz., vinegar 5 oz., spirit of rosemary 1 oz.; mix.

3. Oil of turpentine 1 oz., camphor ¼ oz., Goulard's extract ¼ oz.; mix.

4. Dr. GRAVES'S *Preventive.* Sulphate of copper 10 gr., water 1 oz.; dissolve, brush over the parts with the lotion by means of a camel-hair pencil, and when dry apply a little simple ointment: repeat this for some evenings in succession.

5. LEJEUNE'S *Balsam.* Camphor 1½ dr., tincture of benzoin 1 oz., iodide of potassium 3 dr., extract of lead 2 oz., a mixture of equal parts of rectified spirit and rose water 4 oz.; mix the above with a solution of 2 oz. of soap in 4 oz. of the same diluted spirit; mix the whole, adding a few drops of any essential oil.

6. Sal enixum, alum, and sulphate of zinc, of each ¼ oz., water a pint; apply it frequently.

7. Muriatic acid ½ oz., Friar's balsam 3½ oz.; mix.

8. SWEDIAUR'S *Paste.* Bitter almonds 8 oz., honey 6 oz., powdered camphor ½ oz., flour of mustard ½ oz., burnt alum ¼ oz., olibanum ¼ oz., yelks of 3 eggs; beat together to form a paste; rub a portion of it on the part affected, moistened with water, night and morning, then wash with warm water, and dry with a cloth.

9. WAHLER'S *Ointment for Broken Chilblains.* Black oxide of iron, bole, and oil of turpentine, of each 1 dr.; rub together, and add the mixture to 1 oz. of melted resin cerate.

10. *Another ointment for the same:* Locatelli balsam 1 oz., citrine ointment ¼ oz., balsam of Peru 20 drops; mix.

11. *Russian remedy.* Dry the peelings of cucumbers, and when required for use soften the inner part with water, and apply it to the part affected.

CHING'S WORM LOZENGES. The yellow lozenges contain 1 gr. of calomel in each with sugar, and sufficient mucilage (coloured with saffron) to form a paste. The brown contain ½ gr. of calomel, with 3½ gr. of resinous extract of jalap, according to GRAY; or with 1 gr. of resin of jalap, according to Dr. PARIS and others.

CHOLERA MEDICINES. The following are some of the more popular remedies that have been used during the visitations of this disease.

1. *Liverpool Preventive Powders*. Bicarbonate of soda 1 scruple, ginger 8 gr.; to be taken in a glass of water after breakfast and supper. These powders are said to have been used with good effect among the workmen in the mining and manufacturing districts, during a former visitation of cholera.

2. Dr. STEVENS' *Saline Powders*. Bicarbonate of soda ½ drachm, muriate of soda a scruple, chlorate of potash 7 gr.; mix, for 1 dose.

3. Mr. HOPE'S *remedy*. Nitrous acid (red) 2 dr., peppermint water or camphor mixture 1 oz., tincture of opium 40 minims; dose 1 to 2 teaspoonfuls in a cupful of gruel every 3 or 4 hours.

4. Spirit of wine 1 oz., spirit of lavender ¼ oz., oil of origanum ¼ oz., compound tincture of benzoin ½ oz., spirit of camphor ¼ oz.; twenty drops on moist sugar. To be rubbed outwardly also.

5. *American remedy*. Equal parts of lard, maple-sugar, and charcoal, to be mixed, and the size of a nut swallowed.

6. Remedies recommended by the Board of Health, in premonitory diarrhœa: Chalk mixture 1 oz., aromatic confection 10 to 15 gr., tincture of opium 5 to 15 drops: to be repeated every 3 or 4 hours, or oftener if the attack be severe, until the looseness is stopped.

7. Dr. GRAVES' *Astringent Pills*. Acetate of lead 20 gr., opium 1 gr.: in 12 pills. One every ½ hour till the watery discharges cease.

8. Mr. BUXTON'S *remedy*. Twenty-five minims of diluted sulphuric acid in an ounce of water.

We have inserted the above, not to encourage quackery in reference to this terrible disease, but because the druggist may be called upon to supply these remedies, and expected to know their composition. For Elixir Woroneje, see P. F.

CHIRAYTA PILLS AND MIXTURE. Dr. REECE'S *Pills*. Extract of chirayta 2 dr., dried soda 20 gr., ginger 15 gr., mix, and divide into 36 pills. Two twice a day. *Mixture:* Infusion of chirayta 8 oz., subcarbonate of soda a dr.; two tablespoonfuls 3 times a day.

CLUTTON'S FEBRIFUGE SPIRIT AND TINCTURE. *Spirit:* The original formula is—oil of sulphur by the bell, oil of vitriol, and sea salt, of each 1 oz.; rectified spirit 3 oz.; mix, digest for a month; and distil to dryness. *Tincture:* Febrifuge spirit 8 fluid ounces; angelica root, serpentary, cardamom seed, of each 1½ dr.; digest, and strain. Water acidulated with these and sweetened to the taste, forms a cooling diuretic and diaphoretic julep. Though never admitted into the pharmacopœias, these preparations are favourites with a few practitioners.

COCHRANE'S COUGH MEDICINE. An acidulated syrup of poppies.

COLLIER'S (Dr.) WINE OF QUININE. Disulphate of quinine 18 gr., citric acid 15 gr., sound orange wine 1 bottle, or 24 fluid ounces.

COLLIER'S (Dr.) CREAM OF TARAXACUM. See Cremor Taraxaci, P. F.

COLLINS' DISINFECTING POWDER. See Disinfecting Compounds, among the Trade Chemicals.

CONSUMPTION, *Popular remedies for.* 1. Rum ½ pint, linseed oil, honey, garlic (beaten to a pulp,) and loaf sugar, of each 4 oz., yelks of 5 eggs; mix: a teaspoonful night and morning.

2. *Breastplate.* Dissolve 1 oz. aloes in 12 oz. of a strong decoction of fresh rue; fold a large piece of soft muslin in 8 folds, large enough to cover the chest and part of the stomach; steep it in the solution and dry it in the shade: wear it on the chest constantly.

COUGH LINCTUS. 1. *Rose Linctus.* Confection of roses 3 oz., paregoric elixir 1½ oz., diluted sulphuric acid 1 dr. and a half; mix: a teaspoonful now and then when the cough is troublesome.

2. Dr. LATHAM'S *Cough Linctus.* DOVER'S powder

½ dr., compound powder of tragacanth 2 dr., syrup of tolu ½ oz., confection of hips, and simple oxymel, of each 1 oz.; a teaspoonful 3 or 4 times a day. For other Formulæ, see Linctus; Linctus Oleosus; Linctus Pectoralis, &c.; P. F.

COUGH LOZENGES. See Bath Lozenges, above; also Lozenges, below.

CORN PLASTERS. See KENNEDY'S Corn Plaster,—and Emplastrum Æruginis, Pocket Formulary. Most of the advertised corn plasters contain verdigris. A few additional formulæ are subjoined.

1. Galbanum plaster 1 oz., prepared verdigris 1 scr.; melt, and mix.

2. Galbanum 1 oz., black pitch ½ oz., simple diachylon ¼ oz., verdigris a scruple, sal ammoniac a scruple. Melt together the first three, and add the last two in fine powder.

3. Plaster of ammoniacum with quicksilver 1½ oz., soap plaster ½ oz., opium in fine powder ½ dr.

MECHANICAL CORN PLASTERS. Any suitable adhesive plaster is spread on soft thick leather (buckskin,) which is afterwards cut to a suitable size, and a hole punched in the centre. They are sometimes spread on amadou, or on vulcanized Indian rubber.

CORN SOLVENTS. One of the preparations sold under this name is probably a strong solution of subcarbonate of potash. A powder sold for the same purpose consists of subcarbonate of potash coloured with ochre or bole. A pinch is placed on the corn, and confined by means of a piece of adhesive plaster or rag. Sir Humphry Davy's name has been given to a remedy which consists of subcarbonate of potash and salt of sorrel, similarly applied. The following is one of the advertised Corn and Bunion remedies:—Subcarbonate of soda 1 oz., finely powdered and mixed with ½ oz. of Lard. Applied on linen rag every night: the outer skin to be pared off every 2 or 3 days. It may be varied thus:—Dried soda 4 dr., powder blue (smalts) a scruple, lard 4 dr.; mix.

CAUSTIC FOR CORNS. Tincture of iodine 4 dr., iodide of iron 12 gr., chloride of antimony 4 dr.; mix, and apply with a camel-hair brush, after paring the corn. It is said to cure in 3 times.

COURT PLASTER is made by repeatedly brushing over stretched sarcenet with a solution of 1 part of isinglass in 8 of water, mixed with 8 parts of proof spirit, and finishing with a coat of tincture of benzoin, or of balsam of Peru. See Miscellaneous Preparations.

CUSTARD POWDER. See Dietetic Articles.

DAFFY'S ELIXIR. This is similar to the compound tincture of senna: but different makers have their peculiar formulæ. The following are some of them. Avoirdupois weight seems to be intended.

1. Senna leaves 3¾ ℔, jalap, aniseed, caraway seed, of each 20 oz., rectified spirit 18 pints, sugar 5 ℔. Infuse the senna 2 or 3 times in sufficient boiling water to yield, when strained with pressure, 4 gallons in the whole. Add to this the tincture made with jalap and seeds, digested with the spirit for a week. Pour off the clear liquor, and add the sugar, and brandy colouring if required.

2. DICEY'S, according to GRAY. Senna 5 oz., guaiacum shavings, (some recipes add red sanders,) dried elecampane root, seed of anise, coriander, and caraway, and root of liquorice, of each 2½ oz., stoned raisins 8 oz., proof spirit 6 ℔.

3. SWINTON'S. Jalap 3 ℔, senna 12 oz., coriander seed, aniseed, liquorice root, and elecampane, of each 4 oz.; spirit of wine and water, of each a gallon.

4. Small senna 10 oz., bruised jalap, coriander seed, and aniseed, of each 2½ oz.; proof spirit a gallon. Digest 8 days, frequently shaking, and strain. Pour on the remaining ingredients 6 oz. of boiling water in which 2 dr. of salt of tartar have been dissolved; press strongly, and add the liquid to the tincture, with 3 oz. of treacle. Some recipes add rhubarb, in the proportion of about 4 oz. to the gallon.

DALBY'S CARMINATIVE. 1. Carbonate of magnesia 1 oz., syrup of poppies 5 oz., tincture of wood-soot 1 oz., oil of caraway 25 drops, oil of peppermint 16 drops, water and spirit of wine, each ½ oz. Mix.

2. Carbonate of magnesia 2 scruples, oil of pepper-

mint 1 drop, oil of nutmeg 2 drops, oil of aniseed 3 drops, tincture of castor 30 drops, tincture of assafœtida 15 drops, tincture of opium 5 drops, spirit of pennyroyal 15 drops, compound tincture of cardamom 30 drops, peppermint water 2 oz. Mix.—Dr. PARIS.

DANDELION COFFEE. The roots, collected at the end of the year, are dried at a gentle heat and reduced to powder. Some mix coffee with it. Others *roast* the root in the manner of coffee, but probably at the expense of its medical virtues. The better way is to dry and powder it, and direct it to be mixed with coffee when used. If considered necessary to give it more colour and flavour, it may be previously mixed with a sufficient quantity of roasted chicory, which should not exceed one-eighth of the whole.

DARCET'S ALKALINE LOZENGES, OR VICHY LOZENGES. Bicarbonate of soda 2 dr., refined sugar 14 oz., oil of peppermint 4 drops, mucilage of tragacanth q. s. Mix, and divide into 60 lozenges.

DAWSON'S LOZENGES. See BATH LOZENGES, above.

DELAMOTT'S GOLDEN DROPS. Muriate of iron 1 oz., spirit of sulphuric ether 7 oz.; dissolve and expose to sunshine in a closely-stopped bottle till it becomes divested of colour. See BESTUCHEFF'S Nervous Tincture.

DERBYSHIRE'S PATENT EMBROCATION FOR PREVENTING SEA SICKNESS. Boil 2 oz. of opium, 2 dr. of extract of henbane, 10 gr. of mace, and 2 oz. of mottled soap, in 3 pints of water for ½ hour. When cold add 1 quart of rectified spirit, and 3 dr. of spirit of ammonia.

DESHLER'S SALVE. This is merely resin cerate.

DIGESTIVE PILLS. See BATH DIGESTIVE PILLS, DINNER PILLS, BAILLIE'S PILLS, Lady WEBSTER'S PILLS, Dr. REECE'S CHIRAYTA PILLS.

DINNER PILLS. See BATH DIGESTIVE PILLS, Lady WEBSTER'S Pills, &c. The following are a few additional formulæ:—

1. Rhubarb 30 gr., aloes 60 gr., ipecacuanha 12 gr., tincture of ginger q. s. to form a mass; to be divided into 24 pills.

2. Sir CHARLES BELL'S. Rhubarb 50 gr., mastic 6 gr., sulphate of quinine 4 gr.; in 12 pills.

DIXON'S ANTIBILIOUS PILLS. Equal parts of aloes, scammony, and rhubarb, with the addition of a small quantity of tartar emetic, and made up with Castile soap.

DOVER'S POWDERS. The pulvis ipecacuanhæ compositus of the pharmacopœia. But the original powder consisted of nitre and sulphate of potash, each 4 oz., fused in a red-hot mortar, and afterwards reduced to powder, and mixed with 1 oz. each of ipecacuanha, opium, and liquorice.

DUPUYTREN'S POMMADE. See HAIR COSMETICS.

DUPUYTREN'S EYE SALVE. Nitric oxide of mercury 10 gr., sulphate of zinc 20 gr., lard 2 oz.; rub perfectly smooth.

DUNCAN'S FLUID EXTRACT OF SENNA. See Extractum Sennæ Fluidum, Pocket Formulary.

DR. DUNCAN'S LACTUCARIUM LOZENGES. As the Trochisci Opii (Pocket Formulary,) substituting lactucarium for opium.

DUNCAN'S GOUT REMEDY. A preparation of colchicum, with opium, &c.

DUTCH (or HAERLEM) DROPS. The basis of this popular remedy is said to be the residue which is left in redistilling oil of turpentine. The following is one of the imitations of it made in this country: Linseed oil 1 quart, rosin 2 ℔, sulphur 1 ℔; boil together over a slow fire; when combined remove from the fire, and add 1 pint of oil of turpentine and 50 drops of liquor of ammonia; stir well together, and bottle.

EATON'S STYPTIC. It is similar to that of HELVETIUS, which see below.

EAU DE MAGNANIMITE. A tincture of ants, with aromatics.

EAU MEDICINALE D'HUSSON. It is prepared, according to Dr. Williams, from the juice of colchicum flower with half the quantity of brandy; mix, and after standing a few days, decant into small bottles. But it was more probably made from the root, as prescribed in the following formulæ.—(In one of the French codices.) *Eau Colchique d'Husson.* Dry colchicum 60 parts, in sherry 125 parts. 20 drops for a dose. (According to Mr. Want.)—4 oz. of the fresh root sliced, macerated in ½ a pint of proof spirit.

EAU DE COLOGNE, EAU DE MELISSE, &c. See PERFUMERY.

EAU DE JAVELLE. Dry Chloride of lime 2 oz., carbonate of potash 4 oz., water 2 pints: mix the chloride with 1½ pint of water, dissolve the potash in the remainder; mix the solutions, and filter.

EAU DE LUCE. See PERFUMERY.

EAU DE RABEL. See Acidum Sulphuricum Alcoholisatum, Pocket Formulary.

EDINBURGH OINTMENT. White hellebore powder, sal ammoniac, and lard.

ELLERMAN'S DEODORIZING FLUID. It consists chiefly of persalts of iron. See DISINFECTING COMPOUNDS.

ELIXIR DE GARUS. See Pocket Formulary.

ELIXIR LONGÆ VITÆ. Similar to BAUME DE VIE, above.

ELIXIR OF HALLER. See Elixir Acidum Halleri, Pocket Formulary.

ELIXIR PAREGORIC. See Tinctura Camphoræ Composita, Pocket Formulary.

ELIXIR OF VITRIOL. (Mynsicht's Elixir.) See Acidum Sulphuricum Aromaticum, Pocket Formulary. For common sale druggists frequently keep a more ready and economical preparation, of which the following is one form;—Compound tincture of cardamoms 1 ℔, tincture of cinnamon 3 ℔, cinnamon water 2 ℔; mix, and add gradually 1½ ℔ of pure sulphuric acid.

ERVALENTA; and REVALENTA. See DIETETIC COMPOUNDS.

ESSENCES. Essences of flowers will be found under PERFUMERY. Essences of Celery, and other *culinary essences*, will be found, with allied compounds, in another place. A few concentrated infusions, and other strong preparations of drugs, not sanctioned by the Colleges, but very generally used, may be noticed here.

ESSENCE OF YELLOW BARK. Resinous extract of bark ½ oz., sulphate of quinine 60 gr., rectified spirit 6 oz., tincture of orange peel 2 oz. For Mr. BATTLEY'S preparation, see Liquor Cinchonæ, Pocket Formulary.

ESSENCES OF CALUMBA, RHUBARB, SENNA. See Liquor Calumbæ, Rhei, Sennæ, Pocket Formulary.

ESSENCE OF CAMPHOR. See Liquor Camphoræ, Pocket Formulary.

ESSENCE OF CHAMOMILE. As a substitute for the infusion it may be made as LIQUOR CALUMBÆ, P. F. See CHAMOMILE DROPS for another preparation of this drug.

ESSENCE OF ERGOT. See Essentia Secalis Cornuti, Pocket Formulary.

ESSENCE OF GINGER. Unbleached Jamaica ginger in coarse powder 5 oz., rectified spirit a pint; digest for 8 days, and strain with pressure; or it may be made by percolation. As there is no established form, it varies in strength as prepared by different makers, and often contains cayenne pepper.

ESSENCE OF CUBEBS. Mix powdered cubebs with ether, in a well stopped bottle; in twelve hours put the paste into a percolator, and add ether till the cubebs are nearly exhausted; distil off the ether in a water-bath, and preserve it for the same purpose. Dissolve the extract which remains, in three times as much brandy. One drachm is equal to 2 drachms of the powder. A fluid extract is also made by concentrating the tincture.

ESSENCE OF MINT, PEPPERMINT, AND PENNYROYAL. The strength of these varies as prepared by different makers; some use 1 part of the essential oil to 3 of rectified spirit, but more usually, we believe, 1 part to 7. They are sometimes coloured with the leaves of the plant, or of spinach.

ESSENCE OF MUSTARD. Rectified spirit of turpentine 16 fluid oz., bruised black mustard seed 2 oz., camphor 4 oz., oil of rosemary ½ oz., annotto to colour.

ESSENCE OF SARSAPARILLA. [See also Extractum Sarzæ Fluidum et Liquidum, Liquor Sarzæ, and Essentia Sarsaparillæ, in Pocket Formulary. The latter is an elegant and efficacious preparation.] Jamaica sarsaparilla 16 oz., lukewarm distilled water (100° to 112° F.) sufficient to cover it. Macerate for 6 hours, and strain. Bruise the root, macerate it again in sufficient warm water, and repeat the maceration with fresh water until it ceases to be much coloured. After each straining, let the liquid be immediately heated to 180° F., allowed to cool, and filtered. Evaporate the whole of the filtered liquids by a water or steam-bath, at a heat not above 160°, until reduced to 14 or 15 fluid ounces; add 2 ounces of rectified spirit, and keep it in a close bottle in a cool place for a few days. Then carefully pour off the clear liquid from any sediment into a clear dry bottle. One fluid ounce represents 1 oz. of the root, or 8 ounces of the decoction.

COMPOUND ESSENCE OF SARSAPARILLA. Jamaica sarsaparilla 16 oz.; proceed as above, but reserve the liquor of the last maceration for boiling the other ingredients; namely, guaiacum raspings, bruised liquorice root, sassafras, each 2 oz.; mezereum ¾ oz. Boil them in 4 or more pints of the weak infusion for ½ an hour, and strain; evaporate to 4 fluid ounces; let it cool, stirring it occasionally, and add 2 oz. of rectified spirit in which a few drops of oil of sassafras have been dissolved. Evaporate the sarsaparilla liquid to 11 ounces, and when cool add the other liquid. Proceed as for the former. One measure with 7 of water forms a near approximation to the Pharmacopœia Decoction.

ESSENCES (concentrated infusions) of quassia, cascarilla, chiretta, gentian, &c., may be made as directed for Liquor Calumbæ, P. F. Take 8 times the quantity of ingredients directed in the pharmacopœia for one pint of infusion, and infuse them in one pint of boiling water for the time prescribed; strain with strong pressure, and again infuse the ingredients in nearly as much water as the liquor obtained is short of a pint. Strain again with pressure; mix the products, which should measure 18 or 19 oz., add 2 oz. of rectified spirit, set aside for a few days in a well-closed bottle, and filter. Some substances, as chiretta, senna, calumba, &c., yield their active principles to cold water, which some prefer in these cases; but it is then necessary, before adding the spirit, to place the liquor (in a bottle) in a water-bath, and heat it to 180°, in order to precipitate any albumen it may contain. When cold, filter, and add the spirit. They also may be made by percolation.

VINOUS ESSENCES (by fermentation.) Dr. B. LANE has recently proposed to produce strong and permanent solutions of vegetable medicinal substances, by fermenting concentrated infusions with sugar and yeast. Further experiments are necessary to determine the value of these preparations, and the best means of producing them; an outline of the process is therefore all that can now be given. A strong infusion of the drug, usually 4 times as strong as that of the pharmacopœia, is mixed with lump sugar, usually 3 ℔ to 7 *old wine* pints, and fermented with yeast, at the temperature of 70° to 80° Fahrenheit, for 10 or 20 hours. When the action subsides, the vessels are closed, and placed in a cool cellar, about 55°, till fit for bottling. Wine of senna, gentian, calumba, cascarilla, valerian, &c., are thus made. In making vinous liquor of opium, the opium is macerated in water for some days, strained through coarse canvass, and the liquor submitted to fermentation. It should be made twice the strength of the tincture. A new name would be required to distinguish these preparations from the *Vina* of the pharmacopœias, and the latter also from the *Vinum opii fermentatione paratum* of the French codex.

EXTRACTS, MEDICINAL. See Pocket Formulary.

EXTRACTS OF FLOWERS. See PERFUMERY, in this volume.

EXTRACT OF MALT. Evaporate sweet wort to the consistence of treacle. It is sold as a cough medicine.

FAIRTHORN'S (Dr.) MILD PROVISIONAL PILLS. Sulphate of potash 1 scruple, extract of aloes 2 scruples, extract of senna 1 scruple, compound gamboge pill 50 gr., tartarized antimony 2 gr., compound powder of scammony 12 gr., Peruvian balsam 6 gr.; in 30 pills; one, two, or more, occasionally, when required.

FORD'S BALSAM OF HOREHOUND. It contains the ingredients of paregoric elixir, with squills, honey, and a strong infusion of horehound and liquorice.

FORD'S LAUDANUM. A tincture of opium containing cinnamon and cloves.

FOTHERGILL'S (Dr.) PILLS. Diaphoretic antimony, aloes, scammony, and extract of colocynth.

FRANK'S SOLUTION. See SOLUTION OF COPAIVA.

FREEMAN'S BATHING SPIRIT. Mix water and rectified spirit, of each three gallons, dissolve in them soft soap 6 ℔, and camphor 8 oz.; add Daffy's elixir 8 oz.

FRIAR'S BALSAM. Compound tincture of benzoin. L. P.

GELÉE POUR LE GOITRE. Dissolve 1 oz. of white soap in 2½ oz. of proof spirit by a gentle heat; and add to it whilst still warm, a warm solution of 5 dr. of iodide of potassium in 2½ oz. of proof spirit. A few drops of any fragrant essential oil may be added.

GINGERBREAD, PURGATIVE. Flour 14 oz., butter 4 oz., treacle 8 oz., p. ginger 1¼ oz., jalap 2 oz., caraway ½ oz. Mix the powders, then add the butter, and lastly the treacle, previously warmed. Roll out and divide into cakes of $\frac{1}{4}$ oz. each, containing each 6 or 7 grains of jalap.

GODBOLD'S VEGETABLE BALSAM. An acidulated syrup, or oxymel, of various herbs. The following is an imitation. Dissolve by heat 1 ℔ of lump sugar, in white-wine vinegar 1 quart, in which 3 oz. of garlic have been steeped for 3 days; add tincture of tolu 2 dr.

GODFREY'S CORDIAL. The active ingredient is opium, and there is a great diversity in the strength of the compound as prepared by different makers. Many accidents have arisen from its too general use as a stupefactive for infants, but we believe its sale is now less encouraged by druggists than formerly. The following are some of the more usual formulæ:—

1. Heat together 7 ℔ (avoird.) of treacle, and 8 ℔ of water till united; when nearly cold add the following—rectified spirit 6 fluid ounces, oil of sassafras 40 minims, oil of aniseed 10 drops, laudanum 4 oz. Mix, and make up the weight if necessary to 15 ℔. It contains rather more than 9 minims (equal, according to some authorities, to 16 or 18 drops) of laudanum in each fluid ounce.

2. Treacle $3\frac{1}{2}$ ℔, water 6 ℔, spirit of wine 8 fluid ounces, laudanum 4 fluid ounces, oils of aniseed, sassafras, and caraway, of each $\frac{1}{2}$ dr. Mix. Contains 12 or 14 minims of laudanum in an ounce.

3. Sliced sassafras 2 oz., opium cut small 1 oz., bruised aniseed 8 oz., boiling water a gallon. Infuse, strain, and make the infusion into a syrup with 14 ℔ of treacle. If the whole of the active principles of the opium are extracted, this is much stronger than the preceding.

4. Make a syrup with 3 ℔ (avoird.) each of treacle and coarse sugar, and water sufficient to make up a gallon. Dissolve 24 drops of oil of sassafras, and 16 of oil of aniseed, in 3 fluid ounces of spirit of wine; add 10 fluid drachms of tincture of opium, and mix the whole with 8 pints, o. m., of the syrup. This is weaker than either of the preceding, containing only 5 minims of laudanum in a fluid ounce, or 1 drop in a drachm.

5. The Philadelphia College of Pharmacy to prevent the mischief arising from the different strength of this com-

pound directs it to be prepared as follows:—Dissolve 2½ oz. of carbonate of potash in 26 pints of water, add 16 pints of treacle; heat together over a gentle fire till they simmer, remove the scum, and when sufficiently cool, add ½ ounce of oil of sassafras dissolved in 2 pints of rectified spirit, and 24 fluid ounces of tincture of opium, previously mixed. The old wine measure is here intended. It contains about 16 minims of laudanum, or rather more than 1 gr. of opium, in each fluid ounce.

6. Sassafras 9 oz.; seeds of coriander, caraway, and anise, of each 1 oz.; infuse in 6 pints of water, simmer the mixture till reduced to 4 pints; then add 6 ℔ of treacle, boil the whole for a few minutes, and when cold add 3 fluid ounces of tincture of opium. Nearly the strength of No. 1.—Dr. PARIS.

GODFREY'S SMELLING SALTS. Sesquicarbonate of ammonia resublimed with pearlash, and a little spirit.—Dr. PARIS.

GOLDEN SPIRIT OF SCURVY GRASS. It is said to be coloured with gamboge.

GOLDEN OINTMENT. Singleton's ointment, q. v. The ointment of nitric oxide of mercury is also called golden ointment.

GOULARD'S EXTRACT OF LEAD. Liquor plumbi diacetatis, P. L.

GOUT PAPER. See Charta Antirheumatica, P. F.

GRANVILLE'S (Dr.) COUNTER-IRRITANT LOTIONS. These consist of very strong water of ammonia (sp. gr., 872, being more than 3 times the strength of the Liquor Ammonia of the Pharmacopœia;) of spirit of rosemary (fresh tops of rosemary 2 ℔, alcohol 8 pints; infuse 24 hours, and distil 7 pints;) and spirit of camphor containing 4 oz. camphor in 2 pints of alcohol. The *milder* consists of 4 dr. of the above ammonia, 3 of spirit of rosemary, and 1 of spirit of camphor. The *stronger*, of 5 dr. of ammonia, 2 of spirit of rosemary, and 1 of camphor. The milder is generally sufficient to produce full vesication in from 3 to 10 minutes. The stronger is seldom used except in apoplexy, and to produce cauterization.

GRAVES' (Dr.) GOUT PREVENTIVE. Orange peel 2 oz.,

rhubarb 1 oz., hiera picra 2 oz., brandy a quart. Digest for a week.

GREGORY'S POWDER. Calomel magnesia 2½ oz., powdered Turkey rhubarb 1 oz., powdered ginger ½ oz. Mix. The above is Dr. GREGORY'S formula. Some recipes add powdered chamomile,—Rhubarb 1 oz., ginger ¼ oz., p. chamomile ½ oz., magnesia 2 oz. Mix. Some druggists prepare it with the heavy carbonate of magnesia, instead of the calcined.

GREENOUGH'S TINCTURE. See TOOTH COSMETICS.

GRIFFIN'S TINCTURE, for coughs. Oil of caraway and anise, each 2 dr., saffron ½ oz., benzoic acid ¾ oz., opium 5 dr., camphor ½ oz., spirit 6 oz., honey 6 oz. When mixed and dissolved, colour with burnt sugar.

GRIFFITH'S MIXTURE. This is merely Mistura Ferri Composita of the Pharmacopœia.

GRINROD'S (Dr.) REMEDY FOR SPASMS. Sulphuric ether, aromatic spirit of ammonia, of each ½ oz.; acetate of morphia ½ gr., camphor mixture 2 oz. Mix. A teaspoonful in a little water when required.

GUESTONIAN EMBROCATION. Oil of turpentine 1½ oz., olive oil 1½ oz., dilute sulphuric acid 3 fluid drachms.—Dr. PARIS.

GUTHRIE'S BLACK OINTMENT. 10 grains of nitrate of silver with 1 dr. of spermaceti ointment and 10 drops of a solution of acetate of lead.

GUTHRIE'S EYE OINTMENT. A weaker preparation of the same kind; used in ophthalmia, but causes great pain. See Ung. Hyd. Nit., Pocket Formulary.

HALFORD'S (Sir H.) GOUT PILLS. Acetic extract of colchicum 2½ gr., Dover's powder 1½ gr., compound extract of colocynth 1½ gr., in each pill. One for a dose.

HARROWGATE SALTS (Dr. DUFFIN'S.) Sulphate of magnesia 2 dr., bitartrate of potash 10 gr., sal polychrest (potassæ sulphas cum sulphure, Ph. Ed.) ½ dr.; in a pint of warm water. For another formula *see Mineral Waters (factitious) and salts for producing them*, p. 208.

HELVETIUS' STYPTIC. Melt together equal parts of alum and dragon's blood; when cold, powder the compound.

HENRY'S MAGNESIA. A solution of Epsom salts is precipitated by one of carbonate of potash in the cold; the precipitate is well washed, rose water being used for the last washing; it is then made up while drying into large or small cubes. See Magnes. Carbonas, P. F.

HILL'S BALSAM OF HONEY. Balsam of tolu 2 oz., styrax 2 dr., opium ½ dr., honey 8 oz., spirit of wine 32 fluid ounces.

HOFFMAN'S PILLS contain corrosive sublimate, about ⅛th of a grain in each.

HOULTON'S LAUDANUM. Opium 2½ oz., distilled vinegar 32 fluid oz.; macerate 6 days with a gentle heat, and filter. Evaporate to an extract. Dissolve this in 5 fluid oz. of rectified spirit, and 35 fluid oz. of distilled water.

HOOPER'S FEMALE PILLS. These according to Dr. PARIS, consist of RUFUS' Pill, sulphate of iron, canella, and a portion of ivory black. Mr. GRAY gives two formulæ—

1. Sulphate of iron 8 oz., water 8 oz., dissolve, and add Barbadoes aloes 40 oz., canella 6 oz., myrrh 2 oz., opoponax ½ oz. Make a mass.

2. Sulphate of iron 2 oz., powder of aloes with canella 16 oz., mucilage of tragacanth and tincture of aloes q. s. to form a mass. Divide 60 grains into 18 pills. But, according to a recent analysis, the iron is in a peroxidized state; probably the sulphate is partially calcined.

The Philadelphia College of Pharmacy gives the following formula—

3. Barbadoes aloes 8 oz., dried sulphate of iron 2 oz. 1½ dr., extract of black hellebore 2 oz., myrrh and soap each 2 oz., canella 1 oz., ginger 1 oz., water q. s. to form a mass. Divide into pills of 2½ gr. each.

HOOPING COUGH; popular remedies for. 1. Cochineal and salt of tartar mixture. This appears to have been first introduced by Dr. LOBB, in 1765, and is still a favourite domestic remedy. Salt of wormwood (subcarbonate of potash) 20 gr., powdered cochineal 10 gr., hot water ¼ of a pint; triturate together, strain, and sweeten with white sugar (or sugar candy.) Dose, a teaspoonful to a tablespoonful, according to the age.

2. *Fumigating Powders.* Styrax calamita and gum benzoin, of each a scruple, placed on hot cinders or a heated shovel, in the patient's room every day.

HUXHAM'S TINCTURE OF BARK. The compound Tincture

of Bark of the London Pharmacopœia is precisely that of HUXHAM, except that he used brandy instead of proof spirit.

ISSUE PEAS. Those in general use are unripe oranges (orange berries) turned in a lathe. The unturned berries are also used. Peas are also turned from orris root. NIEMANN gives the following composition for issue peas:—Yellow wax 1½ oz., powdered turmeric 1 oz., powdered orris ½ oz., Venice turpentine q. s. These are more stimulating, and are used to increase the discharge. The following according to Dr. GRAY, will open an issue itself:—Yellow wax 6 oz., verdigris 2 oz., white hellebore 2 oz., cantharides 1 oz., orris 1½ oz., Venice turpentine q. s.

JAMES'S POWDER. It is not known in what respect the mode of preparing this powder differs from the pharmacopœia process for antimonial powder. Dr. JAMES'S specification is vague and impracticable.

JAMES'S ANALEPTIC PILLS. Equal parts of JAMES'S powder, RUFUS' pill, and gum guaiacum, made into pills with tincture of castor. Dr. PARIS has ammoniacum in the place of guaiacum. Another formula is—Compound powder of aloes, aloes and myrrh pill, and JAMES'S powder, in equal quantities, formed into pills with tincture of castor and syrup.

JARAVE, SPANISH. Pour 4 gallons of boiling water on 2 ℔ Rio Negro sarsaparilla, 8 oz. powdered guaiacum bark, 4 oz. each of rasped guaiacum wood, anise seed, and liquorice root, 2 oz. of bark of mezereon root, 2 ℔ of treacle, and 12 bruised cloves. Shake it thrice a day, and keep it in a warm place. When fermentation has set in it is fit for use. Dose, a small tumbler full.

JESUITS' DROPS. WALKER'S. Balsam of capivi 6 oz., gum guaiacum 1 oz., Chio turpentine ½ oz., subcarbonate of potash ½ oz., cochineal 1 dr., rectified spirit 1 quart. See also Elixir Antivenereum, Pocket Formulary.

KENNEDY'S CORN PLASTER. Yellow wax 1 ℔, Venice turpentine 2 oz., verdigris 1 oz., melted together and spread on leather.

KEYSER'S PILLS. See Pilulæ Hydrargyri Acetatis, P. F.

KING'S CORDIAL. Dissolve in ½ pint of proof spirit 1½ dr., each of the oils of caraway and cinnamon; extract the stones from 3 lb of black cherries, and mash the fruit in a pan; grate one nutmeg; take 2 quarts of Madeira wine, 2 quarts of brandy, and 1 gallon of syrup; mix all together, and colour with red sanders wood.

KIRKLAND'S NEUTRAL OINTMENT AND CERATE. See Unguentum Plumbi Compositum and Ceratum Neutrale, P. F.

KITCHENER'S (Dr.) PERISTALTIC PERSUADERS. Turkey rhubarb in powder 2 dr., oil of caraway 10 drops, simple syrup 1 dr. by weight; mix, and divide into 40 pills. Dose, 2, 3, or more. "From 2 to 4 will generally produce one additional motion within 12 hours. The best time to take them is early in the morning."

LARTIGUE'S GOUT PILLS. Compound extract of colocynth 20 gr., extract of colchicum 60 gr., extract of opium 1 gr.; mix, and divide into 18 pills. Dose, one or more, according to their purgative effect.

LEDOYEN'S DISINFECTING FLUID. It consists of about 20 oz. of nitrate of lead in a gallon of water. Its specific gravity should be 1·40.

LEE'S WYNDHAM'S PILLS. Gamboge 3 oz., aloes 2 oz., Castile soap 1 oz., nitre ½ oz., extract of cow-parsnep 1 oz. In pills of 5 gr. each. [Am. Journ. of Pharmacy.]

LEE'S ANTIBILIOUS PILLS. Aloes 12 oz., scammony 6 oz., gamboge 4 oz., jalap 3 oz., calomel 5 oz., soap 1 oz., syrup of buckthorn 1 oz., mucilage 7 oz.; mix, and divide into 5-grain pills. [The same.]

LEROY'S PURGATIVE.

	1.	2.	3.
Scammony	12 dr.	16 dr.	24 dr.
Vegetable turbith .	6 dr.	8 dr.	12 dr.
Jalap	6 oz.	8 oz.	12 oz.
Brandy	10 pints imperial.		

Digest for 12 hours, strain, and add the following syrup:

Senna	6 oz.	8 oz.	12 oz.
Water	24 oz.	32 oz.	48 oz.

Infuse, strain with pressure, and add

Brown sugar	32 oz.	36 oz.	48 oz.

Make a syrup.

No. 4 is stronger than the above.

LEJEUNE'S BALSAM FOR CHILBLAINS. Camphor 1 dr., tincture of benzoin 5 dr.; dissolve, and add iodide of potassium 5 dr., extract of lead 10 dr., spirit of wine reduced to proof with rose-water 2½ oz.; dissolve 10 dr. of white soap in 2½ oz. of the same diluted spirit by a gentle heat, mix the solutions whilst still warm, and add any perfume. Let it cool in wide-mouthed bottles, and cork.

LIEBERT'S COSMETIC. For Chapped Nipples. Dissolve 10 grains of nitrate of lead in 1 oz. of water. A pair of fine lead shields accompany the lotion, to be worn after applying it. The nipples must be carefully washed before the child is put to the breast.

LIGNUM'S ANTI-SCORBUTIC DROPS. These contain bichloride of mercury, and should not therefore be used without great caution.

LIQUEUR DORÉE. Peruvian bark, bitter orange peel, and cinnamon, of each 4 dr., saffron 2 dr., brandy 4 quarts, Malaga wine 2 quarts; digest for 4 days, strain, and add 2½ ℔ of sugar. [*Liqueurs* which are not medicated, but merely alcoholic drams, do not come within the plan of this work.]

LIQUID BLISTER. Powdered cantharides 5 oz., and sulphuric ether 15 ounces.—TOYNBEE.

LISTON'S ISINGLASS PLASTER. Soak 1 oz. of isinglass in 2 oz. of water, and dissolve it in 2 oz. of rectified spirit and 1½ oz. of water, by the heat of a water-bath. Brush it over the surface of oiled silk, properly stretched. An improved kind is made by brushing one side of the peritoneal membrane of the cæcum of the ox (prepared in the same manner as gold-beaters' skin) with the same solution, and the other side with drying oil.

LOCATELLI'S BALSAM. Melt together 4 oz. of yellow wax, 1 ℔ of common oil, and 1 ℔ of Venice turpentine, placing with them 4 oz. of alkanet root wrapped in a linen bag.

LONG'S (ST. JOHN) LINIMENT. See Linimentum Terebinthinæ Aceticum, Pocket Formulary.

LOZENGES. See CHING'S LOZENGES, DAWSON'S, DARCET'S.

The medicated lozenges which are sanctioned by the Pharmacopœias, and employed in practice, will be found under Trochisci and Pasta, in the Pocket Formulary. A few other formulæ are here added:—

Absorbent Lozenges. Precipitated chalk 3 oz., heavy carbonate of magnesia 2 oz., nutmeg in fine powder 1 dr., sugar 6 oz., powdered gum 1 oz., water q. s. to form a stiff paste, which divide by a punch into lozenges of the usual size, and dry them gradually in a warm room.

Aperient Lozenges. Calomel 60 gr., pure scammony, 80 gr., jalap 40 gr. (or jalapine 4 gr.,) ginger 8 gr., cinnamon 4 gr., mucilage of tragacanth q. s. to form a stiff paste; mix the other powders accurately together, then with the sugar, lastly add the mucilage, beat the whole into a uniform mass, and divide it into 40 equal lozenges. Each contains $1\frac{1}{2}$ gr. calomel, 2 of scammony, and 1 of jalap.

Black Currant Paste. Soften 12 ℔ of picked black currants by heating them in a water-bath in a covered earthen vessel, pulp through a hair-sieve, and evaporate to a paste, incorporating with it 1 ℔ powdered sugar; roll it out into a sheet of proper thickness. Mr. Bartlett gives the following formula:—3 ℔ of powdered sugar, 3 ℔ of extract of black currants (the inspissated juice,) 1 oz. tartaric acid, 6 oz. of powdered gum; mixed, rolled out, and cut, when dry, with a large pair of scissors into square pieces.

Black Currant and Ipecacuanha Lozenges. Black currant paste (as above) 8 oz., ipecacuanha 30 gr., tragacanth 90 gr.; in 240 lozenges.

Cough Lozenges (with Lactucarium.) Powdered lactucarium 2 dr., extract of liquorice-root 12 dr., ipecacuanha 30 gr., powdered squill 15 gr., refined sugar 6 oz., mucilage of tragacanth q. s.; mix, and divide into 240 equal lozenges. Each contains $\frac{1}{2}$ gr. lactucarium, $\frac{1}{8}$ gr. of ipecacuanha, $\frac{1}{16}$ gr. of squill.

For other Cough Lozenges, see Trochisci Anticatarrhales, Glycyrrhizæ et Opii, Lactucæ, Morphiæ et Ipecac., Opii, Papaveris, Pectorales, Scillæ, Tolutani, &c., Pocket Formulary.

Digestive or Live-long Candy. 1. Powdered rhubarb 60 gr., heavy magnesia 1 oz., bicarbonate of soda 1 dr., finely-powdered ginger 20 gr., cinnamon powder 15 gr., powdered white sugar 2 oz., mucilage of tragacanth q. s.; beat together, and divide into parallelograms of 20 gr. each.

2. *Caraway Candy.* Rhubarb 60 gr., powdered caraway 60 gr., oil of caraway 10 drops, ginger and cinnamon, each 15 gr., magnesia 6 dr., carbonate of soda 1 dr., sugar 2 oz., mucilage q. s.,—as the last.

Edinburgh Lozenges. Extract of poppies 2 oz., powdered sugar 8 oz., powdered tragacanth 4 oz., water q. s.

Fruit Lozenges. Black currant paste 8 oz., red currant paste (or the juice evaporated to a paste) 4 oz., syrup of raspberries 4 oz.; soften by a gentle heat, and beat in a warm mortar with 2 ℔ of powdered sugar, and a drachm of powdered citric acid, and, if required, a little mucilage of gum tragacanth.

Marshmallow Lozenges. Marshmallow root powdered 2 oz., sugar 14 oz., mixed with some mucilage of tragacanth, and orange flower water.

Peppermint Lozenges. Rub together white sugar 6 oz., oil of peppermint 36 drops, and the whites of 2 eggs. Make into lozenges.

LYNCH'S EMBROCATION. Olive oil coloured with alkanet, perfumed, and rendered stimulating by essential oils.

MADDEN'S ESSENCE. A strongly-acidulated infusion of roses.

MAHOMED'S ELECTUARY. Grocers' currants 1 oz., powdered senna ½ oz., powdered ginger 30 gr., oil of croton 1 drop, syrup of roses sufficient to make an electuary; two teaspoonfuls every morning.—BATEMAN.

MAHY'S PLASTER (American.) Boil 12 oz. of white lead, 32 fluid ounces of olive oil, and a little water, stirring constantly until incorporated. Add yellow wax 4 oz., lead plaster 18 oz., and when these are melted stir in 9 oz. of powdered orris.

MAREDANT'S NORTON'S DROPS. Corrosive sublimate, gentian, ginger, and cochineal.

MARSHALL'S CERATE. Palm oil 5 oz., calomel 1 oz., acetate of lead ½ oz., ointment of nitrate of mercury 2 oz.; mix.—Dr. PARIS.

MARSHALL'S EYE-DROPS. These are said to consist of 2 gr. of nitrate of silver in 1 oz. of decoction of snails.

MARSDEN'S ANTISCORBUTIC DROPS, Morton's, Perry's, Lignum's, and other antiscorbutic drops, contain corrosive sublimate.—DR. PARIS.

MAGNESIA, FLUID. A solution of carbonate of magnesia in water by means of carbonic acid gas, forced into it by pressure. MURRAY'S and DINNEFORD'S should contain from 12 to 15 gr. of the carbonate in each fluid oz. See Liquor Magnesiæ Carbonatis, Pocket Formulary.

MATHIEU'S VERMIFUGE. Tin filings 1 oz., fern root $\frac{3}{4}$ oz., worm seed $\frac{1}{2}$ oz., resinous extract of jalap 1 dr., sulphate of potash 1 dr., honey to form an electuary. A teaspoonful every 3 hours for 2 days: then substitute the following—jalap 2 scruples, sulphate of potash 2 scruples, scammony 1 scruple, gamboge 10 gr.; made into an electuary with honey, and given in the same dose.

MINERAL WATERS, (FACTITIOUS,) AND SALTS FOR PRODUCING THEM. See below, p. 208.

MONTEIN'S BAREGE BALLS (for Sulphur Baths.) Sulphate of lime 8 oz., common salt 2 oz., Flanders glue 1 oz., extract of soapwort 1 oz.; make into 8 balls; to be kept from the air. M. MENIERE recommends,—extract of soapwort $\frac{1}{2}$ oz., water 6 oz., lime in powder 4 oz., sulphur 3 oz., gelatine 1 oz.; dissolve the extract and gelatine in the water, add the lime and sulphur, heat gently, stirring it constantly, till the mass gets detached from the sides of the vessel; then form it into balls of 1$\frac{1}{2}$ oz. each.

MORRISON'S PILLS, No. 1, consist of equal parts of aloes and cream of tartar. No. 2 consist of 2 parts of gamboge, 3 of aloes, 1 of colocynth, and 4 of cream of tartar,—made into pills with syrup.

MORRISON'S ADHESIVE PASTE, for ring-worm. See Pasta Adhesiva, Pocket Formulary.

MOSELEY'S PILLS. Turkey rhubarb 60 gr., Jamaica ginger 24 gr., syrup and tincture of rhubarb q. s. to form a mass, to be divided into 24 pills.

MOXON'S EFFERVESCING MAGNESIAN APERIENT. The

composition, we believe, has not been made public, but the following have been proposed as imitations:—

1. Heavy carbonate of magnesia 2 ℔, bicarbonate of soda 1 ℔, tartaric acid 1½ ℔, refined sugar ½ ℔, essence of lemon 40 minims; the powders to be all separately dried at a moderate temperature.

2. Sulphate of magnesia 1 ℔, bicarbonate of soda 1 ℔, tartaric acid ½ ℔; the ingredients to be well dried separately, at a moderate temperature. (Pharmaceutical Journal.)

3. Carbonate of magnesia 1 ℔, sulphate of magnesia 2 ℔, bicarbonate of soda 2 ℔, potassio-tartrate of soda 2 ℔, tartaric acid 2 ℔; to be separately dried, and mixed.—M. DURANDE.

MUNRO'S COUGH MEDICINE. 4 dr. of paregoric with 2 dr. of sulphuric ether, and 2 drachms of tincture of Tolu. Dose, a teaspoonful in some warm water.

MURRAY'S (Sir J.) FLUID CAMPHOR. Each ounce contains 3 gr. of camphor and 6 gr. of carbonate of magnesia, dissolved by carbonic acid, by pressure.

MURRAY'S GOUT SPECIFIC. It contains iodide of potassium, sulphate of magnesia, and an aromatic tincture. (Pharmaceutical Journal.)

NORRIS'S DROPS. A solution of tartarized antimony, with a tincture of some vegetable substances, not ascertained.

NOUFFLEUR'S (Madame) WORM MEDICINE. Powdered fern root 3 dr., to be given in the morning (the patient being prepared by an emollient clyster, and a supper of panada;) followed in 2 hours by a bolus of calomel, scammony, and gamboge.

OLLIVIER'S BISCUITS. Beat up the white of 2 eggs with 16 oz. of water, and add a solution of 76 gr. of corrosive sublimate; collect, wash, and dry the precipitate, 1-7th of a gr. of which is contained in each biscuit of 2 drachms.

OPODELDOC. Lin. Saponis.

ORMSKIRK MEDICINE, *to prevent hydrophobia.* Elecampane 1 dr., chalk 4 dr., Armenian bole 3 dr., alum 10 grains, oil of aniseed 5 drops.

PALAMOUD. See DIETETIC COMPOUNDS.

PALMER'S AERATED CHALYBEATE. Mix 1½ parts of acetic acid with 40 of water, add 4 of proto-sulphate of iron, and 20 of syrup. Put into 4-ounce bottles, for No. 1 and No. 2 respectively, as much of the above as contains 2 and 4 gr. of sulphate of iron, and fill the bottles with a solution of carbonate of soda or of potash strongly charged with carbonic acid gas. Tartaric acid may be substituted for acetic.

PAPIER EPISPASTIQUE D'ALBESPEYRES. The *Pommade Epispastique* of the French codex, spread on waxed paper. See Unguentum Epispasticum, Pocket Formulary.

PAPIER EPISPASTIQUE, DE VÉE. This is of three strengths, distinguished by the colours white, green, and red. The composition is made by boiling cantharides for an hour with water, and lard, green ointment, or lard coloured with alkanet; adding white wax to the strained fats, and spreading on paper, silk, or linen. No. 1 is made with 10 oz. of cantharides to 4 ℔ of lard; No. 2 of 1 ℔ of flies to 8 ℔ of green ointment; and No. 3 of 1½ ℔ to 8 ℔ of coloured lard; and to each are added 2 ℔ of white wax.—DORVAULT.

PAPIER FAYARD. *Gout Paper.* Euphorbium 3 dr., cantharides 6 dr., powdered and digested with 4 oz. alcohol; and 3 dr. Venice turpentine added to the strained tincture. Fine paper is dipped into it and dried in the air. MOHR directs 4 dr. of cantharides and 1 dr. euphorbium to be digested in 5 oz. of highly rectified spirit; filter and add 1½ oz. Venice turpentine previously liquefied with 2 oz. of resin. To be spread on the paper while warm.

PELLETIER'S ÆTHEREAL OPODELDOC. See Balsamum Aceticum Camphoratum, Pocket Formulary.

PETER'S PILLS. Aloes, jalap, gamboge, and scammony, of each 2 dr.; calomel 1 dr.

PILES, popular remedies for. Dr. WARDLEWORTH'S Pills contain 3½ gr. of pitch in each; 2 every night. For ELECTUARIES for piles see Confectio Resinæ, Confectio Sulphuris Composita, Electuarium Hæmorrhoidale, Electuarium Sulphuris Compositum, in Pocket Formulary.

See also WARD'S PASTE, below. For PILE OINTMENTS see Unguentum Gallæ, Unguentum Gallæ Compositum, Unguentum Gallæ et Opii, Unguentum Hæmorrhoidale, Pocket Formulary. Sir H. HALFORD'S Pile Ointment consists of equal parts of citrine ointment and oil of almonds triturated in a glass mortar till perfectly smooth. Mr. WARE'S is Powdered nut-gall 2 dr., camphor 1 dr., melted wax 1 oz., tincture of opium 2 dr. Mix.

PILLS. See proprietor's names in alphabetical order. A great variety of formulæ for pills of every kind will be found in the Pocket Formulary.

PILLS, TO COAT, WITH GELATINE . } See Pilulæ, Pocket
——, TO SILVER . . . . . . } Formulary.

M. Durden recommends collodion as a covering for pills: others, a solution of gutta percha in chloroform: but the ready solubility of these materials in the stomach may be questioned.

PLUNKET'S OINTMENT FOR CANCER. White arsenic, sulphur, powdered flowers of lesser spearwort and stinking chamomile, levigated together, and formed into a paste with white of egg.

POMMADE DIVINE. Beef marrow 3 ℔; put it into an earthen vessel, and cover it with cold water, and change the water daily for a few days, using rose water the last day. Pour off and press out the water; add to the marrow 4 oz. each of styrax, benzoin, and Chio turpentine, 1 oz. orris powder, ½ oz. each of powdered cinnamon, cloves, and nutmeg. Set the vessel in hot water, and keep the water boiling for 3 hours; then strain. For Pomades for the Hair, see HAIR COSMETICS, after PERFUMERY.

PORTLAND (Duke of) GOUT POWDER. Equal quantities of the roots of gentian and birthwort, tops of germander, ground pine, and lesser centaury: all to be powdered and mixed together.

POWELL'S BALSAM FOR COUGH. Mix together 2 dr. of syrup of Tolu, 1 oz. of paregoric elixir, and 2 oz. of liquorice-juice.

QUEEN OF HUNGARY'S WATER. Tops and flowers of rosemary 2 ℔, rectified spirit 3 ℔; digest in a close vessel for 50 hours in a gentle heat, then distil by water bath.

QUININE AND CAMPHOR PILLS. See Pilulæ Quinæ et Camphoræ, Pocket Formulary.

RADCLIFFE'S Elixir. Aloes 6 dr., cinnamon, zedoary, and cochineal, each ½ dr., rhubarb 1 dr., syrup of buckthorn 2 oz., proof spirit 16 fluid oz., water 5 fluid oz.—Dr. PARIS. According to GRAY, it contains jalap, scammony, and senna.

RASPAIL'S CAMPHOR CIGARETTES. These are merely camphor enclosed in a tube, (a quill or paper tube may be used,) confined by blotting paper, and used cold. Another kind of camphorated cigars is made by saturating dried coltsfoot or other leaves with a strong solution of camphor, and rolling them in the form of cigars.

REECE'S CHIRAYTA PILLS. Extract of chirayta 2 dr., dried carbonate of soda 1 scruple, p. ginger 15 gr. Mix, and divide into 36 pills. Two twice a day.

REGNAULD'S PECTORAL PASTE. Pectoral flowers (mullein, coltsfoot, catsfoot, and red poppies mixed) 16 oz., boiling water 3 ℔; infuse, strain, and add to the clear liquor 6 ℔ of clean gum Arabic; dissolve by a gentle heat, and evaporate to a proper consistence, adding towards the end 6 dr. of tincture of balsam of Tolu.

REYNOLD'S GOUT SPECIFIC. It is supposed to be a wine of colchicum.

REVALENTA. It is said to be prepared from the seeds of the Ervum lens. See Dietetic Articles.

RIGA BALSAM FOR BRUISES. Mix 4 oz. of spirits of wine with 1 dr. of compound tincture of benzoin, and 2 dr. of tincture of saffron.

ROBINSON'S (Dr.) STIMULATING PURGATIVE PILLS. Watery extract of aloes 1 dr., balsam of Peru 10 gr., oil of caraway 10 drops, scammony ½ dr. Mix, and divide into 20 pills: 2 or 3 when required.

ROCHE'S EMBROCATION. Olive oil, with half its weight of oil of cloves and oil of amber.—Dr. PARIS.

ROGÉ'S MAGNESIAN PURGATIVE. Calcined magnesia 1 oz. carbonate of magnesia ½ oz., citric acid 3¼ oz., sugar, rubbed with a few drops of essence of lemon, 6¼ oz. To form Aerated Magnesian Lemonade, put ¼ of the powder into a soda water bottle nearly filled with water, and cork it securely.

ROUSSEAU'S DROPS. See Vinum Opii Fermentatione Paratum, P. F.

RUSPINI'S STYPTIC. It contains (according to Dr. A. T. Thomson) gallic acid, sulphate of zinc, spirit, and rose water.

RYAN'S ESSENCE OF COLTSFOOT. Tincture of balsam of tolu 2 oz., compound tincture of benzoin 2 oz., spirit of wine 4 oz.—GRAY.

RYMER'S TINCTURE. A tincture of capsicum, camphor, cardamom, rhubarb, aloes, and castor, in proof spirit, with a small quantity of sulphuric acid.—Dr. PARIS. (The inventor states that it is impregnated with an aërial acid.)

SALTS, MINERAL. See WATERS, FACTITIOUS MINERAL, page 208.

SCOTT'S PILLS. See ANDERSON'S PILLS.

SCOTT'S PLASTER. It appears to be a carefully prepared Emp. Plumbi, spread on calico. If it contains resin, the quantity is probably less than in Emp. Resinæ.

SEIDLITZ POWDERS (in separate powders.) One contains 2 dr. of powdered Rochelle salts, and 40 gr. of bicarbonate of soda; the other powder is p. tartaric acid 35 gr.

SEIDLITZ POWDER, in one bottle. *Note.*—The powders are all to be thoroughly dried separately, at a gentle heat—the potassio-tartrate of soda at a temperature not exceeding 110° F.; the others not higher than 120°. Take of potassio-tartrate of soda, dried, 15 oz.; tartaric acid, dried, 5 oz. (or citric acid 4¾ oz.,) dry bicarbonate of soda 6 oz. Mix, and keep in a well-closed bottle. Dose, 3 dr. Or, mix two parts of bitartrate of soda with one part of bicarbonate of soda. Keep dry. The above have no resemblance to the natural water of Seidlitz. See WATERS (Mineral,) page 211.

SINGLETON'S GOLDEN OINTMENT. Orpiment mixed with lard to the consistence of an ointment.

SODA POWDERS. These usually contain in one paper 30 gr. of bicarbonate of soda, and in the other 25 gr.

of tartaric acid (or 24 of citric acid.) For sherbet, lemonade, and ginger-beer powders, see BEVERAGES, in another division of this work.

SMELLOME'S EYE-OINTMENT. Prepared verdigris 30 gr.; levigate with 30 drops of olive oil, and add 1 oz. of resinous cerate.

SPEEDIMAN'S PILLS. Rhubarb, aloes, myrrh, and extract of chamomile, of each 60 gr.; oil of chamomile 12 drops. Mix, and divide into 4-grain pills.

SOLOMON'S BALM OF GILEAD. An aromatic tincture, of which cardamoms form a leading ingredient, made with brandy.—Dr. PARIS. It is thought to contain cantharides.

SOLOMON'S ANTI-IMPETIGINES is said to be a solution of corrosive sublimate.

SMITH'S (Dr. HUGH) STOMACHIC PILLS. Aloes, rhubarb, aromatic powder, gum sagapenum, of each 1 dr.; oil of mint and oil of cloves, each 10 drops; balsam of Peru q. s. In 5-grain pills; 2 to 4 every night.

SOLUTION OF COPAIVA. Mix 2 parts of balsam of copaiva with 3 of liquor potassæ, and 7 of water. Boil them for a quarter of an hour, and when a little cooled, add 1 part of spirit of nitric ether. Let the mixture rest for a few hours, then draw off the clear liquor from the lower part of the vessel. This is supposed to resemble FRANK'S Solution. Or copaiva may be boiled in water with an equal weight of carbonate of potash. [For other preparations of copaiva see Gelatina Copaibæ, Electuarium Copaibæ, Elec. Cubebæ et Copaibæ, Syrupus Copaibæ, Mistura Copaibæ, &c., in P. F.]

SPILSBURY'S ANTI-SCORBUTIC DROPS. Corrosive sublimate 2 dr. (not 2 oz., as misprinted in the eighth edition of Dr. PARIS'S Pharmacologia,) precipitated sulphuret of antimony 1 dr., gentian 2 dr., orange peel 2 dr., red sanders 1 dr., proof spirit 16 fluid oz.; digest and strain. —Dr. PARIS. But we are informed that this is incorrect. Another formula is—Levigated crocus metallorum 18 dr., corrosive sublimate 135 gr., red sanders 1½ dr., gentian 6 dr., orange-peel 6 dr., brandy 48 fluid oz.; digest for 10 days, shaking frequently, and strain; dose 5 to 60 drops.

SQUIRE'S ELIXIR. Opium 1 oz., camphor 1 oz., spirit of aniseed (compound) 4 pints, tincture of serpentaria 1 pint, water 4 pints, tincture of ginger ½ oz. Some recipes add a little aurum musivum.

STANDERT'S RED MIXTURE. Carbonate of magnesia 4 dr., powdered rhubarb 2 dr., tincture of rhubarb 1½ oz., tincture of opium 1 dr., oil of aniseed 24 drops, essence of peppermint 30 drops, water 1½ pint; mix. A popular remedy for bowel complaints in the west of England.

STANDERT'S STOMACHIC CANDY. Cardamom seed, ginger, rhubarb (all in fine powder,) each 4 dr., lump sugar 4 oz., water 6 dr.; boil together, stirring constantly till the sugar is dissolved, then pour it into a proper mould.

STEERS' OPODELDOC. 1. Rectified spirit a quart, Castile soap 5 oz., camphor 2½ oz., oil of rosemary 2½ dr., oil of origanum 5 dr., weaker ammonia 4 oz.; digest till dissolved, and pour while warm into wide-mouthed bottles.

2. Rectified spirit 8 pints o. m., white soap 20 oz., camphor 8 oz., water of ammonia 4 oz., oil of rosemary 1 oz., oil of horsemint 1 oz.; dissolve the soap in the spirit by a gentle heat, and add the other ingredients. Bottle whilst warm.—PHIL. COLL. OF PHARMACY.

STOUGHTON'S ELIXIR. 1. Gentian 36 oz., serpentary 16 oz., dried orange-peel 24 oz., calamus aromaticus 4 oz., rectified spirit and water, of each 6 gallons old measure.

2. Gentian 4 ℔, orange-peel 2 ℔, cochineal 2 dr., cardamom seed 1 oz., rectified spirit 8 gallons.

STOREY'S WORM CAKES. Calomel 1 scruple, jalap 1 dr., ginger 2 scruples, sugar 1 oz., cinnabar to colour, syrup q. s. to form 10 cakes.

STRUVE'S LOTION FOR HOOPING COUGH. Emetic tartar 60 gr., water 2 oz., tincture of cantharides 1 oz.

SWAIM'S VERMIFUGE. Worm seed 2 oz., valerian, rhubarb, pink root, white agaric, of each 1½ oz.; boil in sufficient water to yield 3 quarts of decoction, and add to it 30 drops of oil of tansy, and 45 drops of oil of cloves, dissolved in a quart of rectified spirit. (American remedy.)

SYDENHAM'S LIQUID LAUDANUM. See Vinum Opii, Pocket Formulary.

TANJORE PILLS. See Pilulæ Arsenici, Pocket Formulary.

THIBAUT'S BALSAM for wounds. Digest flowers of St. John's wort, one handful, in ½ pint rectified spirit, then express the liquor, and dissolve in it myrrh, aloes, and dragon's-blood, of each 1 dr., with Canada balsam ½ oz.

TINCTURE OF QUININE. (AROMATIC.) See Tinct. Quinæ Co., and Tinct. Quinæ Sulphatis Acida, Pocket Formulary.

TISSOT'S PURGATIVE POWDERS. Jalap, rhubarb, senna, and soluble cream of tartar, equal quantities. Dose, 2 to 6 drachms. Used in Normandy.

TURLINGTON'S BALSAM. Rectified spirit 8 old wine pints, benzoin 12 oz., liquid styrax 4 oz., socotrine aloes 1 oz., balsam of Peru 2 oz., myrrh 1 oz., angelica-root ½ oz., balsam of tolu 4 oz., extract of liquorice 4 oz.; digest 10 days and strain.—PHIL. COLL. of PHARM. The certified copy of the original recipe is more complex, containing three times as many ingredients.

VALANGIN'S SOLUTION OF SOLVENT MINERAL. Arsenious acid (which has been mixed with muriate of soda, and resublimed) 30 gr., hydrochloric acid 90 gr., distilled water 1 oz.; dissolve, and add distilled water to make up 30 fluid oz. Dose, from 3 drops, increased very gradually to 10. See Liquor Arsenici Chloridi, P. F.

VENLO'S VEGETABLE SYRUP. It is supposed to be a decoction of burdock, mint, dandelion, senna, &c., boiled with sugar, and a small portion of solution of sublimate added.

WALKER'S JESUIT'S DROPS. See Jesuit's Drops, above.

WARBURG'S FEVER TINCTURE. M. FUCHS gives the following recipe for imitating this secret remedy: Hepatic aloes and zedoary root, of each 1 dr., angelica-root and camphor, of each 2 gr., saffron 3 gr., proof spirit 3 oz. In 25 dr. of the filtered tincture dissolve 30 gr. of sulphate of quinine. Put it up in 5-drachm bottles, containing a dose. Sold at about 5 shillings each bottle.

WARD'S PASTE. The same as Confectio Piperis Nigri of the London Pharmacopœia.

WARD'S WHITE DROPS. To 16 oz. of strong nitric acid add gradually 7 oz. of subcarbonate of ammonia; let it stand 2 or 3 hours, then put it into a bolt-head which it will only half fill, and to each 16 oz. put 4 oz. of pure quicksilver, and digest in a sand heat till the solution is complete; then gently increase the heat, and add a little more quicksilver at intervals till it will dissolve no more; then evaporate it in a glass or earthen dish placed in sand, till a pellicle appears, and set it aside to crystallize. Dissolve 1 ℔ of the drained salt in 3 ℔ of rose water by the heat of a sand-bath.

WARD'S ESSENCE FOR THE HEADACHE. Spirit of wine 2 ℔, roche alum in fine powder 2 oz., camphor 4 oz., essence of lemon ½ oz., strong water of ammonia 4 oz.; stop the bottle close, and shake it daily for 3 or 4 days.

WARD'S RED PILL. Glass of antimony levigated with a fourth of its weight of dragon's-blood, made into a mass with wine, and divided into pills of a grain and a half each; one pill is a dose, on an empty stomach. In foulness of the stomach and bowels, and obstinate rheumatic disorders.

WARD'S DROPSY PURGING POWDER. Jalap 1 ℔, cream of tartar 1 ℔, red bole 1 oz.; mix; dose, from 30 to 40 gr., in broth or warm beer, repeated for 2 or 3 days, or oftener if necessary.

WARD'S SWEATING POWDER. Similar to Dover's Powder.

WARD'S WASHING POWDER. See Washing Compounds, Trade chemicals.

WARNER'S CORDIAL. Rhubarb 1 oz., senna ½ oz., saffron 1 dr., liquorice ½ oz., raisins 1 ℔, brandy 3 pints; digest for a week, and strain.

WARWICK'S (Countess of) POWDERS. Scammony 2 oz., calx of antimony 1 oz., cream of tartar ½ oz. Mix.

WEBSTER'S DIET DRINK. A decoction or syrup of sarsaparilla, betony, dulcamara, guaiacum, liquorice, sassafras, turmeric, and thyme.

WEBSTER'S (Lady) PILLS. See Pilulæ Aloes cum Mastiche.—P. F.

WHITEHEAD'S ESSENCE OF MUSTARD. See ESSENCE OF MUSTARD for an imitation of it.

WHITEHEAD'S MUSTARD PILLS. Dr. PARIS says they consist of balsam of tolu and resin.

WHITELAW'S ETHEREAL TINCTURE OF LOBELIA. See Tinctura Lobeliæ Etherea, Pocket Formulary.

WILSON'S GOUT TINCTURE. A vinous infusion of colchicum.

WISDOM'S (Dr.) EYE-WATER. Bole 2 oz., sulphate of zinc ¼ oz., camphor (dissolved in 1½ oz. of rectified spirit) ¼ oz., water a gallon.

WRIGHT'S PEARL OINTMENT. White precipitate 8 oz., extract of lead a pint, rub together, and add 7 ℔ of white wax melted with 16 ℔ of olive oil.—PHARM. JOURNAL.

WORM LOZENGES. See CHING'S LOZENGES, and STOREY'S WORM CAKES, above; see also Trochisci Anthelmintici, and Trochisci Santoninæ, Pocket Formulary.

YOUNG'S PURGING DRINK. Carbonate of soda in crystals 2½ dr., cream of tartar in crystals 3 dr., water 8 oz.; put it into a stone bottle, and secure the cork.

FACTITIOUS MINERAL WATERS,

AND

Salts for Producing them.

AERATED OR CARBONATED WATERS.

THESE require the aid of the powerful machine employed by soda-water manufacturers, to charge the waters strongly with carbonic acid gas. The gas is made from whiting, and diluted sulphuric acid, and is forced by a pump into the watery solution. Sometimes the gas is produced by the mutual action of the ingredients introduced into the bottle of water, which must be instantly closed: but this method is found practically inconvenient, and is only adopted in the absence of proper apparatus. The quantity of gas introduced is directed, in the French and American pharmacopœias, in most cases, to be 5 times the volume of liquid. For chalybeate and sulphuretted waters, the water should be previously deprived of the air it naturally contains, by boiling it, and allowing it to cool in a closed vessel.

BAKEWELL'S apparatus will be found very convenient for making small quantities of aërated waters; and the syphon bottles suitable for holding them.

SIMPLE AERATED WATER. Carbonic acid gas water. Water charged with 5 or more volumes of carbonic acid gas, as above.

ALKALINE AERATED WATERS. Aërated soda and potash waters should be made by dissolving a drachm of the carbonated alkali in each pint of water, and charging it strongly with carbonic acid gas. But the soda water of the shops generally contains but little soda.

AERATED MAGNESIA WATER. This is made of various strengths.

MURRAY'S and DINNEFORD'S FLUID MAGNESIA may be thus made:—To a boiling solution of 16 oz. of sulphate of magnesia in 6 pints of water, add a solution of 19 oz. of crystallized carbonate of soda in the same quantity of water; boil the mixture till gas ceases to escape, stirring constantly; then set it aside to settle; pour off the liquid, and wash the precipitate on a cotton or linen cloth, with warm water, till the latter passes tasteless. Mix the precipitate, without drying it, with a gallon of water, and force carbonic acid gas into it under strong pressure, till a complete solution is effected. The *Eau Magnésienne* of the French codex is about a third of this strength; and we have met with some prepared in this country not much stronger.

CARBONATED LIME WATER. *Carrara Water.* Lime water (prepared from lime made by calcining Carrara marble) is supersaturated, by strong pressure, with carbonic acid; so that the carbonate of lime at first thrown down is re-dissolved. It contains 8 gr. of carbonate of lime in 10 fluid oz. of water.

AERATED LITHIA WATER. This may, probably, be most conveniently made from the fresh precipitated carbonate, dissolved in carbonated water as directed for fluid magnesia. Its antacid and antilithic properties promise to be useful; but we have not yet heard of its being prepared in this form. [See page 214.]

SALINE CARBONATED WATERS.

THE following afford approximate imitations of these waters. The earthy salts, with the salts of iron, should be dissolved together in the smallest quantity of water. The other ingredients to be dissolved in the larger portion of the water, and the solution impregnated with the gas. The first solution may be then added, or be previously introduced into the bottles. The salts, unless otherwise stated, are to be crystallized.

BADEN WATER. Muriate of magnesia 2 gr., muriate of

lime 40 gr., muriate of iron ¼ gr., (or 3 minims of the tincture,) muriate of soda 30 gr., sulphate of soda 10 gr., carbonate of soda 1 gr., water 1 pint, carbonic acid gas 5 volumes.

CARLSBAD WATER. Muriate of lime 8 gr., tincture of muriate of iron 1 drop, sulphate of soda 50 gr., carbonate of soda 60 gr., muriate of soda 8 gr., carbonated water 1 pint.

EGER. Carbonate of soda 5 gr., sulphate of soda 4 scruples, muriate of soda 10 gr., sulphate of magnesia 3 gr., muriate of lime 5 gr., carbonated water a pint. (Or it may be made without apparatus thus:—Bicarbonate of soda 30 gr., muriate of soda 8 gr., sulphate of magnesia 3 gr., water a pint; dissolve, and add a scruple of dry bisulphate of soda, and close the bottle immediately.)

EMS. Carbonate of soda 2 scruples, sulphate of potash 1 gr., sulphate of magnesia 5 gr., muriate of soda 10 gr., muriate of lime 3 gr., carbonated water a pint.

MARIENBAD. Carbonate of soda 2 scruples, sulphate of soda 96 gr., sulphate of magnesia 8 gr., muriate of soda 15 gr., muriate of lime 10 gr., carbonated water a pint. (Or, Bicarbonate of soda 50 gr., sulphate of soda 1 dr., muriate of soda 15 gr., sulphate of magnesia 10 gr.; dissolve in a pint of water, add 25 gr. of dry bisulphate of soda, and cork immediately.)

MARIENBAD PURGING SALTS. Bicarbonate of soda 5 oz., dried sulphate of soda 12 oz., dry muriate of soda 1½ oz., sulphate of magnesia, dried, 2 oz., dried bisulphate of soda 2½ oz. Mix the salts, previously dried, separately, and keep them carefully from the air.

PULLNA WATER. Sulphate of soda 4 dr., sulphate of magnesia 4 dr., muriate of lime 15 gr., muriate of magnesia (dry) a scruple, muriate of soda a scruple, bicarbonate of soda 10 gr., water slightly carbonated, a pint. One of the most active of the purgative saline waters.

PULLNA WATER, WITHOUT THE MACHINE. Bicarbonate of soda 50 gr., sulphate of magnesia 4 dr., sulphate of soda 3 dr., muriate of soda a scruple; dissolve in a pint of water; add, lastly, 2 scruples of bisulphate of soda, and close the bottle immediately.

SALTS FOR MAKING PULLNA WATER. Dry bicarbonate of soda 1 oz., exsiccated sulphate of soda 2 oz., exsiccated sulphate of magnesia 1½ oz., dry muriate of soda 2 dr., dry tartaric acid ¾ oz. (or rather, dry bisulphate of soda 1 oz.)

SEIDLITZ WATER. This is usually imitated by strongly aerating a solution of 2 dr. of sulphate of magnesia in a pint of water. It is also made with 4, 6, and 8 dr. of the salts to a pint of water.

SEIDLITZ POWDER. The common seidlitz powders (as given p. 202) do not resemble the water. A closer imitation would be made by using effloresced sulphate of magnesia instead of the potassio-tartrate of soda. A still more exact compound will be the following:—Effloresced sulphate of magnesia 2 oz., bicarbonate of soda ½ oz., dry bisulphate of soda ½ oz.; mix and keep in a close bottle.

SEIDSCHUTZ WATER. Sulphate of magnesia 3 dr., muriate of lime, nitrate of lime, bicarbonate of soda, of each 8 gr., sulphate of potash 5 gr., aerated water 1 pint.

SELTZER WATER. Muriate of lime and muriate of magnesia, of each 4 gr.; dissolve these in a small quantity of water, and add it to a similar solution of 8 gr. bicarbonate of soda, 20 gr. muriate of soda, and 2 gr. of phosphate of soda: mix, and add a solution of ¼ of a gr. of sulphate of iron; put the mixed solution into a 20-oz. bottle, and fill up with aerated water. But much of the Seltzer water sold is said to be nothing more than simple carbonated water. An imitation of Seltzer water is also made by putting into a stone Seltzer bottle, filled with water, 2 dr. bicarbonate of soda, and 2 dr. of citric acid in crystals, corking the bottle immediately. Sodaic powders are sometimes sold as Seltzer powders.

VICHY WATER. Bicarbonate of soda 1 dr., muriate of soda 2 gr., sulphate of soda 8 gr., sulphate of magnesia 3 gr., tincture of muriate of iron 2 drops, aerated water a pint. DORVAULT directs 75 grains of bicarbonate of soda, 4 grains of chloride of sodium, ⅕ gr. sulphate of iron, 10 gr. sulphate of soda, 3 gr. sulphate of magnesia, to a pint of water. By adding 45 grains (or less) of citric acid an effervescing water is obtained.

VICHY SALTS. Bicarbonate of soda 1½ oz., muriate of soda 15 gr., effloresced sulphate of soda 1 dr., effloresced sulphate of magnesia 1 scruple, dry tartarized sulphate of iron 1 gr., dry tartaric acid 1 oz. (or dry bisulphate of soda;) mix the powders, previously dried, and keep them in a close bottle.

SALINE WATERS, &c., NOT CARBONATED.

SEA WATER. Muriate of soda 4 oz., sulphate of soda 2 oz., muriate of lime ¼ oz., muriate of magnesia 1 oz., iodide of potassium 4 gr., bromide of potassium 2 gr., water a gallon. A common substitute for sea water as a bath is made by dissolving 5 or 6 oz. of common salt in a gallon of water.

The following mixture of dry salts may be kept for the immediate production of a good imitation of sea water. Muriate of soda (that obtained from evaporating sea water and not recrystallized, in preference) 85 oz.; effloresced sulphate of soda 15 oz., dry muriate of lime 4 oz., dry muriate of magnesia 16 oz., iodide of potassium 2 dr., bromide of potassium 1 gr. Mix, and keep dry. Put 5 or 6 oz. to a gallon of water.

BALARUC WATER. Muriate of soda 1 oz., muriate of lime 1 oz., muriate of magnesia ½ oz., sulphate of soda 3 dr., bicarbonate of soda 2 dr., bromide of potassium 1 gr., water a gallon. Chiefly used for baths.

SULPHURETTED WATERS.

SIMPLE SULPHURETTED WATER. Pass sulphuretted hydrogen into cold water (previously deprived of air by boiling, and cooled in a closed vessel,) till it ceases to be absorbed.

AIX-LA-CHAPELLE WATER. Bicarbonate of soda 12 gr., muriate of soda 25 gr., muriate of lime 3 gr., sulphate of soda 8 gr., simple sulphuretted water 2½ oz., water slightly carbonated 17½ oz.

BAREGES WATER. (Cauterets, Bagneres de Luchon, Bonnes, St. Sauveur, may be made the same.) Crystallized hydrosulphate of soda (see Sodæ Hydrosulphas, P. F.,) crystallized carbonate of soda, and muriate of soda, of each 2½ gr., water (freed from air) a pint. A stronger solution for adding to baths is thus made:—Crystallized hydrosulphate of soda, crystallized carbonate of soda, and muriate of soda, of each 2 oz., water 10 oz. Dissolve. To be added to a common bath at the time of using.

NAPLES WATER. Crystallized carbonate of soda 15 gr., fluid magnesia 1 oz., simple sulphuretted water 2 oz., aerated water 16 oz. Introduce the sulphuretted water into the bottle last.

HARROGATE WATER. Muriate of soda 100 gr., muriate of lime 10 gr., muriate of magnesia 6 gr., bicarbonate of soda 2 gr., water 18½ oz. Dissolve, and add simple sulphuretted water 1½ oz.

HARROGATE SALTS. See Dr. DUFFIN'S, above.

CHALYBEATE WATERS.

SIMPLE CHALYBEATE WATER. Water freed from air by boiling 1 pint, sulphate of iron ½ gr.

AERATED CHALYBEATE WATER. Sulphate of iron 1 gr., carbonate of soda 4 gr., water deprived of air, and charged with carbonic acid gas, a pint. Dr. PEREIRA recommends 10 gr. each of sulphate of iron and bicarbonate of soda to be taken in a bottle of ordinary soda water. This is equivalent to 4 gr. of carbonate of iron.

BRIGHTON CHALYBEATE. Sulphate of iron, muriate of soda, muriate of lime, of each 2 gr., carbonate of soda 3 gr., carbonated water 1 pint.

BUSSANG, FORGES, PROVINS, and other similar waters may be imitated by dissolving from ½ to ⅔rds of a grain of sulphate of iron, 2 or 3 gr. of carbonate of soda, 1 gr. of sulphate of magnesia, and 1 of muriate of soda, in a pint of aerated water.

MONT D'OR WATER. Bicarbonate of soda 70 gr., sulphate of iron ⅔ gr., muriate of soda 12 gr., sulphate of soda ½ gr., muriate of lime 4 gr., muriate of magnesia 2 gr., aerated water a pint.

PASSY WATER. Sulphate of iron 2 gr., muriate of soda

3 gr., carbonate of soda 4 gr., muriate of magnesia 2 gr., aerated water a pint.

PYRMONT WATER. Sulphate of magnesia 20 gr., muriate of magnesia 4 gr., muriate of soda 2 gr., bicarbonate of soda 16 gr., sulphate of iron 2 gr., Carrara water a pint.

The mineral waters prepared by Messrs. Struve, of Brighton, are stated to be very exact imitations of the natural springs.

VARIOUS AERATED MEDICINAL WATERS, NOT RESEMBLING ANY NATURAL SPRING.

MIALHE'S AERATED CHALYBEATE WATER. Water a pint, citric acid 1 dr., citrate of iron 15 grains; dissolve, and add 75 grains of bicarbonate of soda.

TROUSSEAU'S MARTIAL AERATED WATER. Potassio-tartrate of iron 10 grains, artificial Seltzer water a pint.

BOUCHARDAT'S GASEOUS PURGATIVE. Phosphate of soda 1½ oz., carbonated water a pint.

MIALHE'S IODURETTED GASEOUS WATER. Iodide of potassium 15 grains, bicarbonate of soda 75 grains, water a pint; dissolve and add sulphuric acid diluted with its weight of water 75 grains. Cork immediately.

DUPASQUIER'S GASEOUS WATER OF IODIDE OF IRON. Solution of iodide of iron (containing $\frac{1}{10}$ of dry iodide) 30 grains, syrup of gum 2½ oz., aerated water 17½ oz.

[See also Magnesian, Carrara, and Lithia Waters, page 209; Bewley's Chalybeate Water, page 174. Also Aqua Benzoata Aerata, and Aqua Magnesiæ Citratis, P. F.]

PERFUMERY.

DISTILLED WATERS.

THE simple distilled waters (without spirit) used in perfumery are chiefly those of rose, elder, and orange-flower, cinnamon, &c. The points requisite to be attended to are, that the flowers be fresh, gathered after the sun has risen and the dew exhaled, and that sufficient water be used to prevent the flowers being burned, but not much more than is sufficient for this purpose. The quantities usually directed are—Roses 15 ℔, water 40 ℔: distil 15 ℔, for *single*, and the same water with 15 ℔ of fresh roses for *double* rose water.

Orange-flowers 12 ℔, water 36 ℔: distil 24 ℔ for *double* orange-flower water; this with an equal quantity of distilled water forms the *single*. The flowers should not be put into the still till the water nearly boils.

ELDER-FLOWER WATER, ACACIA-FLOWER WATER, and BEAN-FLOWER WATER, are prepared in the same manner as rose water.

CINNAMON WATER. A gallon should be distilled from 20 oz. of fine cinnamon (bruised) and 2 gallons of water.

STRAWBERRY WATER. Bruised strawberries 4 ℔, water a gallon; macerate for 12 hours, and distil 6 pints.

The waters prepared without distillation (by diffusing the essential oils through water, after mixing them with chalk or magnesia, or dissolving them in spirit,) are seldom so proper for perfumery purposes as those distilled from the flowers, &c. Rose water, made from the otto (8 drops of otto, previously mixed with a drachm of precipitated chalk, diffused in a quart of distilled water, and afterwards distilled or simply filtered,) is to most persons very agreeable; but that distilled from the flowers should also be kept, as it is by others greatly preferred.

Musk Water, Violet Water, Jessamine Water, and some others, are made by mixing the *spirituous essences* with distilled or pure soft water. A usual proportion is 2 drachms to a pint.

SPIRITUOUS WATERS.

The spirit employed in perfumery should be selected with great care; it should be perfectly free from grain-oil and other impurities. It should be 60 over-proof, unless otherwise directed.

Simple Spirit of Lavender. Lavender-flower (free from stalks) 2 ℔, rectified spirit 8 pints, water 16 pints; distil 8 pints.

Smyth's Distilled Essence of Lavender. Essential oil of English lavender 4 oz., rectified spirit (60° over-proof) 5 pints, rose water 1 pint. Mix, and distil 5 pints for sale.

Essence of Lavender (by mixture.) Essential oil of lavender 3½ oz., rectified spirit 2 quarts, rose water ½ pint, tincture of orris ½ pint.

Lavender Water. English oil of lavender 4 oz., spirit 3 quarts, rose water 1 pint. Mix and filter. (A commoner and cheaper preparation may be made with the French oil.)

Odoriferous Lavender Water. 1. Rectified spirit 5 gallons, essential oil of lavender 20 oz., oil of bergamot 5 oz., essence of ambergris ½ oz. Sometimes 4 oz. of orris-root are digested with the above.—Mr. Brande.

2. Oil of lavender, oil of bergamot, of each 3 dr.; otto of roses and oil of cloves, of each 6 drops; musk 2 gr., true oil of rosemary 1 dr., honey 1 oz., benzoic acid 2 scruples; rectified spirit a pint, distilled water 3 oz. —Dr. Pereira.

3. Oil of lavender 2 oz., essence of ambergris 1 oz., eau de Cologne a pint, rectified spirit a quart.

4. Oil of lavender 4 dr.; essence of bergamot, essence of lemon or cedrat, and otto of roses, of each 20 minims; essence of ambergris a dr., rectified spirit 3 pints, orange-

flower water 4 oz., rose (or distilled) water 12 oz., burnt alum 20 gr. Agitate frequently, then let it stand in a cool place for some days before filtering.

5. Oil of lavender 3 dr., oil of bergamot 20 drops, neroli 6 drops, otto 6 to 12 drops, essence of cedrat 8 or 10 drops, essence of musk 20 drops, rectified spirit 28 fluid oz., distilled (or orange-flower) water 4 oz.

6. *Eau de Lavande au Millefleurs.* Oil of lavender 4 dr.; essence of bergamot, essence of lemon, otto of roses, of each 12 drops; essence of millefleurs 3 dr., essence of ambergris 1 dr., rectified spirit a pint and half.

Note.—The oil of lavender in the above should be the finest English oil: that which first comes over is said to be the most fragrant. It should be kept for 12 months before using, either alone or mixed with an equal quantity of alcohol. Some makers prefer a mixture of old and new oil. The lavender water improves by age.

Eau de Cologne—Cologne Water. 1. English oil of lavender, oil of bergamot, oil of lemon, oil of neroli, of each 1 oz.; oil of cinnamon ½ oz.; spirit of rosemary, and spirit of balm (*eau des Carmes*) of each 15 oz.; highly rectified spirit 7½ pints. Let them stand together for 14 days, then distil in a water-bath.—Dr. Granville.

2. Oil of bergamot, citron, and lemon, of each 3 oz.; oils of rosemary, neroli, and lavender, of each 1½ oz.; oil of cinnamon 6 dr., rectified spirit 24 pints; compound spirit of balm (*eau des Carmes*, below) 3 pints, spirit of rosemary 2 pints. Mix, and after standing a week, distil 24 pints.—French Pharmacopœia.

3. Essential oils of bergamot, of lemon, of neroli, of orange-peel, and of rosemary, each 12 drops; cardamom seeds a dr.; rectified spirit a pint. It improves by age.—Trommsdorf.

4. Essence of bergamot 40 minims, essence of lemon 45 minims, oil of rosemary 6, oil of orange 22, neroli 12 minims, highly rectified spirit 6 oz.

5. Alcohol a pint, oil of bergamot, oil of orange-peel, true oil of rosemary, cardamom seeds, of each a drachm; orange-flower water a pint. Mix, and distil a pint by water-bath.—Dr. A. T. Thomson.

EAU DES CARMES—EAU DE MELISSE. Fresh flowering balm 24 oz.; yellow rind of lemon, cut fine 4 oz.; cinnamon, cloves, and nutmeg (bruised,) of each 2 oz.; coriander seed (bruised) 1 oz., dried angelica root 1 oz., rectified spirit a gallon. Macerate for 4 days, and distil in a water-bath.

ARQUEBUSADE WATER. 1. Sage, angelica, wormwood, savory, sweet fennel, hyssop, balm, sweet basil, rue, thyme, marjoram, rosemary, angelica seed, origanum, red calamint, creeping thyme, lavender flowers, of each 10 oz.; sweet flag root 5 oz., rectified spirit 2 gallons, water q. s. Distil 3 gallons.

2. (Simplified.) Balm, rosemary, thyme, calamus root, angelica seeds, lavender flowers, of each 4 oz.; rectified spirit 3 pints, water q. s. Macerate for a day, and distil 4 pints.

QUEEN OF HUNGARY'S WATER. Spirit of rosemary. 1. Rosemary tops 2 ℔, rectified spirit a gallon, water q. s. Distil carefully one gallon.

2. Spirit of rosemary (as No. 1) 4 pints, orange-flower water ¼ pint, essence of neroli 4 drops.

3. Simple spirit of rosemary 3 pints, simple spirit of lavender a pint, rose water 8 oz.

EAU D'ANGE. Flowering tops of myrtle 16 oz., rectified spirit a gallon; digest, and distil to dryness in a water-bath. Or dissolve ¼ oz. essential oil of myrtle in 3 pints of rectified spirit. Mr. GRAY gives under this name a water without spirit—Water 2 pints, benzoin 2 oz., storax 1 oz., cinnamon 1 dr., cloves 2 dr., calamus a stick, coriander seeds a pinch; distil.

HONEY WATER. *Eau de Miel.* 1. Rectified spirit 8 pints, oil of cloves, oil of lavender, oil of bergamot, of each ½ oz., musk 15 gr., yellow sanders shavings, 4 oz.; digest for 8 days, and add 2 pints each of orange-flower and rose water.

2. Oil of santal 20 drops, tincture of musk 2½ oz., essence of bergamot 2½ oz., oil of cloves 5 dr., oil of lavender 5 dr., rose water 2 pints, orange-flower water 2 pints, spirit of wine a gallon; mix and filter.

3. (With honey.) White honey 8 oz., coriander seed

8 oz., fresh lemon-peel 1 oz., cloves ¾ oz., nutmeg, benzoin, styrax calamita, of each 1 oz.; rose and orange-flower water, of each 4 oz., rectified spirit 3 pints; digest for a few days and filter. Some recipes add 3 dr. of vanilla, and direct only ½ oz. of nutmeg, storax, and benzoin.

4. Coriander seeds 7 ℔, cloves 12 oz., storax 8 oz., nutmeg 8 oz., fresh lemon-peel 10 oz., calamus root 6 oz., rectified spirit 15 pints; macerate for a month, add water q. s. Distil 22 pints, and add to the distilled spirit 5 pints of orange-flower water, 24 drops otto of roses, a dr. of ambergris, and 2 oz. of fine vanilla; macerate for a week, and filter. The dry ingredients to be bruised or cut small.

LISBON WATER. To rectified spirit 1 gallon add the essential oils of orange-peel and lemon-peel, of each 3 oz., and of otto of rose ¼ oz.—PIESSE.

EAU DE PORTUGAL. To rectified spirit 1 gallon add the following essential oils: of orange-peel 6 oz., of lemon-peel 1 oz., of lemon-grass ¼ oz., of bergamot 1 oz., and of otto of rose ¼ oz.—PIESSE.

EAU D'ELEGANCE. Spirit of jessamine 2 ℔, spirit of styrax 1 ℔, spirit of hyacinth 1 ℔, spirit of star aniseed 4 oz., tincture of balsam of Tolu 4 oz., tincture of vanilla 2 oz.

EAU DE MARESCHALE. Spirit of wine 1½ pint, spirit of jessamine 1 oz., essence of bergamot ¼ oz., essence of violets 1 oz.

EAU ROMAINE. Spirit of jessamine 3 quarts, tincture of vanilla 1 quart, spirit of acacia flowers 1 quart, spirit of tuberose a pint, essence of ambergris 2 oz., tincture of benzoin 8 oz.

EAU DE MILLEFLEURS. Rectified spirit 2 pints, balsam of Peru ¼ oz., essence of bergamot ½ oz., oil of cloves ¼ oz., essence of neroli ½ dr., essence of musk 1 dr., orange-flower water 2 oz.

EAU SPIRITUEUSE D'HELIOTROPE. Vanilla 3 dr., double orange-flower water 6 oz., rectified spirit a quart; macerate for 3 days, and distil in a water-bath. It may be coloured with cochineal. But the essence d'heliotrope of some perfumers appears, by the colour, not to have been distilled.

Eau d'Ispahan. Essential oil of bitter orange-peel 4 oz., oil of rosemary 3 dr., oil of mint 1 dr., oil of cloves 7 scruples, neroli 7 scruples, spirit of wine 14 pints. It is used for the same purposes as Eau de Cologne.

Eau sans Pareille. Essential oil of lemon ½ oz., of bergamot 2½ dr., of cedrat, ¼ oz., rectified spirit 6 pints, spirit of rosemary 8 oz.; mix. Some authorities state that it is improved by distillation.

Eau de Bouquet de Flore. 1. Honey water 2 oz., tincture of cloves 1 oz., tincture of calamus, of lavender, and of long cyperus, each ½ oz.; eau sans pareille 4 oz., spirit of jessamine 9 dr., tincture of orris 1 oz., spirituous essence of neroli 20 drops.

2. Essence of violets ½ oz., spirit of rosemary ½ oz., essence of lemon 1 dr., rectified spirit 24 oz., rose water 8 oz.

3. Spirit of rosemary 8 oz., rectified spirit 8 oz., lavender water 2 oz., oil of neroli 5 drops, cloves 1 dr., orris root 2 dr., rose water 2 oz.; digest for a few days, and filter.

Esprit de Bouquet. English oil of lavender, oil of cloves, and of bergamot, of each 2 dr.; otto of rose, and oil of cinnamon, of each 20 drops; essence of musk 1 dr., rectified spirit a pint; mix.

Eau de Rosieres. Spirit of roses 4 pints, spirit of jessamine a pint, spirit of orange-flowers a pint, spirit of cucumber 2¼ pints, spirit of celery seed 2¼ pints, spirit of angelica-root 2¾ pints, tincture of benzoin (simple) ¾ of a pint, balsam of Mecca a few drops.

Eau d'Ambre Royale. Rectified spirit 2 ℔, tincture of musk seed 1 ℔, essence of ambergris 1 oz., tincture of musk 1 oz., reduced with a proper proportion of orange-flower water.

Esprit de Suave. Spirit of jessamine 1½ pint, spirit of acacia flowers 1½ pint, spirit of wine 12 oz., spirit of tuberose 8 oz., oil of cloves 1½ dr., oil of neroli 30 drops, essence of bergamot 1½ dr., tincture of musk 1 oz., rose-water 12 oz.

Parfum des Rois. Spirit of wine 2 gallons, styrax 6 oz., benzoin 16 oz., aloes wood 8 oz., spirit of rose 2 pints, spirit of orange-flowers 2 pints, essence (tincture) of ambergris 8 oz., tincture of musk 8 oz., tincture of vanilla 16 oz.

ODOR DELECTABILIS. Rose water, orange-flower water, each 4 oz.; oil of lavender, oil of cloves, each 1 dr., oil of bergamot 2 dr., musk 2 gr., rectified spirit a pint.

NEW VICTORIA PERFUME. Cloves, bruised, 2 scruples; vanilla, cut small, 1 dr.; oil of cedrat 4 drops, oil of santal 1 dr., cinnamon 12 gr., oil of verbena 8 drops, otto of roses 8 drops, oil of neroli 20 drops, oil of lavender 1 dr., ambergris 16 gr., tincture of musk 1 dr., rectified spirit 16 fluid oz.; digest for a few days, and filter. Or the whole except the musk and ambergris may be distilled in a water-bath, and these added to the distilled spirit.

Another similar perfume is—Vanilla ½ dr., yellow sanders 6 dr., cloves No. 16, neroli 3 drops, oil of lavender 6 drops, rectified spirit 4 oz.: digest for 3 days, and add 4 oz. of orange-flower water, water q. s.; distil 6 oz., and add essence of musk 1 drachm.

ESPRIT DE ROSE. 1. Macerate the fresh and picked flowers of the most fragrant varieties of the rose, with half their weight of rectified spirit, and distil in a water-bath to dryness.

2. Dissolve from 20 to 30 drops of otto in a pint of rectified spirit. A stronger solution, 6 or 8 drops of otto to an ounce of alcohol, forms essence of roses, or *esprit de rose triple.*

3. It is also made by agitating and digesting the spirit with the perfumed oil or pomade of roses. (See EXTRACTS, below.)

ESPRIT DE JASMIN. *Eau de Jasmin.* It is prepared by digesting and agitating pure spirit with oil or pomade of jessamine made with the flowers. (See EXTRACTS, below.) Spirit of jonquil, tuberose, violet, &c., may be obtained by the same process.

ESPRIT DE VIOLETTE. *Eau de Violette.* Macerate 5 oz. of fine orris root in a quart of rectified spirit for some days, and filter. It may also be obtained by the method just mentioned, or by mixing the product of both processes.

Eau odorante de Jasmin. Compound spirit of jessamine; for the handkerchief. Spirit of jessamine 1 pint, rectified spirit 1 pint, essence of ambergris a dr., simple tincture of benzoin a dr.

Spirit of Orange-flowers, Spirit of Elder-flowers, and Spirit of Acacia-flowers. Fresh flowers 1 ℔, rectified spirit 4 pounds, or pints, water 2 ℔; distil 4 ℔, or pints.

Spirit of Orange-peel, or Lemon-peel, of Citron, and of Bergamot. Fresh peel 1 ℔, rectified spirit 6 ℔; macerate for 2 days, and distil in a water-bath to dryness. Or, 1 oz. of the essential oil to 2 pints of spirit.

Spirit of Cinnamon, of Cloves, of Nutmeg, and of Calamus Root. Macerate 1 ℔ of the bruised drug with 8 ℔, or a gallon, of rectified spirit, and distil as the last.

Spirit of Cucumbers. Cucumbers grated 8 ℔, rectified spirit 1 ℔; distil 2 ℔.

Spirit of Rosewood. Rosewood shavings 1 ℔, spirit 6 ℔, water 2 ℔; distil 6 ℔. It is also made by adding the essential oil of rhodium to spirit.

Spirit of Angelica. Dried angelica root 1 ℔, rectified spirit a gallon. Macerate, and distil by water-bath to dryness.

Spirit of Balsam of Peru. Balsam 3 parts, spirit 15 parts, carbonate of potash 1 part; macerate for 3 days, and distil by water-bath.

Spirit of Strawberries, and of Raspberries. Fresh fruit 3 ℔, rectified spirit 1 ℔; macerate 24 hours, and distil 2 ℔.

The following tinctures are chiefly used in the compound perfumes:—

Tincture of Balsam of Peru, and of Tolu. Digest 1 oz. of the balsam with 8 of rectified spirit for some days, shaking it occasionally, then filter. Tincture of benzoin in the same manner.

Tincture of Angelica. One part of the dried root to 8 of rectified spirit; as the last.

Tincture (common spirituous essence) of Lemon, Citron,

ORANGE, AND BERGAMOT. An ounce of the fresh peel to ½ pint of spirit; as above.

TINCTURE OF MUSK SEED. *Essence d'Ambrette.* Digest 16 oz. of bruised musk seed with 3 pints of rectified spirit for a month, and filter.

TINCTURE OF MUSK. China musk 2 dr., rectified spirit 16 oz. For more compound tinctures of musk, see ESSENCE OF MUSK, below.

TINCTURE OR ESSENCE OF AMBERGRIS. GUIBOURT directs 1 dr. of ambergris to be digested with a gentle heat in 3 oz. of rectified spirit. Another form is—Ambergris 1 dr., subcarbonate of potash 1 dr., spirit of roses 4 oz., (or rectified spirit 4 oz., otto 6 drops.) Some recipes direct a weaker tincture—24 gr. of ambergris to 8 oz. of spirit. For other formulæ, see ESSENCE, below.

TINCTURE OF CIVET. Bruise ½ oz. of civet, ¼ oz. of ambergris, and the same of sugar-candy, and macerate in a quart of rectified spirit for 6 weeks, in a warm place; then filter.

TINCTURE OR ESSENCE OF VANILLA. Vanilla cut very small 2 oz., rectified spirit a pint; infuse for 2 or 3 weeks. This is sometimes distilled, forming spirit of vanilla.

TINCTURE OF RHODIUM. Rosewood 1 ℔, rectified spirit 3 or 4 pints; macerate for 3 or 4 weeks, and filter.

ESSENCE (OR TINCTURE) OF VETIVER. Take 2 ℔ of the root of vittie vayr cut small, and moisten it with a little water; let it macerate for 24 hours, then beat it in a marble mortar. Macerate it in sufficient spirit to cover it for 8 or 10 days, and strain with pressure; filter through paper, and in a fortnight repeat the filtration. Sometimes the root is moistened with diluted sulphuric acid, which, after maceration, is neutralized by adding a sufficient quantity of chalk, and the whole digested with spirit. The tincture, when strained off, is distilled, and forms (with the addition of essence of balm and of roses) Essence de Vetiver double.

ESSENCE OF PATCHOULI. Dried patchouli (pucha pat) 1 oz., rectified spirit a pint. It is generally combined with other perfumes.

EXTRACTS (extraits) are spirituous solutions of the odorous principle of flowers, obtained, indirectly, by agitating and digesting oils and pomatums which have been perfumed by the flowers (see HUILES ANTIQUES, under HAIR COSMETICS) with pure spirit. This is repeated with fresh oil until the spirit is sufficiently perfumed. When the same oil or pomade is treated with fresh spirit, inferior extracts, numbered 2, 3, &c., are obtained. These preparations are chiefly made in France.

EXTRACTS (EXTRAITS, or ESPRITS) OF JESSAMINE, VIOLETS, LILY OF THE VALLEY, are prepared by the process just mentioned.

EXTRAIT DE BOUQUET. Spirit (extrait) of jessamine 2 quarts, extract of violets 2 quarts, spirit of acacia-flowers, of rose, and of orange-flowers, each a quart, spirit of carnations a quart, flowers of benzoin ½ oz., essence of ambergris 8 oz.

EXTRAIT DE MARESCHALE. Essence of millefleurs 1½ oz., essence of jessamine 1 oz., essence of musk ½ oz., essence of ambergris ½ oz., essence of cedrat 20 drops, essence of violets 1 oz., sweet spirits of nitre 50 drops, true oil of rosemary 20 drops, rectified spirit 6 oz., oil of neroli 48 drops. Set aside for some time.

COMPOUND ESSENCES. Some of these contain a preparation of the substances whose name they bear, while others are fictitious or imitative, being made up of a variety of other essences and volatile oils. Several of the formulæ are those of M. PIESSE.

ESSENCE OF AMBERGRIS. This name is applied both to the simple and more compound tinctures of ambergris. See TINCTURE OF AMBERGRIS, above. Other formulæ may here be given.

1. Ambergris 4 oz., musk 2 oz., tincture of musk seed 7 pints. Digest with a gentle heat.

2. Ambergris 1 dr., musk ½ dr., oil of cinnamon 18 drops, oil of rhodium 12 drops, rectified spirit 8 oz., spirit of roses 4 oz., carbonate of potash 1½ dr.; digest in a warm place for a few days, and strain. See also ESSENCE ROYALE.

ESSENCE OF CEDRAT. Dissolve 2½ oz. of oil of cedrat in 1 gallon of spirit, and add bergamot ½ oz.

ESSENCE OF CLOVE PINK. Esprit de rose ½ pint, de fleur d'orange and de fleur de cassie, each ¼ pint, esprit de vanille 2 oz., oil of cloves 10 drops.

COLOGNE ESSENCE. Oil of bergamot 2 dr., essence of lemon ½ dr., essence of cedrat ½ dr., true oil of rosemary 15 drops, rectified spirit (or spirit of balm) 1½ oz.

ESSENCE OF HELIOTROPE. Spirituous extract of vanilla ½ pint, of French rose-pomatum ¼ pint, of orange-flower pomatum 2 oz., of ambergris 1 oz.; add 5 drops of the essential oil of almonds.

ESSENCE OF HONEYSUCKLE. Spirituous extract of rose-pomatum 1 pint, of violet 1 pint, of tuberose 1 pint; extracts of vanilla and tolu, of each ¼ pint; oil of neroli 10 drops, essential oil of almonds 5 drops.

ESSENCE OF HOVENIA. Rectified spirit 1 quart, rose-water ½ pint, essential oil of lemons ½ oz., otto of roses 1 dr., oil of cloves ½ dr., oil of neroli 10 drops.

ESSENCE OF JONQUIL. Spirituous extract of jasmine pomade 1 pint, of tuberose 1 pint, of orange-flower ½ pint; add extract of vanilla 2 oz.

ESSENCE OF LILY OF THE VALLEY. Mix the following extracts—of tuberose ½ pint, of jasmin 2 oz., of orange-flower 2 oz., of vanilla 3 oz., of cassia ¼ pint, of rose ¼ pint; add 3 drops of hydrocyanic acid. Keep together for a month, then bottle.

ESSENCE OF MAGNOLIA. Spirituous extract of orange-flower pomatum 1 pint, of rose pomatum 2 pints, of tuberose pomatum ½ pint, of violet pomatum ½ pint; essential oil of citron 2 drachms, and essential oil of almonds 10 drops.

ESSENCE OF MIGNONETTE. Digest 1 ℔ of pommade de rézéda in rectified spirit 1 pint for 14 days; filter off, and add 1 oz. of extrait d'ambré.

ESSENCE OF MOSS ROSE. Spirituous extract of French rose pomatum 1 quart, esprit de rose triple 1 pint, extract of orange-flower pomatum 1 pint, of ambergris ½ pint, and of musk 4 oz.

ESSENCE OF MYRTLE. Take the following extracts—of

vanilla ½ pint, of roses 1 pint, of orange-flower ½ pint, of tuberose ½ pint, of jasmin 2 oz. Mix, and allow to stand for a fortnight.

Essence of Musk. A tincture of musk, of various strength. The formula given above (tincture of musk) is that of the Dublin Pharmacopœia, 1826. Guibourt directs 1 part of musk to 12 of proof spirit. Other authorities direct a smaller quantity of musk. A French work gives the following—Musk in the bag cut small 6 oz., civet 1 oz., tincture of musk seed 7 pints; digest in the sun, or in a warm place for 2 months.

Essence of Patchouli. Oil of patchouly 1¼ oz., otto of rose ¼ oz., rectified spirit 1 gallon.

Essence of Rondeletia. Essence of bergamot, essence of lemon, oil of cloves, each 1 drachm, otto of roses 6 drops, rectified spirit a pint.

Essence Royale. Ambergris 1 dr., civet 15 gr., musk 30 gr., carbonate of potash 20 gr.; triturate together, and add oil of cinnamon 10 drops, oil of rhodium, and of neroli, 6 drops, otto of roses 6 drops, rectified spirit ¼ pint; digest, and filter.

Essence of Sweet Brier. Spirituous extracts of French rose-pomatum 1 pint, of cassia and orange-flowers, each ¼ pint, esprit de rose ¼ pint, with oils of neroli and lemon-grass, of each ½ dr.

Essence of Sweet Pea. Essences of tuberose, orange-flower, and rose-pomatum, each ½ pint, with essence of vanilla 1 oz.

Essence of Verbena. Essential oil of verbena 2 dr., rectified spirit 4 oz., essence of ambergris ½ dr., orange-flower water ½ oz.; mix. Another form is—Oil of verbena ½ oz., essence of vanilla 40 drops, rectified spirit 4 oz. Mix, and filter.

Essence of White Lilac. Spirituous extract of tuberose pomade 1 pint, of orange-flower pomade ¼ pint; add essential oil of almonds 3 drops, and extract of civet ½ oz.

Essences for Scenting Pomatums. *Millefleur:* Oil of lemon 3 oz., essence of ambergris 4 oz., oil of cloves 2 oz., oil of lavender 2 oz.—*Cowslip:* Essence of bergamot 16 oz., essence of lemon 8 oz., oil of cloves 4 oz., oil of orange-peel 2 oz., oil of jessamine 2 dr., eau de bouquet 2 oz., oil of bitter almonds 16 drops.—*For general use:* Essence of bergamot 16 oz., essence of lemon 8 oz., true oil of origanum and oil of cloves, each 2 oz., oil of orange-peel 1½ oz.

MISTURA ODORATA. Rectified spirit 48 oz., tincture of benzoin 4 oz., tincture of vanilla ¼ oz., tincture of musk ½ oz., balsam of Peru ½ oz., oil of cloves, of mace, and of cinnamon, each ½ oz., oil of bergamot 1 oz., oil of cedrat 2 oz.—GIESKE.

SCENT FOR SNUFF. Oil of lavender 2 dr., essence of lemon 4 dr., essence of bergamot 1 oz.; mix. [1 drachm with 8 oz. of fine Scotch snuff constitutes Queen's Snuff.]

[The following Essences, Spirits, and Waters, are given as specimens of some of the cheaper perfumes, as made in France.

ESSENCES (SPIRITUOUS.)

Essence (Spirituous) of Neroli. Spirit of wine ½ pint, orange-peel cut small 3 oz., orris-root in powder, 1 dr., musk 2 gr.; let it stand in a warm place for 3 days, and filter.

Essence of Lemon. Spirit of wine ½ pint, fresh lemon-peel 4 oz.; as above.

Essence of Bergamot. Spirit of wine ½ pint, bergamot-peel 4 oz.; as above.

Essence of Violets. Spirit of wine ½ pint, orris-root 1 oz.

Essence of Cedrat. Essence of bergamot (as above) 1 oz., essence of neroli 2 dr.

Essence of Jessamine. Essence of violets 1 oz., essence of cedrat 2 dr.

Essence of Musk. Spirit of wine ½ pint, musk 16 gr.

Essence of Ambergris. Spirit of wine ½ pint, ambergris 24 gr.

Essence of Cloves. Spirit of wine ½ pint, bruised cloves 1 oz.

Other essences in the same manner.

SPIRITS.

Spirit of Rose. Spirit of wine ½ pint, otto 6 drops.

Spirit of Jessamine. Spirit of wine ½ pint, essence of jessamine (as above) a drachm.

Spirit of Orange. Spirit of wine, essence of orange, or neroli, a drachm.

Spirit of Lavender. Spirit of wine ½ pint, essential oil of lavender a drachm.

Spirit of Musk. Spirit of wine ½ pint, essence of musk a drachm.

Others in a similar manner.

Simple Waters.

Rose Water. Distilled or rain water ½ pint, spirit of roses a drachm.

Jessamine Water, Musk Water, Violet, Orange-flower Water, &c., by adding a dr. of the above spirits to ½ pint of water.

AMMONIATED PERFUMES.

Ammoniated Cologne Water. A fragrant and reviving substitute for Spirit of Sal Volatile. Muriate of ammonia 5 dr., subcarbonate of potash 8 dr., eau de Cologne 12 oz., essential oil of cedrat and of bergamot, of each 15 drops (dissolved in an oz. of rectified spirit,) orange-flower water 8 oz.; mix, and carefully distil 15 or 16 oz.

Eau de Luce. Mastic 2 dr., rectified spirit 9 dr.; dissolve and add to the clear tincture 30 drops of oil of lavender, 10 drops of bergamot, and a pint of strong water of ammonia. This is more agreeable than the compound of the Pharmacopœia, which, however, should always be used when prescribed medicinally.

Essence for Smelling Bottles. 1. English oil of lavender and essence of bergamot, of each a dr., oil of orange-peel, or of cedrat, 8 drops, oil of cinnamon 4 drops, oil of neroli 2 drops, alcohol, and strongest water of ammonia, of each 2 oz. (or 4 oz. of strong ammoniated alcohol.)

2. Ammoniated alcohol 12 fluid oz., English oil of lavender, essence of bergamot and essence of lemon, of each a dr., cloves ½ dr., camphor ½ oz., macerate for a week, and filter.—Mr. Maggs.

3. Essence of ambergris and musk 4 dr., otto of rose

20 drops, oil of lavender 1 dr., ammoniated alcohol 10 oz.; mix, and add strongest liquor ammoniæ 10 oz.—PHARM. JOURNAL.

GODFREY'S SMELLING SALTS. Dr. PARIS says it is prepared by resubliming volatile salts with subcarbonate of potash and a little spirit of wine. It is usually scented with an alcoholic solution of essential oils.

ACETIC PERFUMES.

AROMATIC SPIRIT OF VINEGAR. 1. Strong acetic acid 16 oz.; camphor 1 oz.; when dissolved, add 1 oz. each of essential oils of cloves, lavender, and lemon. This is said to resemble HENRY'S.

2. Glacial acetic acid 8 oz., true oil of rosemary 20 gr., of bergamot 15 gr., of lavender 9 gr., of cloves 24 gr., neroli 4 gr., cinnamon 20; dissolve the oils in 2 dr. of rectified spirit. For another formula, see Pocket Formulary.

AROMATIC VINEGARS are made in France by infusing various flowers, &c., in distilled or finest wine vinegars, with or without the addition of spirit. Others are made by distillation. As they are seldom required in this country, a few examples will suffice.

ROSE VINEGAR. Red roses, picked and dried, ½ ℔, best vinegar 8 ℔; macerate for a fortnight, with occasional stirring, and strain; then filter.

LAVENDER VINEGAR. Fresh lavender-flowers 1 ℔, vinegar 12 ℔. Macerate as above. It is sometimes distilled, drawing off 8 ℔.

DISTILLED ROSE VINEGAR. Pale roses dried 2 ℔, distilled vinegar 8 ℔. Distil three-fourths by sandbath, and add 2 ℔ of spirit of roses. It is occasionally coloured with cochineal, and used as a cosmetic.

ORANGE-FLOWER VINEGAR. Fresh orange-flowers 1½ ℔, distilled vinegar 8 ℔, spirit of orange-flowers 1 ℔. Macerate for 12 days, strain, and filter.

VINAIGRE VIRGINAL. Benzoin in powder 2 oz., rectified spirit 8 oz., white vinegar 2 ℔. Digest the benzoin in the spirit for 6 days, strain, and add the vinegar to the residue; macerate for 6 days, decant, and add to it the tincture. The next day filter. It is chiefly used as a cosmetic.

Vinaigre de Cologne. To each pint of eau de Cologne add an ounce of strong acetic acid.

Vinaigre de Jouvence. Spirit of cucumber 4 oz., spirit of storax 2 ℔, strong vinegar 8 ℔.

Vinaigre de Flore. Equal parts of rose vinegar, vinaigre virginal, and orange-flower vinegar.

Vinaigre de quatre Voleurs. Thieves' vinegar. Dried tops of large and small (pontic) wormwood, rosemary, sage, mint, rue, lavender flowers, of each 2 oz.: calamus root, cinnamon, cloves, nutmeg, garlic, of each ¼ oz.; camphor ½ oz., concentrated acetic acid 2 oz., strong vinegar 8 ℔. Macerate the herbs, &c., in the vinegar for a fortnight, strain, press, and add the camphor dissolved in the acetic acid.

POT POURRI; SCENTED POWDERS; SACHETS OR SCENT BAGS; SCENT BALLS; PASTILS, &c.

Pot Pourri. 1. Gather in the season the petals of the most fragrant kinds of roses (with which other flowers may be mixed, at pleasure, in smaller proportion;) spread them out to dry in the sun, or in a warm room, sprinkle a little salt on them, and put them into a jar, in which they are to be kept covered up till wanted for use. Take of these rose leaves 4 oz.; dried lavender flowers 8 oz.; vanilla, cloves, storax, and benzoin, all bruised, of each 1 dr.; ambergris 20 gr., otto of rose 20 drops. Mix.

2. Calamus root, yellow sanders, of each 1 oz., vanilla 1 dr., musk 8 gr., ambergris 8 gr., cascarilla 1 oz., orris root 3 oz., cinnamon 1 oz., lavender flowers 1 oz., styrax 2 dr., benzoin 2 dr., cloves 2 dr., coriander seeds 1 oz., nutmegs 2 dr., otto of rose 20 drops, oil of neroli 10 drops. The dry ingredients to be coarsely bruised. Mix.

3. French. Take the petals of the pale and red roses, pinks, violets, moss rose, orange-flower, lily of the valley, acacia flowers, clove-gilliflowers, mignionette, heliotrope, jonquils; with a *small* proportion of the flowers of myrtle, balm, rosemary, and thyme; spread them out for some days, and as they become dry, put them into

a jar with alternate layers of dry salt, mixed with orris powder, till the vessel is full. Close it for a month, then stir the whole up, and moisten it with rose water.

4. Orris-root 16 oz., dried acacia flowers 8 oz., dried bergamot-peel 2 oz., musk seed ¼ oz., cloves ¼ oz.; pound them together.

5. Dry rose leaves quickly on a wicker tray, in a warm place. To a pint of the petals add powdered orris 2 oz., pimento ½ oz., cascarilla ¼ oz., musk 2 grs., otto of rose 2 drops, bruised cloves ¼ oz.

Sachets or Scent Bags. The pot pourri No. 2 or 4 may be put into bags, alone, or with any perfume to increase the strength. Or coarsely powdered patchouli (an herb of the Pogostemon genus) may be used, with any other perfume. Or the bags may be filled with carded cotton mixed with any of the following scented powders.

Scented Powders, Balls, &c.

Rose. Powdered starch 3 oz., carmine to colour, otto of roses 8 drops, orris powder 1 oz.

Violet. Orris powder 4 oz., essence of bergamot 20 drops, essence of ambergris 20 drops.

Poudre de Chypre. Oak moss is macerated in clean water for a day or two, and strongly pressed in a cloth; it is then moistened with rose water mixed with a third of orange-flower water for two days, pressed, and pulverized. It serves as a basis for other perfumes, the power of which it is said to increase.

Poudre à la Mousseline. Orris 16 oz., coriander-seed 8 oz., musk-seed 2 oz., cinnamon, cloves, and sandal-wood, each 1 oz., star aniseed ¼ oz., mace, ginger, and violet ebony, of each 2 oz.; beat them to a powder, and pass through a sieve.

Poudre à l'Œillet. Red roses 48 oz., orris 48 oz., cloves 6 oz., bergamot peel 20 oz., musk seed 24 oz., cinnamon 6 oz., long cyperus 6 oz., pale roses 26 oz., dried acacia flowers, orange flowers, and clove stalks, of each 8 oz.

Poudre à la Marechale. Oak-moss in powder 2 ℔, plain starch powder 1 ℔, cloves 1 oz., calamus 2 oz., cyperus 2 oz., rotten oak-wood powder 2 oz.; mix.—Gray.

Portugal. Dried orange-peel 1 oz., dried bergamot peel ½ oz., cloves 4 oz., storax 1 dr., ambergris 8 gr., benzoin a drachm, musk-seed a scruple, musk 4 gr.

SCENTED BALLS, MEDALLIONS, &c. *Pastilles de Toilette odorantes.* These consist of perfumed powders made into a paste, and moulded to any desired form before drying. The above scent powders beaten up with mucilage of tragacanth will answer the purpose; or the following:—

1. Beat the fresh petals of red roses in an *iron* mortar to a smooth paste, with a few drops of essence of ambergris, or other suitable perfume. It becomes sufficiently smooth to take a polish.

2. Powdered orris, oak-moss, and poudre de mousseline, of each 1 oz.; lamp black, or other colour, q. s. Form into a stiff paste with a jelly made of 6 dr. of isinglass, 2 of tragacanth, and boiling water q. s. Make it into beads by means of a pill-machine, or into any ornamental form by moulds.

3. Jessamine flowers 1 oz., powdered gum tragacanth ½ oz., vermilion 2 oz.

4. Yellow sanders, cyperus, cloves, balsam of Peru, of each 2 dr., benzoin and styrax, of each ½ oz., musk and civet, of each 10 gr., oil of cinnamon 5 drops, oil of rhodium 15 drops, essence of jessamine 1 dr., neroli 20 drops, ivory black 1½ oz., Paris plaster 2 oz., mucilage of tragacanth, made with rose-water q. s. As the last.

PASTILS FOR BURNING. 1. Yellow sanders 3 oz., styrax 4 oz., benzoin 3 oz., olibanum 6 oz., cascarilla 6 oz., ambergris 1 dr., Peruvian balsam 2 dr., myrrh 1½ oz., nitre 1½ oz., oil of cinnamon 20 drops, oil of cloves ½ dr., otto 30 to 60 drops, oil of lavender 1½ dr., balsam of Tolu 1½ oz., camphor ½ oz., strong acetic acid 2 oz., charcoal 3 ℔; mix, s. a., and beat into a paste with mucilage of tragacanth, and form into conical pastils. A second and third quality may be made by using, respectively, 4 and 5 ℔ instead of 3 ℔ of charcoal. These are highly approved, but rather expensive.

2. (*Clous fumans* of the French Codex.) Benzoin 2 oz., balsam of Tolu ½ oz., labdanum 1 dr., yellow

sanders ½ oz., light charcoal 6 oz., nitre ¼ oz., mucilage of tragacanth q. s. Reduce the substances to powder, and form into a paste with the mucilage, and divide into small cones with a tripod base.

3. Powdered cascarilla 8 oz., benzoin 4 oz., yellow sanders 2 oz., styrax calamita 2 oz., olibanum 2 oz., charcoal 3 ℔, nitre 1½ oz., mucilage of tragacanth q. s.

4. Benzoin 1 oz., cascarilla 1 oz., myrrh 8 scruples, oil of nutmeg 4 scruples, oil of cloves 4 scruples, nitre ½ oz., charcoal 6 oz., mucilage of tragacanth q. s.—Dr. Paris.

Incense. 1. Styrax 2½ oz., benzoin 12 oz., musk 15 grains, burnt sugar ½ oz., frankincense 2½ oz., gum tragacanth 1½ oz., rose water sufficient to form a mass; to be divided into small tablets.—Mr. Astley.

2. Powdered cascarilla 2 oz., myrrh, styrax, benzoin, thus, Burgundy pitch, each 1 oz. Mix.—Mr. Atkins (Ph. Journal.)

Mouth Pastils. Dry compounds for perfuming or correcting the breath.

Cachou Aromatisé. The basis of these compounds, as the name implies, was originally *catechu*, with which various odoriferous substances were combined. The catechu, however, is now often omitted. The following are some of the most approved forms:—

1. Extract of liquorice 3 oz., oil of cloves 1½ dr., oil of cinnamon 15 drops; mix, and divide into one-grain pills, and silver them.

2. (M. Chevallier's.) Chocolate powder, and ground coffee, of each 1½ oz., prepared charcoal 1 oz., sugar 1 oz., vanilla (pulverized with the sugar) 1 oz., mucilage q. s. Make into lozenges of any form, of which 6 to 8 may be used daily to disinfect the breath.

3. *Cachou de Bologne.* Bologna Catechu. Extract of liquorice, 3 oz., water 3 oz.; dissolve by heat in a water-bath, and add catechu 1 oz., gum Arabic ½ oz.; evaporate to the consistence of an extract, and add (in powder) ½ dr. each of mastic, cascarilla, charcoal, and orris: remove from the fire, and add oil of peppermint ½ dr., essence of ambergris and essence of musk each 5 drops;

roll it flat on an oiled marble slab, and cut it into very small lozenges. [Or it may be rolled into small pills, and silvered. They are chiefly used by smokers.]

4. Catechu 7 dr., orris powder 40 grains, sugar 3 oz., oil of rosemary (or of peppermint, cloves, or cinnamon,) 4 drops, or q. s. Proceed as for the last.

5. *Cachou Aromatisé.* Extract of liquorice and water, of each 3½ oz.; dissolve in a water-bath, and add Bengal catechu in powder, 462 grains, and gum Arabic in powder 231 grains; evaporate to an extract, and then incorporate the following substances, first reduced to a fine powder:—Mastic, cascarilla, charcoal, and orris root, of each 30 grains; melt the mass to a proper consistence, remove it from the fire, and then add English oil of peppermint 30 drops, tinctures of ambergris and musk, of each 5 drops; pour it now on an oiled slab, and spread it out, by means of a roller, to the thickness of a sixpenny piece. When cool, apply some folds of blotting paper to absorb any adherent oil, moisten the surfaces with water, and cover it with sheets of silver leaf. Allow it to dry, and finally divide into thin strips and these again into small pieces, about the size of a fenugreek seed.—(JOURNAL DE PHARMACIE.)

PASTILS OR LOZENGES, with chlorine, for disinfecting the breath. 1. Sugar flavoured with vanilla 1 oz., powdered tragacanth 20 gr., liquid chloride of soda q. s., any essential oil 2 drops. Form a paste, and divide into lozenges of 15 gr. each.

2. Dry chloride of lime 2 dr., sugar 8 oz., starch 1 oz., gum tragacanth 1 dr., carmine 2 gr. Form into small lozenges.

SKIN COSMETICS.

WASHES FOR THE FACE, &c.

Aqua Cosmetica. Cosmetic Lotion. 1. Emulsion of bitter almonds 3 oz.; rose and orange-flower water, of each 4 oz.; borax 1 dr., tincture of benzoin 2 dr.; mix.—Dr. Copland.

2. Elder-flower water a pint, borax ½ oz., eau de Cologne 1 oz.; mix.

Kalydor. The following is said to resemble Kalydor and Gowland's lotion. Bitter almonds blanched 1 oz., corrosive sublimate 8 gr., rose-water 16 oz.

Milk of Roses. Sweet almonds 5 oz., bitter almonds 1 oz., rose-water 2½ pints, white curd soap ½ oz., oil of almonds ½ oz., spermaceti 2 oz., white wax ½ oz., English oil of lavender 20 drops, otto of roses 20 drops, rectified spirit a pint. Blanch the almonds, and beat them with the soap and a little of the rose-water. Melt together the oil of almonds, spermaceti, and white wax, and mix with the former into a cream, and strain it through fine muslin. Then add gradually the remaining rose-water, and lastly the spirit, with the essential oils dissolved therein.

2. A common kind is made by mixing 1 oz. of fine olive oil with 10 drops of oil of tartar, and a pint of rose-water.

3. Bitter almonds 6 dr., sweet almonds 12 dr., blanch, dry, and beat up with 1 dr. of Castile soap; gradually adding 15 gr. of spermaceti, 30 gr. of white wax, and a dr. of almond oil, melted together. When thoroughly incorporated add gradually six drops of otto of roses dissolved in 6 oz. of rectified spirit, and 14 oz. of distilled water.

Milk of Cucumbers. In the same manner as milk of roses, substituting juice of cucumbers for the rose-water.

Milk of Houseleek. As milk of roses, No. 1, substituting expressed juice of houseleek for a pint of the rose water.

Alibert's Cosmetic. Cucumber pomade (see below) 3 oz., almond soap, 1 oz., rose-water a quart. Mix the pomade and soap, and add the rose-water gradually.

Siemmerling's Cosmetic. Make an emulsion with 1 oz. of sweet almonds, ½ oz. bitter almonds, black-cherry-water 10 oz.; and add bichloride of mercury 5 gr., tincture of benzoin 5 dr., lemon juice ½ oz.

Withering's (Dr.) Cosmetic. An infusion of horseradish in milk.

Lait Virginal. Virgin's Milk. Simple tincture of benzoin 2 dr., orange-flower water 8 oz. It may be varied by using rose or elder-flower water.

Lait de Fraicheur. Double rose-water 8 oz., tincture of benzoin 4 dr., balsam of Mecca ½ oz.

Schubarth's Cosmetic Emulsion. Almond emulsion (made with rose-water) 8 oz., tincture of benzoin 3 dr.

Italian Cosmetic Wash. Melilot water 12 oz., tincture of benzoin 2 dr.

Augustin's. Rose water 8 oz., salt of tartar 2 dr., tincture of benzoin 3 dr.

Kittoe's Lotion for Freckles. Muriate of ammonia 1 dr., spring water a pint, lavender-water 2 dr. Apply with a sponge 2 or 3 times a day.

Lemon Cream for Sunburns, Freckles, &c. Sweet cream 1 oz., new milk 8 oz., juice of 1 lemon, brandy, or eau de Cologne 1 oz., alum 1 oz., sugar 1 dr. Boil and skim. Buttermilk is used for the same purpose.

Lemon Embrocation, for Freckles, &c. Borax 15 gr., lemon juice 1 oz., sugar candy ½ dr.; mix the powders with the juice, and let them stand in the bottle, shaking occasionally, till they are dissolved.

PASTES, POMMADES, COLD CREAM, LIP-SALVE, &c.

Pommade de Beauté. Melt together, in an earthen vessel placed in hot water, white wax 1½ dr., spermaceti

2 dr., oil of sweet almonds ½ oz., virgin olive oil ½ oz., oil of poppies ½ oz.; beat them with a few drops of balsam of Peru.

CUCUMBER POMATUM, for softening and cooling the skin. Clarified lard 4 ℔, veal suet 1 ℔, juice of cucumbers 3 ℔; melt the two former together, then beat it up assiduously with the juice. Next day, pour off the juice that has separated, and add the same quantity of fresh to the melted pomade. Repeat this six times, or until the pomade is sufficiently imbued with the odour of cucumbers. Then melt the pomade by a water-bath, and mix with it 3 dr. of powdered white starch; let it settle, and before it is too cold, pour it off into small pots, taking care not to disturb the dregs.

POMMADE D'HEBE. Incorporate together juice of lily-bulbs 2 oz., Narbonne honey 2 oz., white wax 1 oz., rose-water 3 dr.; melt the wax with a gentle heat, and add the other ingredients. To be applied at night, and not wiped off till morning. To remove wrinkles. Probably cod-liver oil, used externally and internally, would be a more successful though less agreeable remedy.

PATE DIVINE DE VENUS. Mix equal parts of washed lard, fresh butter, and white honey; add balsam of Mecca and otto of roses, to perfume.

POMMADE DE NINON. Oil of sweet almonds 4 oz., washed lard 3 oz., juice of houseleek 3 oz.; mix. Softening and cooling.

POMMADE EN CREME. Melt together 1 dr. each of white wax and spermaceti, and add oil of sweet almonds 2 oz.; pour it into a warm mortar, and gradually stir in ½ oz. of rose or other perfumed water, and 1 dr. of tincture of tolu.

LEMON CREAM. Melt together 2 dr. of spermaceti and 1 oz. of oil of almonds; and as it cools stir in 16 drops of essence of lemon.

COLD CREAM. 1. Oil of Almonds 16 oz., white wax, 4 oz.; melt together in an earthen vessel, and when nearly cold, stir in, by little and little, 12 oz. of rose-water.

2. Melt together white wax 2 oz., oil of almonds 8 oz., and stir in 4 oz. of rose-water. Next day, add 6 drops of otto of roses.

3. White wax and spermaceti, of each ½ oz., oil of almonds 4 oz., orange-flower water 2 oz.; mix, s. a.

4. As No. 3, but without the orange-flower water.

5. Lard 16 oz., white wax 2 oz., olive oil 1 oz., magistery of bismuth 1 oz.

6. White wax 1 oz., almond or olive oil 4 oz., rose-water 1 oz., glycerine 2 dr.

N. B. Those cold creams are generally preferred for present use which contain rose or other water, but they keep longer without them.

GRANULATED COLD CREAM. Melt together 1 oz. each of white wax and spermaceti, with 3 oz. of almond oil; when a little cooled, pour the mixture into a large Wedgewood mortar previously warmed, and containing about a pint of warm water. Stir briskly until the cream is well divided, add sufficient otto of rose to scent it, and pour the whole suddenly into a clean vessel containing 8 or 10 pints of cold water. Throw the whole on muslin, and shake out as much water as possible.—Mr. OWEN, Dublin.

POMMADE DIVINE. Put 3 ℔ of beef marrow into an earthen vessel, and cover it with cold water, changing the water daily for a few days, and using rose water the last day; press out the water and add to the marrow styrax calamita, benzoin, Chio turpentine, each 4 oz.; orris powder 1 oz.; powdered cinnamon, cloves, nutmeg, of each ½ oz. Place them in a well-tinned vessel in a water-bath, and keep the water boiling for 3 hours; then strain.

ALMOND PASTE, for the skin. 1. Powdered bitter almonds 4 oz., white of egg 1 oz., beat them well together to a smooth paste, with equal parts of spirit of wine and rose-water.

2. Sweet and bitter almonds, blanched, of each 2 oz.; spermaceti 2 dr.; oil of almonds ½ oz.; Windsor soap ½ oz. rose-water 1 oz. or q. s.; otto of roses, and oil of bergamot, of each 12 drops.

3. (Camphorated.) To either of the above add 2 dr. of powdered camphor. A few drops of oil of bitter almonds may be substituted for the otto and bergamot.

4. (French.) Blanch 12 oz. of bitter almonds, and

beat them in a mortar with a small quantity of rose or other water to a smooth paste; then add 7 oz. of rice flour, 3 oz. of bean flour, 1 oz. of orris powder, and when perfectly mixed, ½ oz. of carbonate of potash dissolved in rose-water; again beat together, and add 3 oz. of spirituous essence of jessamine, and 2 drops of oil of rhodium, and one of neroli.

ALMOND AND HONEY PASTE. Fine honey may be added to either of the preceding; or mix 16 oz. of clarified honey with 16 oz. of bitter almond powder; and add gradually, in alternate portions, 32 oz. of oil of almonds, and the yolks of 5 eggs.

HONEY PASTE. *Pâte au Miel.* It is sometimes made as the last; or by mixing clarified honey with cold cream, or some similar compound.

CAMPHOR BALLS, for rubbing on the hands, after washing them, to prevent chaps, &c. 1. Melt 3 dr. of spermaceti, and 4 dr. of white wax, with 1 oz. of almond oil, and stir in 3 dr. of powdered camphor. Pour the compound into small gallipots, so as to form hemispherical cakes. They may be coloured with alkanet, &c.

2. Lard 2 oz., white wax 2 oz., camphor ½ oz.

3. Spermaceti 3 oz., white wax 1 oz., olive oil 4 oz.; melt together, and add 1½ oz. of powdered camphor, and stir it well.

4. Melt 3 dr. of spermaceti, and 4 dr. of white wax, with 1 oz. of almond oil, and stir in 3 dr. of powdered camphor.

CAMPHOR ICE. Melt 1 dr. of spermaceti with 1 oz. of almond oil, and add 1 dr. of powdered camphor.

ALMOND POWDER. (Cosmetic.) This is prepared by grinding the marc or cake left after expressing the oil from sweet or bitter almonds. It is sometimes perfumed, and mixed with other ingredients. It is used for cleaning the skin, and is less irritating than soap.

ALMOND WASH POWDER. 1. Almond powder (from expressed bitter almonds) 16 oz., rice flour 2 oz., powdered soap 1 oz., orris powder 1 oz., bergamot or other scent q. p.

2. Almond powder (as above) 16 oz., powdered ben-

zoin ¼ oz., oil of bitter almonds 10 drops. For cleaning the hands and removing any unpleasant smell. To render it more detergent 4 oz. of fine sand, or powdered pumice-stone, may be added.

ROSE LIP SALVE. 1. Oil of almonds 3 oz., alkanet ½ oz.; digest with a gentle heat, and filter. Melt 1½ oz. white wax and ½ oz. spermaceti with the filtered oil, stir it until it begins to thicken, and add from 12 to 36 drops of otto of roses.

2. White wax 1 oz., oil of sweet almonds 2 oz., alkanet 1 dr.; digest till coloured, strain, and add 6 drops of otto of roses.

PERUVIAN LIP SALVE. As either of the above, substituting 20 or 30 drops of Peruvian balsam for the otto; 8 drops of oil of lavender may be added.

GRAPE LIP SALVE. *Pommade au raisin pour les levres.* Put into a glazed earthen pipkin ½ ℔ of fresh butter, ¼ ℔ fine yellow wax, 1 oz. of alkanet, and 3 bunches of black grapes; boil together, and strain without pressure through linen.

FRENCH LIP SALVE. Lard 16 oz., white wax 2 oz., nitre and alum in fine powder, of each ½ oz., alkanet to colour.

GERMAN LIP SALVE. Butter of cacao ½ oz., oil of almonds ¼ oz.; melt together with a gentle heat, and add 6 drops of essence of lemon.

GANTS COSMETIQUES. These are white kid gloves, which have been turned inside out, and brushed over with a melted compound of wax, oil, lard, balsam, &c. The Peruvian lip salve, without the alkanet, may answer the purpose. *For softening the hands.*

FACE PAINTS. FARDS.

FINE CARMINE (prepared from cochineal) is used alone, or reduced with starch, &c. And also the colouring matter of safflower, and other vegetable colours, in the form of pink saucers, &c.

ROUGE is prepared from carmine, and the colouring matter of safflower, by mixing them with finely levigated French chalk or talc, generally with the addition of a few drops of olive or almond oil. Sometimes fine white starch is used as the reducing ingredient. It is used in the form of powder, pomade, and *crepons*,—the latter being pieces of crape imbued with the colouring matter. For common purposes vermilion is used; and it is sometimes prepared for this purpose by mixing with a few drops of almond oil and of mucilage of tragacanth, placing the mixture in rouge pots, and drying it by a very gentle heat.

ALMOND BLOOM. Boil 1 oz. of Brazil dust in 3 pints of distilled water, and strain; add 6 dr. of isinglass, 2 dr. of cochineal, 1 oz. of alum, and 3 dr. of borax; boil again, and strain through a fine cloth.—GRAY'S SUPPLEMENT.

FACE WHITES. One of most innocent kind is prepared from Venetian talc, or French chalk, finely levigated. These are sometimes calcined, to increase their whiteness; but this diminishes their unctuosity and adhesiveness. Digestion with vinegar, and subsequent washing, are practised for the same purpose. Flake white (a fine variety of white lead) was formerly much used; but is now generally condemned as unsafe; it is also liable to become brown under certain circumstances. Pearl or bismuth white (magistery of bismuth*) is less injurious when pure, but is subject to the latter inconvenience. M. THENARD recommends oxide of zinc, with an equal weight of French chalk prepared by vinegar. Magnesia is said to be employed by the American ladies. White starch is used for the same purpose.

TOILET SOAPS, &c.

As the retail druggists and perfumers do not generally make their own soap in the first instance, it is only

* For this purpose a little muriatic acid is added to the solution of the metal in nitric acid, and the magistery is precipitated by a small quantity of water; or the nitric solution is mixed with a weak solution of sea salt. Dr. Ure states that the precipitate thus acquires a more pearly lustre.

necessary to mention the means by which the soap, as it comes from the manufacturers, is prepared for the toilet.

SCENTED SOAPS, in general. Cut the best white curd soap (or, for some kinds, palm soap) into thin shavings and place it in a copper-vessel, with sufficient distilled water, and heat it by a water-bath till the whole is uniformly liquefied. Let it cool to 135 F.; then add the colouring matters and perfumes. On the large scale these additions may be mixed with the liquid soap at the maker's, before it is poured into the frames. The quantity of perfume used must depend on the price at which it is to be sold.

ALMOND SOAP. To one hundred weight of the best hard white soap, melted as above, add 20 oz. of essential oil of bitter almonds. (Soap really made from expressed almond oil is, we apprehend, rarely met with in commerce.)

SAVON AU BOUQUET. Melt 60 ℔ of white curd soap as above, and 8 oz. of oil of bergamot, 1½ oz. each of oils of cloves, sassafras, and thyme, ¾ oz. of neroli, and 14 oz. or q. s. brown ochre.

ROSE SOAP. Put into a copper vessel, placed in boiling water, 20 ℔ of white curd soap, and 30 ℔ of olive oil soap, both in thin shavings; add 5 ℔ of soft water, or rose-water; keep the heat below boiling till the soap is uniformly liquefied, then add 12 oz. of finely sifted vermilion, or enough to produce the required tint. Withdraw it from the fire, and when sufficiently cool add 3½ oz. of otto of roses, ½ oz. of oil of cloves, ½ oz. of oil of cinnamon, and 2½ oz. bergamot. For a cheaper article use less perfume.

WINDSOR SOAP. This is said to be made with lard. In France they use lard with a portion of olive or bleached palm oil. Dr. PEREIRA states that it is made with one part of olive oil to nine of tallow. But a great part of what is sold is probably only curd (tallow) soap, scented with oil of caraway and bergamot. The brown is probably coloured with burnt sugar, or umber.

HONEY SOAP. White curd soap 1½ ℔, brown Windsor soap ½ ℔; cut them into thin shavings, and liquefy as directed above for scented soaps; then add 4 oz. of honey, and keep it melted till most of the water is evaporated; then remove from the fire, and, when cool enough, add any essential oil. According to Piesse, the *honey soap* usually sold consists of fine yellow soap perfumed with oil of citronella.

FLOATING SOAPS. These are made by liquefying, as described above, 30 ℔ of oil soap with about 5 ℔ of water; and agitating the mixture, by a suitable wooden apparatus turned by a handle till the froth rises to the top of the vessel. It is then poured into frames to cool. They are variously perfumed and coloured.

TRANSPARENT SOAP. Cut fine white curd soap into thin shavings, and dry them with a gentle heat till they can be reduced to powder. Put 2 ℔ of this powder into a water-bath with 5 or 6 pints of rectified spirit of wine, and heat it gently (taking care that the water does not quite boil) till the solution is complete; add the perfume, and pour into the frames. When cold, cut it into squares. They must be kept some time in a dry place before they can attain their full degree of transparency. By using a still, most of the spirit may be recovered for future use.

WASH BALLS. *Savonettes.* These are made from various kinds of soap, usually with the addition of powdered starch or hair powder, or of rice flour, together with perfuming and colouring ingredients. They are formed into spherical balls by taking a mass of the prepared soap in the left hand, and a conical drinking glass with rather thin edges in the right. By turning the glass and ball of soap in every direction the rounded form is soon given; when dry the surface is scraped to render it more smooth and even. One or two examples of this kind of soap will suffice.

COMMON, OR LEMON WASH BALLS. Cut 6 ℔ of soap into very small pieces; melt it with a pint of water in which 6 lemons have been boiled. When melted, withdraw the soap from the fire, and add 3 ℔ of powdered starch, and a little essence of lemon: knead the whole into a paste, and form into balls of the desired size.

CREAM WASH BALLS. White curd soap 7 ℔, powdered starch 1 ℔; water, or rose-water, q. s. Beat the whole together, and form into balls.—GRAY'S SUPPLEMENT.

CAMPHOR WASH BALLS. White soap 1 lb, spermaceti 1 oz., water q. s.; melt together, and add 1 oz. of powdered camphor.

MRS. SYMOND'S SOAP PASTE, for the hands. Best soft soap (from olive oil and potash if procurable) 16 oz., spermaceti 4 oz., best olive oil 1 oz., camphor ¼ oz., rectified spirit ½ oz., soft water 1 pint, essence of lemon ½ oz., M. S. A. With 8 oz. of pumice-stone, powdered and sifted through fine book muslin, it forms sand soap paste.

POWDERED SOAP. Any of the hard soaps may be pulverized, if first cut into thin shavings, and kept at a gentle heat till sufficiently dry. This process renders the soap more mild.

SHAVING POWDER. Melt together in a water-bath 1 lb of white soap with 1 oz. of powdered spermaceti and ¼ oz. of chlorate of potash dissolved in a little water, or rose water. Pour the liquefied soap into a shallow mould; when solidified shave it fine and dry as above.

SHAVING PASTE. 1. Melt together 1 dr. each of spermaceti, white wax, and almond oil; beat it up with 2 oz. of the best white soap, and a little lavender or Cologne water.

2. Naples soap, beaten up with sufficient powdered soap to form a stiff paste.

3. White soft soap 4 oz., powdered Castile soap 1 oz., oil of olives or almonds ¼ oz.

SHAVING LIQUID. Essence of soap. 1. White soap 3 oz., proof spirit 8 oz., distilled water 4 oz., carbonate of potash 1 dr., essence of lemon q. s. Dissolve the soap without heat, and add the potash and essence.

2. (Italian essence of soap.) White curd or Windsor soap 10 parts, rectified spirit 34 parts, rose or orange-flower water 34 parts. Digest with a gentle heat and filter.

3. Naples soap, or white soft soap, 16 oz., oil of olives ½ oz., gum benzoin 1 dr., rectified spirit 24 oz. Digest. Rub a few drops on the beard, followed by warm water.

HAIR COSMETICS.

HAIR POWDER. The basis of hair powder is finely powdered starch. It is variously scented, and was formerly tinted with various colours. The plain and violet hair powders are now principally used. The latter is perfumed with orris powder, or essence of violets, usually with the addition of bergamot, &c. GRAY gives the following species for scenting hair powder:—Powdered orris 1 ℔, essence of bergamot 12 oz., oil of neroli 1 dr., musk 1 scruple. Hair powder is also perfumed with jessamine, roses, &c., by mixing the flowers with plain powder for 2 or 3 days, stirring the mixture twice or thrice a day, and then sifting out the powder from the flowers.

COMPOUNDS TO PROMOTE THE GROWTH OF THE HAIR.

POMADES FOR THE CURE OF BALDNESS.

1. DUPUYTREN'S POMADE. The recipe given by BATEMAN and RENNIE for this celebrated preparation—viz., Almond oil, lard, suet, and essential oils, is remarkable as entirely omitting the active ingredient. It is probable that the preparation first employed by M. DUPUYTREN was more simple in its form than what he subsequently adopted, but *cantharides* was always the essential constituent. The first formula we met with was—Tincture of cantharides (made according to the Paris Codex, 1 part of flies to 8 of proof spirit) 1 part, lard 9 parts. The following are said more nearly to represent the compound in its improved and more elegant form. M. CAP prescribes—Beef marrow 2 oz., spirituous extract of cantharides (made by evaporating the above tincture) 8 gr., rose oil 1 dr., essence of lemon 50 drops. M. FONTAINE

directs—Beef marrow 4 oz., calomel 2½ dr., extract of cantharides 18 gr., attar of roses 2 drops. But the following, by M. RECLUZ, is said to have been acknowledged by DUPUYTREN as the true formula:—Beef marrow 6 oz., nervine balsam* 2 oz., Peruvian balsam 2 oz., oil of almonds 1½ oz., extract of cantharides 16 gr.; melt the marrow and nervine balsam with the oil, strain, add the balsam of Peru, and lastly the extract, dissolved in a drachm of rectified spirit. M. GUIBOURT says that no better than the following can be used:—Beef marrow 1 oz., nervine balsam 1 oz., rose oil 1 dr., extract of cantharides (dissolved in spirit) 6 gr. These pomades should be rubbed on the scalp once or twice a day for some weeks. If any soreness is produced, it should be less frequently applied.

2. POMMADE CONTRE L'ALOPÉCIE. Fresh lemon juice 1 dr., extract of bark (by cold water) 2 dr., marrow 2 oz., tincture of cantharides (as above) 1 dr., oil of lemon 20 drops, oil of bergamot 10 drops; mix. First wash the head with soap and water, with a little eau de Cologne; then rub it dry. Next morning rub in a small lump of pomade, and repeat it daily. In 4 or 5 weeks the cure of baldness is effected.—Dr. SCHNEIDER.

3. CAZENAVE'S REMEDY FOR BALDNESS. Beef marrow 1 oz., tincture of cantharides (as above) 1 dr., powdered cinnamon 1 dr. To be applied night and morning, the head being first washed with salt and water. Keep the hair short.

4. Dr. CATTELL'S is the same, substituting 10 drops each of oils of origanum and bergamot for cinnamon.

5. Beef marrow 1 oz., castor oil ½ oz., tincture of cantharides 1 dr., essential oil of bitter almonds and of lemon, each 12 drops.

6. Beef marrow 3 dr., almond oil 1 dr., sulphate of quinine 15 gr., otto 2 drops.—SOUBEIRAN.

7. Prepared lard 2 oz., white wax 2 dr.; melt together, remove from the fire, and add 2 dr. balsam of Tolu,

* This is made by melting together 4 oz. each of beef marrow and oil of mace, and adding 2 dr. of Balsam of tolu, and 1 dr. each of oil of cloves and camphor, dissolved in ½ oz. rectified spirit.

20 drops of oil of rosemary: and in chronic cases 1 dr. of tincture of cantharides.—Dr. Neligan.

8. Camphor 1 scruple, citrine ointment 2 dr., spermaceti cerate 6 dr.; mix. To be applied every night.

9. Bate's *Unguentum Criniscum.* Labdanum 6 dr., bear's-grease 2 oz., honey ½ oz., powdered southernwood 3 dr., ashes of reed-root 1½ dr., oil of nutmeg 1 dr., balsam of Peru 3 dr.; mix. Let the bald part be first rubbed with an onion till it is red, then apply the ointment. It should be used daily, or oftener, for 5 or 6 weeks.

10. Box leaves 2 oz., southernwood 2 oz., lard, marrow, or bear's-grease 8 oz.; digest together by the heat of a water-bath, and strain.

11. *Bear's-grease.* The most approved consists of 2 parts of prepared bear's fat, with one of beef marrow, scented at pleasure. We have placed this, on the ground of common report, among the preparations which may possess some efficacy, but reserve the compounds usually sold under this name for the Pomatums. See below.

12. *Pommade Philocome.* Powdered cinchona ½ dr.; oil of almonds 2 dr., beef marrow 6 dr., oil of bergamot 6 drops, balsam of Peru 20 drops; mix.—Dorvault.

LIQUID COMPOUNDS FOR THE CURE AND PREVENTION OF BALDNESS.

1. Dr. Locock's *Lotion.* Oil of mace (expressed oil of nutmeg) ½ oz., olive oil 2 dr., water of ammonia ½ dr., spirit of rosemary 1 oz., rose-water 2½ oz.; mix. [Mr. Astley recommends the following modification: Oil of mace ½ oz., olive oil 2 dr., oil of rosemary 4 drops; incorporate them carefully, then add gradually 3¼ oz. of rose-water, 2 dr. of solution of carbonate of ammonia, and 2 dr. of rectified spirit.]

2. Mr. Erasmus Wilson's. Eau de Cologne 2 oz., tincture of cantharides 2 dr., oil of rosemary and oil of lavender, of each 10 drops.

3. Mr. Acton's. Equal parts of rectified spirit, castor oil, and eau de Cologne.

4. Mr. ACTON'S, *stronger*. Equal parts of honey-water and tincture of cantharides.

5. Tincture of cantharides 3 dr., acetate of copper 3 gr., oil of almonds and castor oil, of each a fluid oz., with any essential oil to scent it. A small quantity to be applied to the roots of the hair every morning.

6. Vinegar of cantharides (Lond. Pharm.) ½ oz., eau de Cologne 1 oz., rose-water 1 oz.; mix.

7. Castor oil, lavender-water, and tincture of cantharides, in equal quantities.

8. *American Shampoo Liquor*. Rum 3 quarts, spirit of wine 1 pint, water 1 pint, tincture of cantharides ½ oz., carbonate of ammonia ½ oz., salt of tartar 1 oz. Rub it on, and afterwards wash with water. By omitting the salt of tartar it nearly resembles balm of Colombia.

9. Dr. LANDERER'S. Bay leaves 2 oz., cloves ¼ oz., spirit of lavender 4 oz., spirit of thyme 4 oz.; digest for 6 days, filter, and add ½ oz. of ether. To be rubbed on every morning.

10. Put into a still 4 ℔ of honey, 12 handfuls of the tendrils of vine, and the same of rosemary tops; distil very slowly till the liquor begins to taste sour.

11. Dr. CATTELL'S. See WASHES FOR THE HAIR, below.

Note.—The above ointments and liquids require to be used for some weeks, in order to produce a decided effect, either in curing or preventing baldness. Those which contain cantharides in any form are the most active, and must be used with caution. They should be applied once or twice a day, according to the effect produced; but if the scalp become sore, their use must be intermitted for a time, or longer intervals allowed, as the case may require. When employed to prevent the hair falling off or becoming gray, they need not be applied so frequently as for baldness.

The following require no particular caution, being less active than the preceding:—

POMATUMS, LOTIONS, &c.

FOR EMBELLISHING, STRENGTHENING, AND CLEANSING THE HAIR.

Pomatums, or Pommades.

These are composed usually of animal fats, variously perfumed. The lard, veal fat, beef and mutton suet, bear's fat, and beef marrow, employed for this purpose, require to be prepared with great care. The following is, perhaps, the best mode:—Cut the raw fat into pieces, carefully removing the fleshy and bloody portions of membrane, &c., and beat it in a marble mortar; melt it in a well-tinned vessel placed in boiling water, and strain the melted fat through a hair-sieve without pressure (reserving the residue to be heated again and pressed for more fat, to be used for commoner purposes.) Keep the melted fat for some time gently warm, without disturbing it; remove any scum which may have arisen, and pour off the clear fat, taking care that none of the dregs or watery liquid which have subsided pass with it. A mixture of these fats forms the basis of many varieties of pomades. Sometimes a little white wax is added. A greater degree of whiteness is said to be given by adding to the liquefied fat a few grains of citric acid. The same end is promoted by assiduously beating the pomade, while cooling, with a wooden spatula.

To perfume pomatums, various essential oils, &c., are added (see COMMON POMATUM;) but the finer sorts are perfumed by infusing fresh flowers in the melted fats for some hours, and straining; or, in other cases, the simple pomade is thinly spread on plates of glass set in frames, and the fresh flower stuck in the scored surface of the fat; changing the flowers daily till the pomatum is sufficiently perfumed. As these compounds can seldom be prepared to advantage by the retailer, a few varieties only require to be noticed here.

COMMON POMATUM. Mutton suet (prepared as above) 1 ℔, prepared lard 3 ℔; melt together in a water-bath, pour it into an earthen basin, and beat it assiduously with a wooden spatula. When sufficiently cool, add 2 oz. or q. s. of essence of bergamot, or of lemon, and continue the stirring till nearly cold.

ROSE POMATUM. Prepared lard 16 oz., prepared suet 2 oz.; melt with a gentle heat, and add 2 oz. of rose-water, and 6 drops of otto of roses. Beat them well together, and pour it into pots before it is too cold. For making jessamine, violet, and orange pomade, put the same quantity of water, and 1 drachm of the essence.

MARROW POMATUM. Beef marrow and beef suet, coloured with a little annotto, may be employed for this and other yellow pomatums. For the perfumes employed for these and other pomatums, see *Essence for scenting Pomatums*, under PERFUMERY.

POMADE FOR BEAUTIFYING THE HAIR. Oil of sweet almonds a pint, spermaceti 1½ oz., purified lard 2 oz.; melt with a gentle heat; when nearly cold add any agreeable scent, and pour it into pots or wide-mouthed bottles.

BEARS' GREASE (ARTIFICIAL.) Bears' grease is imitated by a mixture of prepared veal suet and beef marrow. It may be scented at pleasure; oil of lavender, with a very little oil of thyme, is sometimes used. The following are some of the compounds sold under this name:

1. Prepared suet 3 oz., lard 1 oz., olive oil 1 oz., oil of cloves 10 drops, compound tincture of benzoin 1 dr.; mix.

2. Lard 1 ℔, solution of carbonate of potash 2 oz.

3. Olive oil 4 flasks, white wax 4 oz., spermaceti 2 oz.; scented with otto of roses and oil of bitter almonds.

GREEN BEARS' GREASE. Bears' grease digested with fresh walnut leaves, and strained. This is repeated with more leaves till the pomade is sufficiently coloured; it is then scented with oil of rosemary, thyme, and bergamot.

GERMAN POMADE, FOR STRENGTHENING THE HAIR. Take 8 oz. of purified marrow, melt it in a glass or stoneware vessel, and add 1½ oz. of fresh bay leaves, 1 oz. of orange leaves, 1 oz. of bitter almonds, ½ oz. of nutmegs,

½ oz. of cloves, and 1 dr. of vanilla, all bruised; cover the vessel, and let the whole digest for 24 hours, with a gentle heat; strain while warm through linen, and stir it as it cools.

HARD, OR ROLL POMATUM. 1. Suet 5 ℔, white wax 8 oz., spermaceti 2 oz., oil of lavender and essence of ambergris, each ½ oz.

2. Beef suet 16 oz., white or yellow wax 1 oz., with 1 dr. of oil of lavender or of bergamot.

3. Lard melted with one-third or half its weight of white wax, and poured into semi-cylindrical paper moulds when nearly set. This is sold under the name of *cosmetique.* It is sometimes coloured to match the hair. See after HAIR DYES, below.

COLOURED POMATUMS. The colouring matters employed are annotto, alkanet, marigold, carmine, indigo, cobalt blue, umber, ivory black, &c.

CIRCASSIAN CREAM. Two flasks of oil, 3 oz. of white wax, 2 oz. of spermaceti, ½ oz. of alkanet root. Digest the oil with the alkanet till coloured, strain, melt the wax and spermaceti with the oil, and when sufficiently cool add 2½ dr. of English oil of lavender, and ½ dr. of essence of ambergris.

CRYSTALLINE CREAM. Oil of almonds 8 oz., spermaceti 1 oz.; melt together; when a little cooled add ½ oz. or less of essence of bergamot, or other perfume; put it into wide-mouthed bottles, and let it stand till cold.

Camphorated crystalline cream may be made by using camphorated oil (Lin. Camphoræ) instead of oil of almonds.

CASTOR OIL POMADE. Castor oil 4 oz., prepared lard 2 oz., white wax 6 dr., essence of bergamot 2 dr., oil of lavender 20 drops, eau de Cologne ½ dr.; stir till cold.

CRYSTALLINE CASTOR OIL POMADE. Castor oil 16 oz., spermaceti 1¾ oz.; melt together, and when a little cool add 1 oz. of essence of bergamot, ½ dr. oil of verbena, ½ dr. oil of lavender; pour it into wide-mouthed bottles, and let it stand till cold.

FOX'S CREAM. Marrow pomatum 2 oz., oil of almonds 2 oz.; melt, and add while cooling, with constant stirring, essence of jessamine or of bergamot 2 dr.—BATEMAN.

HUILES ANTIQUES.

PERFUMED OILS FOR THE HAIR.

The basis of these oils is either almond oil, olive oil, or oil of ben; whichever is used should be perfectly fresh, and of the finest quality. The perfume is communicated in three ways: by infusing the flowers in the oil at a gentle heat; by placing layers of flowers alternately with folded cotton soaked in the oil, in proper frames, and pressing out the oil when sufficiently imbued with the odour of the flowers; or simply by adding essential oils, &c., to the fixed oil. An example or two of each method will be sufficient.

Oil of Roses, by Infusion. Heat in a water-bath 1 ℔ of virgin oil, and add 1 ℔ of picked fresh petals of Provence roses. Let these remain together in the water-bath for half an hour; then remove from the bath, and leave them together for 24 hours, stirring them twice during the time. Strain through a cloth, and express all the oil. To this oil add fresh roses, and proceed as before; repeating this for 5, 6, or 7 times, till the oil is sufficiently perfumed.

Oil of Jessamine, Perfumed with the Flowers. Fold pieces of white cotton cloth twice or four times; moisten them with fine olive oil, slightly pressing them, and place them in proper frames. Then place on the cloths a rather thick layer of fresh-gathered and dry jessamine flowers, carefully deprived of all green parts. In 24 hours carefully remove the flowers, and replace them by fresh ones, till the oil is sufficiently perfumed. The oil is then expressed. The same method is employed in preparing oils from other delicate flowers; as violet, lily of the valley, &c.

Oil of Roses, Common. Fine olive or almond oil a pint, otto of roses 16 drops. If required red, colour the oil with alkanet root, and strain before adding the otto. For common sale, essence of bergamot or of lemon is often substituted, wholly or in part, for the more expensive otto.

PERFUMED OIL OF BERGAMOT, LEMON, ORANGE, &c. To oil of ben, or finest almond or olive oil, add essential oil of bergamot, lemon, &c., q. s. For common purposes a drachm of the essential oil may be added to 16 oz. of oil. Some recipes, however, direct as much as 1½ oz. or 2 oz.

OIL OF AMBERGRIS AND MUSK. Ambergris 2 dr., musk ½ dr.; grind them together in a mortar, then with a small quantity of oil; add more oil to make up a pint, and let them stand together for 12 days, stirring them occasionally. Then decant or filter. Add half a pint of oil to the residue for an oil of second quality.

COMMON OIL OF MUSK, OIL OF BENZOIN, OIL OF STYRAX, &c., may be obtained by mixing a strong tincture of these drugs with fine oil, agitating them frequently together, and, after remaining some hours at rest, decanting the clear oil.

HUILE COMOGENE. Mix equal parts of oil and spirit of rosemary with a few drops of oil of nutmeg. To be used daily.

HUILE DE PHÉNIX. Clarified beef marrow 4 oz., lard 2 oz., oil of mace 4 oz.; melt together and strain through linen into a warm mortar; stir, and when it begins to cool add the following solution, and stir constantly till it is quite cold:—Oil of cloves, lavender, mint, rosemary, sage, and thyme, of each ½ dr.; balsam of tolu 4 dr., camphor 1 dr., rectified spirit 1 oz. Put the spirit and balsam in a phial, and place it in warm water till the solution is complete, then add the camphor and essential oils.

HUILE PHILOCOME D'AUBRIL. Triturate together, without heat, equal parts of cold-drawn nut oil, almond oil, and prepared beef marrow, adding any essential oil as a perfume.

HUILE VERTE. Macerate 1 dr. of guaiacum with 1 ℔ of olive oil; strain, and add any essential oil to perfume it.—GRAY.

MARROW OIL. Clarified beef marrow, or marrow pomatum, with enough almond or olive oil to bring it to the desired consistence.

FLUIDE DE JAVA. This consists of beef marrow, white wax, fine olive oil, and essential oils at pleasure.

MACASSAR OIL. The oil made by the natives in the island is obtained by boiling the kernel of the fruit of a tree resembling the walnut, called in Malay, *badeau*. The oil is mixed with other ingredients, and has a smell approaching to that of creasote. But the Macassar oil sold in this country has probably no relation to the above, except in name. The following is given by GRAY:—Olive oil 1 ℔, oil of origanum 1 dr.; others add 1¼ dr. of oil of rosemary. The following French compound is probably named Macassar oil rather to denote its properties than from any resemblance either to the product of Macassar, or to the oil sold under this name in England:—

HUILE DE MACASSAR, DE NAQUET. Oil of ben 14 pints, nut oil 7 pints, spirit of wine 1 quart, essence of bergamot 3 oz., tincture of musk 3 oz., spirit of orange (*esprit de Portugal*) 2 oz., otto of roses 2 dr., alkanet to colour it. Digest them together with a gentle heat for an hour, and shake frequently for a week.

WASHES FOR THE HAIR.

VEGETABLE EXTRACT FOR CLEANSING AND STRENGTHENING THE HAIR. 1. Southernwood 2 oz., box leaves 6 oz., water 4 pints. Boil gently in a saucepan for ¼ of an hour, strain, and to each pint of the liquid add 2 oz. of spirit of rosemary and ½ dr. of salt of tartar (or 1 dr. of Naples soap.)

2. Boil 1 ℔ of rosemary in 2 quarts of water, and add to the filtered liquor 1 oz. of spirit of lavender, and ¼ oz. of Naples soap, or salt of tartar.

3. Incinerate 2 oz. each of rosemary, maidenhair, southernwood, myrtle berries, and hazel bark; make a strong solution of the ashes, with which wash the hair at the roots every day. Keep the hair short.—Dr. CATTELL.

4. Borax 1 oz., powdered camphor ½ oz., boiling water a quart. When cold, filter for use. Damp the hair with it frequently.

WASH FOR REMOVING SCURF, AND PROMOTING THE CURLING

OF THE HAIR. 1. Beat up the yolk of an egg with a pint of clean rain water. Apply it warm, and afterwards wash the head with warm water.

2. Lime water a pint, distilled vinegar ¼ of a pint. Mix.

COMPOUNDS FOR STIFFENING THE HAIR.

EAU COLLANTE. Dissolve, without heat, 8 oz. of clear gum in 2 ℔ of distilled or rose water, and filter through coarse filtering paper.

BANDOLINE, OR FIXATEUR. Vegetable mucilage, with sufficient spirit to preserve it. Mucilage of quince seed is used; mucilage of picked Irish moss, carefully strained, is said to answer still better. But the following is employed by some London perfumers:—Finest picked gum tragacanth, reduced to a coarse powder, 1 oz., rose-water a pint; put them into a wide-mouthed vessel, and shake them together daily for 2 or 3 days; then strain with gentle pressure through fine linen or cambric. If required to be coloured, infuse cochineal in the water employed before making the mucilage. Another form is—linseed (not bruised) a tablespoonful, water ½ a pint; boil for 5 minutes, and strain.

POMMADE COLLANTE, FOR FALSE CURLS. Melt together in an earthen pipkin 24 oz. of fine Burgundy pitch, and 8 oz. of white wax, and add 1 oz. of pomatum; remove from the fire, and add 4 oz. of brandy or other spirit, replace it on the fire till it boils slightly, then strain through linen, adding bergamot or other perfume, and cast it into moulds.

HAIR DYES.

ORFILA'S HAIR DYE. Take 3 parts of litharge and 2 of quicklime, both in an impalpable powder, and mix them carefully. When used, a portion of the powder is mixed with hot water or milk, and applied to the hair, the part being afterwards enveloped in oil-skin, or a cabbage-leaf, for 4 or 5 hours.

2. Litharge 2 parts, slaked lime 1 part, chalk 2 parts, all finely powdered, and accurately mixed. When re-

quired for use, mix the powder with warm water, and dip a brush in the mixture, and rub the hair well with it. After 2 hours, let the hair be washed.

3. Litharge 4½ oz., quicklime ¾ oz.; reduce to an impalpable powder, and pass it through a sieve. Keep it in a dry, close bottle. Wash the hair first with soap and water, then with tepid water; wipe it dry, and comb with a clean comb. Mix the dye in a saucer with hot water to the consistence of cream, and apply it to the hair, beginning at the roots. Place over it four folds of brown paper, saturated with hot water, and drained till cool; and over this an oil-skin cap and a nightcap. Let it remain from 4 to 8 hours, according to the shade required. When removed, oil the hair, but do not wet it for 3 or 4 days.

4. CHEVALLIER'S. Mix 5 dr. of fresh slaked lime with 1½ oz. of water, and strain through silk; put the milk of lime into a 4-oz. bottle. Dissolve 5 dr. of acetate of lead in sufficient water, and add enough slaked lime to saturate the acetic acid (a drachm, or rather more,) let it settle, pour off the supernatant liquor, wash the precipitate with water, and add it to the milk of lime.

5. Dr. HANMANN'S. Levigated litharge 11 oz., powdered quicklime 75 oz., hair powder 37 oz.; mix. When used, a portion of the powder is mixed with warm water in a saucer, and applied to the hair with the fingers, taking care to cover the hair to the roots. Cover the whole with a sheet of cotton wadding moistened with water, and this with a folded cloth. Let it remain on for 3 hours; or better, for the night.

6. WARREN'S. Sifted lime 16 oz., white lead 2 oz., litharge in fine powder 1 oz.; mix well together, and keep dry. To dye *black*, mix a little powder with water to the consistence of cream. To dye *brown*, use milk instead of water. Apply with a small sponge to every hair.

ESSENCE OF TYRE. GRECIAN WATER. EAU D'EGYPT. EAU DE CHINA. These are solutions of nitrate of silver: in applying them it must be remembered that they stain the *skin* as well as the hair. Hence there is more difficulty in applying than in the preceding; but they are considered to impart a finer colour to the hair, with the disadvantage, however, of rendering it dry and crisp. The following are some of the most approved formulæ:

1. Dr. Cattel's. Nitrate of silver 11 dr., nitric acid 1 dr., distilled water 1 pint, sap green 3 dr., gum Arabic 1 dr.; mix.

2. Nitric acid 1 dr., nitrate of silver 10 dr., sap green 9 dr., mucilage 5 dr., distilled water 37½ fluid oz.

3. Silver 2 dr., iron filings 4 dr., nitric acid 1 oz., distilled water 8 oz. Digest, and decant the clear solution. To be carefully applied with a close brush.

4. Hydrosulphuret of ammonia 1 oz., liquor of potash 3 dr., distilled water 1 oz. Mix. Apply this with a tooth brush for 15 or 20 minutes, then brush the hair over with the following:—Nitrate of silver 1 dr., distilled water 2 oz., using a clean comb to separate the hair.

Pyrogallic Stain. Distil coarsely powdered nutgalls in a retort, dissolve the solid acid which sublimes in a little hot water, add the solution to the acid liquid which passes over, separate the floating oil, shake the liquid with charcoal, filter, and add a little spirit.

La Forest's Cosmetic Wash for the Hair. Red wine 1 ℔., salt 1 dr., sulphate of iron 2 dr. Boil for a few minutes, and add common verdigris 1 dr.; leave it on the fire 2 minutes, withdraw it, and add 2 dr. of powdered nut gall. Rub the hair with the liquid; in a few minutes dry it with a warm cloth, and afterwards wash with water.

Pomatums, or Cosmetiques, in sticks, for the hair.

Black Pomatum, in sticks, for the eyebrows, whiskers, &c. Prepared lard melted with a third of its weight of wax in winter, or half in summer, and coloured with levigated ivory black, and strained through tammy, or any material which will permit the fine particles of ivory black to pass through. Stir it constantly, and when it begins to thicken pour it into paper moulds.

Brown and Chestnut Pomatums are prepared in the same way, but coloured with umber, &c. White, as Hard Pomatum.

EBONY POMATUM, in pots. Melt 4 oz. of white wax with 12 oz. of any kind of pomatum, and add 2 oz. of levigated ivory black. Proceed as above, and pour into pots.

POMMADE DE JEUNESSE. Pomatum mixed with magistery of bismuth. It is said to turn the hair black.—GRAY.

DEPILATORIES.

FOR REMOVING SUPERFLUOUS HAIRS.

These require caution, as they are apt to injure the skin. We have omitted those which contain sulphuret of arsenic (orpiment) as there is danger of its being absorbed; and the object can be accomplished without its use. The powders require to be kept in close bottles or boxes, and no more should be mixed with liquid than is required to be used at once.

1. Mix lime and water to a thick cream, and pass through the mixture 25 or 30 times its volume of sulphuretted hydrogen gas. When the gas escapes, stop the process. The pulpy mass is spread on paper, and applied for 12 or 15 minutes, and then washed off with a sponge and water. The only objection to this is its disgusting smell.

2. CHINESE. Quick lime 16 oz., pearlash 2 oz., liver of sulphur 2 oz. Reduce to a fine powder, and keep it in a close bottle. Use it as No. 4.

3. Mr. REDWOOD recommends a strong solution of sulphuret of barium, with sufficient powdered starch to form a paste: to be left on for a few minutes, then scraped off with the back of a knife.

4. BOUDET'S DEPILATORY. Crystallized hydrosulphate of soda 3 parts, quicklime in powder 10 parts, starch 10 parts. Mix. To be mixed with water, and applied to the skin, and scraped off in 2 or 3 minutes with a wooden knife.

TEETH AND MOUTH COSMETICS.

TOOTH POWDER.

General Directions.—The dry ingredients should be finely pulverized, and the whole well mixed; which is best effected by triturating the powders together, or agitating them in a bottle, and afterwards passing the whole through a sieve. Some ingredients are usually *levigated*, or ground with water, as prepared chalk, coral, &c. The tooth powders which contain acids and acid salts should not be frequently used. For children those only which contain very soft powders should be permitted; the heavy carbonate of magnesia is very suitable for them.

AMERICAN TOOTH POWDER. Coral, cuttle-fish bone, dragon's blood, of each 8 oz., burnt alum and red sanders, of each 4 oz., orris 8 oz., cloves and cinnamon, of each ½ oz., vanilla 2 dr., rosewood ½ oz., rose pink 8 oz.

ANTISEPTIC TOOTH POWDER. Prepared or precipitated chalk 2 oz., dry chloride of lime 10 gr., oil of cassia or of cloves 5 drops; mix. It may be coloured, if preferred, by a little levigated bole.

ANTISCORBUTIC TOOTH POWDER. Extract of rhatany ½ oz., prepared charcoal 2 oz., cinnamon ¼ oz., cloves ¼ oz.

AROMATIC TOOTH POWDER. Calamus aromaticus 4 dr., charcoal 1 dr., soap 1 dr., oil of cloves 12 drops.—PITTSCHAFT.

ASIATIC TOOTH POWDER. Prepared coral 4 oz., Venetian red 3 dr., ochre 5 dr., pumice 5 dr. musk 1 gr.; mix. Or, Bole 3 parts, chalk 2, ochre 1, pumice 1, musk to scent.

CADET'S, or DR. COOMBE'S. Sugar 1 oz., charcoal 1 oz.,

Peruvian bark ½ oz., cream of tartar 1½ dr., cinnamon 24 gr.

CAMPHORATED CHALK. Camphor (pulverized by the aid of a few drops of spirits) 1 oz., prepared or precipitated chalk 3 oz. Some makers put only 1 part of camphor to 7 of chalk.

COMPOUND CAMPHORATED TOOTH POWDER. Camphor 1 oz., precipitated chalk 2 oz., cuttle-fish bone ½ oz., myrrh 2 dr., borax 2 dr., lake or rose pink 1 dr., or q. s.

CARTWRIGHT'S DENTIFRICE. Prepared chalk 1 oz., orris 1 oz., Castile soap ½ dr.

CARABELLI'S. Cuttle-fish bone 1½ oz., prepared shells 1½ oz., cinnamon, orris, and lime-tree charcoal, of each 3 dr., vanilla 10 gr.

CHARCOAL, PREPARED. The charcoal, made in iron cylinders, from willow, is preferred. It should be reduced to an impalpable powder, and kept from the air. Charcoal of areka nut is highly commended. That of the shells of cocoa nuts is said to be used for the same purpose. Dr. HEIDER prefers the charcoal of the lime tree.

CHARCOAL TOOTH POWDER (Grey.) Prepared charcoal 1 oz., prepared chalk 3 oz.

CHARCOAL TOOTH POWDER (French.) Prepared charcoal 1 oz., sugar 1 oz., oil of cloves 3 drops; mix.

CHARCOAL WITH BARK. Charcoal 1 oz., red cinchona 1 oz., powdered sugar ½ oz., with a few drops of some essential oil. See also RIGHINI'S, below.

CHARCOAL WITH BARK (French recipe.) Charcoal 1 oz., Peruvian bark ½ oz., oil of cinnamon, mint, or other oil, 2 drops, essence of ambergris 30 drops.

CHARCOAL WITH QUININE. Charcoal 1 oz., sulphate of quinine 2 to 4 gr., magnesia 4 to 8 gr., otto of rose (or other perfume) 2 drops.

CARBONIC DENTIFRICE (DESFORGES'.) Willow charcoal 4 oz., cinchona bark 4 oz., cloves ½ dr.

CIRCASSIAN DENTIFRICE (Dr. HALIFAX'S.) Prepared hartshorn 2 oz., sulphate of potash 2 oz., cuttle-fish bone 8 oz., orris 4 oz., yellow sandal wood 1 oz., rose-pink 3 oz., oil of rhodium 30 drops. Mix the dry ingredients, previously reduced to a fine powder, and add the oil of rhodium.

CORAL DENTIFRICE (*Poudre Dentifrice* of the French Pharmacopœia.) Red coral, bole, cuttle-fish bone, of each 3 oz., dragon's blood 1½ oz., cochineal 3 dr., cream of tartar 4½ oz., cinnamon 6 dr., cloves 1 dr.; reduce, separately, to powder, mix, and grind on porphyry.

DESCHAMP'S ALKALINE DENTIFRICE. Venetian talc 4 oz., bicarbonate of soda 1 oz., carmine 4 or 5 grains, oil of mint (or other perfume) 15 drops.

DESCHAMP'S ACID DENTIFRICE. Venetian talc 4 oz., cream of tartar 1 oz., carmine 4 or 5 grains, oil as the last.

DESFORGES'. See CARBONIC DENTIFRICE.

DETERGENT TOOTH POWDER. Bicarbonate of soda 1 oz., powdered Castile soap ½ oz., sulphate of potash ½ oz., sugar of milk ½ oz., orris root 4 oz., oil of bitter almonds 4 drops. Coloured at pleasure.

ELEPHANT'S (Mrs.) TOOTH POWDER. Bole 1 oz., myrrh, bark, and orris, each ¼ oz. All to be finely powdered, and mixed.

FLORENTINE DENTIFRICE. Prepared shells 14 dr., orris 6 dr., cream of tartar 3 dr., lake to colour.

FRENCH TOOTH POWDER. (See CORAL TOOTH POWDER, above; also GALVANIC, DESCHAMP'S, &c.) Peruvian bark, burnt crust of bread, and sugar, in equal proportions.

GALVANIC DENTIFRICE. Triturate 2 leaves of gold-leaf and 3 of silver with 2 dr. of sulphate of potash and 1 dr. of alum; then add white sugar 2 dr., common salt 1 dr., pellitory of Spain ½ dr., prepared hartshorn 1 oz., sulphate of quinine 10 grains. Mix. Colour with finest smalts (powder blue,) rose pink, or lake. FOZEMBAS' recipe is—2 leaves of gold, 2 of silver, alum 3 dr., salt 1½ dr., white sugar 1½ dr., pepper 15 gr., opium 5 gr., coral 3 dr., Peruvian bark 3 dr. Grind the gold and silver with the salt and alum, and add the last. For the *double* galvanic tooth powder, put twice the above quantities of gold, silver, alum, salt, pepper, and opium. The galvanic action of the metals is thought to stimulate the gums.

GERMAN TOOTH POWDER. Peruvian bark 6 dr., red sanders 2 dr., oil of cloves and of bergamot 3 drops.

GROSVENOR'S TOOTH POWDER. Prepared shells and coral, of each 12 oz., orris root 2 oz., oil of rhodium 6 drops.

HEMET'S DENTIFRICE. It is said to consist of cuttle-fish bone 6 oz., cream of tartar 1 oz., orris ½ oz.; mix.

JAMES'S. Orris 16 oz., magnesia 4 oz., pumice-stone 8 oz., cuttle-fish bone 8 oz., sulphate of quinine 4 oz., cascarilla 1 oz., sugar of milk 16 oz., oil of mint 1 oz., oil of cinnamon 2 dr., oil of neroli 1 dr., essence of ambergris 1 dr.

KEMMERER'S. Wood-soot 1½ oz., strawberry root ½ oz., and a few drops of eau de Cologne.

LAVENDER TOOTH POWDER. Crimson lake 1 drachm, Chinese blue (or Turnbull's blue) a scruple; mix, and add bicarbonate of soda ½ oz., cuttle-fish bone 2 oz., precipitated chalk 6 oz., oil of lavender 8 drops.

LARDNER'S TOOTH POWDER. See CHARCOAL TOOTH POWDER (*gray.*)

LEFOULON'S TOOTH POWDER. Scurvy-grass, horse-radish, guaiacum, cinchona, mint, pellitory root, calamus, rhatany, of each equal quantities. Reduce to an impalpable powder. A little calcined magnesia is sometimes added.

MAURY'S CARBONIC TOOTH POWDER. Charcoal 8 oz., cinchona 4 oz., sugar 8 oz., oil of mint ½ oz., oil of cinnamon ¼ oz., tincture of ambergris ½ drachm.

METGES' TOOTH POWDER. Prepared chalk 3½ ℔, lake or rose pink 1 ℔, orris 2 ℔, cream of tartar 12 oz., levigated pumice 1 oz., sugar 9 oz., oil of cloves 1 dr.

MIALHE'S RATIONAL DENTIFRICE. Sugar of milk 3 oz., pure tannin 3 dr., lake 1 dr., oil of mint 8 drops, oil of aniseed 8 drops, neroli 4 drops.

MYRRH DENTIFRICE. Myrrh 1 oz., cuttle-fish bone 4 oz., orris 3 oz.; mix.

NICHOLS' TOOTH POWDER. Cuttle-fish bone, prepared chalk, orris, of each 1 oz.; cassia ½ oz., myrrh ½ oz.; mix.

PALMER'S TOOTH POWDER. Prepared chalk 1 ℔, camphor 1 oz., orris 1 ℔, cuttle-fish bone 4 oz., rose pink 1 oz.

PEARL DENTIFRICE. Precipitated chalk 16 oz., talc 8 oz., finest smalts ½ oz., or q. s. to give it a slight tint.

PELLETIER'S QUININE DENTIFRICE. Sulphate of quinine 4 gr., prepared red coral 1 oz., myrrh a scruple. For the coral may be substituted levigated bole 2 dr., precipitated chalk 6 dr.

REGNAUD'S DENTIFRICE. Calcined magnesia ½ oz., sulphate of quinine 8 gr., carmine (or cochineal) ½ dr., oil of peppermint 3 drops.

RHATANY TOOTH POWDER. Rhatany root 2 oz., cuttle-fish bone 4 oz., prepared chalk 8 oz., borax 1 dr.

RIGHINI'S CHARCOAL AND BARK. Charcoal 4 parts, yellow bark 1 part.

ROSE DENTIFRICE. Lake ½ dr., myrrh 2 dr., bicarbonate of soda 2 dr., orris 2 oz., cuttle-fish bone 2 oz., precipitated chalk 6 oz., otto of rose 16 drops; or it may be coloured with rose pink to any desired shade.

RUSPINI'S DENTIFRICE. Cuttle-fish bone 8 oz., prepared hartshorn 2 oz., alum 1 oz., cream of tartar 2 oz., orris 1 oz., oil of rhodium 6 drops.

RUSSIAN TOOTH POWDER. Peruvian bark 2 oz., orris root 1 oz., sal ammoniac ½ oz., catechu 6 dr., myrrh 6 dr., oil of cloves 6 or 8 drops.

SAUNDERS' DENTIFRICE. Prepared chalk 2 oz., cuttle-fish bone 1 oz., orris 1 oz., myrrh ½ oz., sulphate of quinine 10 gr.

DR. SCHOEPF'S TOOTH POWDER, *against mercurial salivation.* Alum 2 scruples, cinchona bark 1 oz.

VIOLET TOOTH POWDER. Orris root 2 oz., cuttle-fish bone 4 oz., precipitated chalk 12 oz., bicarbonate of soda ½ oz., essence of violets 1 dr., pure percyanide of iron and crimson lake or rose pink, enough to give it a pale violet colour.

TOOTH PASTES.

Any of the above tooth powders may be formed into a paste with honey, clarified honey, or honey of roses. A little perfumed spirit may be added. A common objection to these pastes or electuaries, is their liability to fermentation, or effervescence. Some makers keep the paste in the bulk for a considerable time, till the effervescence has completely subsided, and then put it up in pots for sale. Others heat the honey, stir in the powders, and keep the mixture warm till any effervescence produced by the action of the acidity of the honey on the cretaceous powders has subsided. It would perhaps be preferable in all cases to use the *prepared* honey (see Mel Preparatum, Pocket Formulary) for these purposes. Electuaries of this kind are termed by the French *opiats*, although they may contain no opium in any form.

CORAL TOOTH PASTE. *Opiat dentifrice.* 1. Prepared coral 5 oz., cream of tartar 3 oz., cuttle-fish bone 3 oz., cochineal ½ dr., Narbonne honey 16 oz.—DESFORGES.

2. *Opiat Dentifrice Rouge.* Prepared coral 8 oz., cochineal 1 oz., cinnamon 2 oz., alum 3 dr., honey 20 oz., water 1 oz.; triturate the cochineal with the alum and water, add the honey, then the coral and cinnamon; leave the whole for 24 hours, or till the effervescence has subsided; then rub it up with a few drops of oil of cloves, or other aromatic oil, and put it into covered pots for sale.

DYON'S CHARCOAL PASTE. Triturate ½ dr. of chlorate of potash with ½ oz. of mint water, and add gradually 1 oz. of powdered charcoal.

METGES' TOOTH PASTE. Metges' tooth powder (as above) 48 oz., Narbonne honey 32 oz., syrup 64 oz., cochineal 1 oz., alum 1 oz., water 4 oz.; triturate the cochineal and alum with the water, add the honey and syrup, and lastly the powder.

PELLETIER'S ODONTINE. This is said to consist of magnesia and butter of cacao, aromatized with some essential oil.

ROSE TOOTH PASTE. Cuttle-fish bone 3 oz., prepared or precipitated chalk 2 oz., orris 1 oz., lake or rose pink to give it a pale rose colour, otto of roses 16 drops, honey of roses q. s.

RED OR CHERRY PASTE. See CORAL PASTE, No. 2.

ROSEMARY PASTE. Levigated bole 4 oz., myrrh 1 oz., oil of rosemary 2 dr. (dissolved in 1 oz. rectified spirit,) clarified honey q. s.

SALINE TOOTH PASTE. Sulphate of potash 1 oz., bay salt ½ oz., clarified honey q. s. eau de Cologne 2 dr. (or essence of ambergris 30 drops.)

VANILLA TOOTH PASTE. (French.) Charcoal 1 oz., white honey 1 oz., vanilla sugar 1 oz., Peruvian bark ½ oz., and a few drops of any essential oil. The vanilla sugar may be made by triturating a drachm of saturated tincture of vanilla with 1 oz. of pure sugar, and drying the mixture with a gentle heat.

WHITE TOOTH PASTE. 1. (French.) Orris, sal ammoniac, cream of tartar, of each 2 oz., tincture of cinnamon and tincture of vanilla of each ½ oz., oil of cloves 60 drops, clarified honey and syrup to form a paste.

2. Precipitated chalk 4 oz., sulphate of potash ½ oz., prepared honey sufficient to form a paste; to be flavoured with a few drops of otto of roses, or oil of cinnamon, &c.

LIQUID PREPARATIONS FOR THE TEETH AND GUMS.

ASTRINGENT TINCTURE FOR THE TEETH AND GUMS.

1. Borax, alum, bay salt, of each a dr., spirit of camphor, tincture of myrrh, of each 1 oz., spirit of scurvy-grass (or of horseradish) 4 oz., tincture of rhatany 2 oz.; mix, and shake occasionally for a day or two, then filter. A teaspoonful in a wine-glassful of water, to rinse the mouth after cleaning the teeth, or at any other time.

2. Tannin 1 dr., rose-water 4 oz., spirit of wine 2 oz., spirit of scurvy-grass (or of horseradish) 2 oz., essence of bitter almonds a few drops.

ODORIFEROUS TINCTURE OF MYRRH. 1. Choice Turkey myrrh 3 oz., eau de Cologne a quart; digest for 7 days, and filter.

2. To 18 fluid oz. of tincture of myrrh, add 2 oz. of essence of Cologne. (See PERFUMERY, p. 225.) If the tincture should not be quite clear, add a few gr. of burnt alum, shake frequently, and filter in a day or two.

BORATED TINCTURE OF MYRRH. 1. Myrrh 1 ℔, eau de Cologne 16 ℔, borax 1 ℔, distilled water 3 ℔, syrup 3 ℔, essence (or tincture) of roses 6 dr., rhatany root 4 oz.; digest for 10 or 12 days, and filter.—Mr. COCKLE.

2. Borax 1 oz., shell-lac ½ oz., myrrh 2 oz., spirit of camphor 2 oz., honey of roses 2 oz., rectified spirit a pint, Cologne essence 2 dr., orange-flower or rose-water 4 oz.;

digest for a few days in a warm place, shaking occasionally, and filter.

3. Borax 1 oz., shell-lac ½ oz., water 8 oz.; boil together to 4 oz., and add spirit of scurvy-grass a pint, camphor ½ oz., myrrh 2 oz.; digest, and filter.

ANTISCORBUTIC ELIXIR. Cinchona 3 oz., guaiacum 5 oz., pellitory 3 oz., orange-peel 2 dr., cloves 5 dr., saffron ½ dr., benzoin 2 dr., spirit of wine or brandy 32 oz.; digest and filter.—DESFORGES.

DESFORGES' EXTRACT OF PELLITORY. Pellitory root 5 oz., cinchona 1 oz., benzoin 1½ dr., essence of peppermint 3 dr., brandy a quart.

ELIXIR OF ROSES. Cloves 1 dr., cinnamon 3 oz., ginger 2 oz., spirit of wine 2½ pints, oil of orange-peel 1 dr., otto of roses 15 drops, essence of peppermint 1 oz.; mix, digest for 15 days, and filter.

LEFANDINIÈRE'S ELIXIR. Rasped guaiacum wood ½ oz., pellitory 1 dr., nutmegs 1 dr., cloves ½ oz., oil of rosemary 10 drops, oil of bergamot 4 drops, brandy a pint; macerate for a fortnight, and filter.

EAU DE BOTTOT. Aniseed 4 oz., cinnamon 1 oz., cloves 1 oz., cochineal 2 dr., oil of mint 2 dr., spirit of wine or brandy 8 ℔; macerate 8 days and filter.

2. Tincture of cedar wood 1 pint, tincture of myrrh 1 oz., mixed with the following essential oils—of peppermint ½ dr., of spearmint ¼ dr., of cloves 10 drops, of roses 10 drops.—PIESSE.

EAU DENTIFRICE DE STAHL. Spirit of wine or brandy 2 gallons, rose-water 3 quarts, pellitory 5 oz., cypress root 3 oz., tormentil 3 oz., balsam of Peru 3 oz., cinnamon 5 dr., goat's rue 1 oz., rhatany 1 oz.: macerate for 6 days, shaking it occasionally; let it rest 24 hours, and pour off the clear. Add to the clear liquor, oil of mint 1½ dr., cochineal 4 dr.; in 3 or 4 days filter.

EAU DU DR. O'MEARA. It is a tincture of pellitory, vetiver, cloves, orris, and coriander, with creasote, &c.

BORIES' ODONTALGIC ELIXIR. Pellitory root 2 oz., simple spirit of lavender 16 oz., muriate of ammonia ½ dr.; digest 24 hours, and filter.

GREENOUGH'S Tincture. Bitter almonds 2 oz., Brazil wood

½ oz., cinnamon ½ oz., orris root ¼ oz., cochineal, alum, salt of sorrel, each 1 dr., spirit of wine 32 fluid oz., spirit of scurvy-grass 1 oz.

HUDSON'S PRESERVATIVE. Tincture of myrrh, tincture of bark, cinnamon water, of each 3 oz., arquebusade water 1 oz., powdered gum ½ oz.

CHELTENHAM DENTAL TINCTURE. Camphor 4½ oz., myrrh 2 oz., bark 5 oz., rectified spirit 36 fluid oz., distilled water 8 oz.

LEFOULON'S ELIXIR FOR THE TEETH. Fresh roots of horse-radish, fresh leaves of scurvy-grass and of mint, of each 6 dr., guaiacum, cinchona, pellitory, calamus, and rhatany, each 5 dr., proof spirit a quart; macerate 16 days, and strain.

EAU DE MADAME DE LA VRILLIERE POUR LES DENTS. Cinnamon 2 oz., cloves 6 dr., fresh lemon-peel 1½ oz., dried rose petals 1 oz., scurvy-grass 8 oz., spirit 3 ℔.; macerate 24 hours, and distil in a water-bath.

RUSPINI'S TINCTURE. Orris 8 oz., cloves 1 oz., spirit 32 fluid oz., essence of ambergris 1 oz. (or ambergris a scruple;) macerate 14 days, and filter.

FRENCH ELIXIR FOR THE TEETH. Rose-water 16 oz., spirit of scurvy grass 2 oz., tincture of galbanum 1 oz; colour with cochineal.

ALKALINE LOTION, for preventing injury to the teeth from acid medicines. Bicarbonate of soda 4 dr., distilled water 8 oz., eau de Cologne 2 dr., aromatic spirit of ammonia 1 dr. The mouth to be rinsed out with the lotion *immediately* after swallowing any medicine containing an acid.

LOTION OF CHLORINATED SODA, for purifying the breath, cleansing the mouth, removing unpleasant odours, &c. Liquid chlorinated soda 1 oz., distilled water 19 oz.; mix. A teaspoonful in a glass of water. The same direction applies to most of the above.

STRONGER TINCTURES, SOLUTIONS, OR ESSENCES, FOR TOOTHACHE.

THESE are applied by moistening a little cotton wool or lint with the liquid, and introduced into the cavity of the decayed and aching tooth. Where there is no cavity, they are sometimes applied to the gums surrounding the affected tooth. Most of them are stated by their several inventors or patrons to give "immediate relief." The cavity should be dried with lint before applying the remedy.

1. M. PIESSE'S. Water of ammonia, with half the quantity of tincture of opium; applied as above.

2. Creasote 1 dr., spirit of camphor 2 dr., laudanum 1 dr. Creasote is also used alone: so is *carvacrol*, a liquid of similar properties. LAENNEC prescribes 1 part of creasote and 10 of alcohol. See also No. 14.

3. M. COTTEREAU'S. Ether saturated in the cold with camphor, and then a few drops of ammonia added.

4. Mr. BLAKE'S. Finely-powdered alum 1 dr., spirit of nitric ether 7 dr.

5. *Paraguay-roux, or Compound Tincture of Para Cress.* Flowers of Para cress 4 parts, Italian elecampane (*inula bifrons*) 1 part, pellitory root 1 part, rectified spirit 8 parts; macerate 14 days, express, and filter.

6. Mr. BRANDE'S *Tincture.* Bruised pellitory ½ oz., camphor 3 dr., opium 1 dr., oil of cloves ½ dr., rectified spirit 6 oz.; digest for 10 days, and strain.

7. Pellitory, ginger, cloves, camphor, of each 1 oz., tincture of opium 4 oz., spirit of wine 16 oz.; macerate for 8 days, and strain.

8. Camphor 1 dr., ether 4 dr.; dissolve.

9. Camphor 2 dr., chloroform 1 dr., spirit of sal volatile ½ dr.

10. Opium 2 oz., mastic ½ oz., balsam of tolu 1 dr., camphor 1 oz., oil of cloves 1 dr., rectified spirit 16 fluid oz., oil of bitter almonds 8 drops.

11. BOERHAAVE'S *Odontalgic.* Rectified spirit 1 oz., camphor ½ oz., opium 1 scruple, oil of cloves 80 drops.

12. LEMAZURIER'S *Odontalgic*. Cherry-laurel water 2 oz., acetate of morphia 1 gr. Wash the mouth with warm water to a glass of which a few drops of this mixture have been added.

13. Oil of rosemary 2 oz., tincture of galbanum 1 oz.; mix. Cotton wet with this is to be introduced into the ears.

14. RIGHINI'S. Alcohol 4 dr., creasote 6 dr., tincture of cochineal 2 dr., oil of peppermint 3 drops.

15. Mr. DRUITT'S. Tannin 20 gr., mastic 5 gr., ether 2 dr. Wash the mouth with warm water containing a little carbonate of soda; lance the gums, and apply the tincture to the cavity of the tooth on cotton.

16. Mr. TOMES recommends a solution of mastic in chloroform. The mastic serves to retain the chloroform, but the latter may be used alone on cotton or lint. Mr. BEATSON uses a solution of copal in chloroform.

HENBANE FUMIGATION FOR TOOTHACHE. A popular remedy is to throw henbane seed on hot cinders, inverting a cup over them to receive the smoke and empyreumatic oil produced. The cup is then filled with hot water, and the steam conveyed to the affected side of the mouth. Dr. DOWNING'S Aneuralgicon would probably prove a more effective means of applying remedies of this kind.

PILLS, OR PASTES, FOR TOOTHACHE.

MASSES ODONTALGIQUES.

1. DE HANDEL'S. Opium 12 gr., camphor 24 gr., cajeput oil 4 drops, tincture of cantharides 4 drops, extract of henbane and of belladonna, of each 24 gr., distilled water of opium q. s.

2. VOGLER'S. Powdered opium 1 oz., mastic 2 dr., sandarach 2 dr., dragon's blood ½ dr., oil of rosemary 8 drops, spirit to form a paste; to be applied near the affected tooth.

3. Powdered alum 1 dr., powdered mastic ½ dr., spirit of nitric ether q. s. to form a paste.

4. RUST'S. Opium 5 gr., oil of cloves 3 drops, extract of henbane 5 gr., extract of belladonna 10 gr., powdered pellitory sufficient to form a paste.

CEMENTS, &c., FOR STOPPING THE CAVITIES OF TEETH.

THESE are harder than the preceding, and intended to remain in the tooth for an indefinite time. In all cases the cavity should be previously cleared from all extraneous matters, and wiped perfectly dry with a piece of lint or blotting paper.

1. SOUBEIRAN'S. Powdered mastic and sandarach, of each 4 drachms, dragon's blood 2 dr., opium 15 gr.; mix with sufficient rectified spirit to form a stiff paste. A solution of mastic, or of mastic and sandarach, in half the quantity of alcohol, is also used, applied with a little cotton or lint.

2. Sandarach 12 parts, mastic 6 parts, amber in powder 1 part, ether 6 parts. Applied with cotton. Or simply a paste of powdered mastic and ether. Or a saturated ethereal solution of mastic, applied with cotton.

3. TAVEARE'S CEMENT is made with mastic and burnt alum. BERNOTH directs 90 parts of powdered mastic to be digested with 40 of ether, and enough powdered alum added to form a stiff paste.

4. Gutta-percha, softened by heat, is recommended. Dr. ROLLFS advises melting a piece of caoutchouc at the end of a wire, and introducing it while warm.

5. GAUGER'S CEMENT. Put into a quart bottle 2 oz. of mastic and 3 oz. of absolute alcohol; apply a gentle heat by a water-bath. When dissolved, add 9 oz. of dry balsam of tolu, and again heat gently. A piece of cotton dipped in this viscid solution, becomes hard when introduced into the tooth, previously cleaned and dried as above.

6. Mr. ROBINSON'S. After washing out the mouth with warm water, containing a few grains of bicarbonate of soda, and cleaning the cavity as above directed, he drops into it a drop of collodion, to which a little

morphia has been added, fills the cavity with asbestos, and saturates with collodion, placing over all a pledget of blotting paper.

7. OSTERMAIER'S CEMENT. Mix 12 parts of dry phosphoric acid with 13 of pure and pulverized quick-lime. It becomes moist in mixing, in which state it is introduced into the cavity of the tooth, where it quickly becomes hard. [In some hands this has failed, from what cause we are not aware.] The acid should be prepared as directed under Trade Chemicals (Acid, Phosphoric.)

8. SILICIA. This name has been given to a mixture of Paris plaster, levigated porcelain, iron filings, and dregs of tincture of mastic, ground together.

9. WIRTH'S CEMENT. It is said to consist of a viscid alcoholic solution of resins, with powdered asbestos.

10. METALLIC CEMENTS. Amalgams for the teeth are made with gold or silver, and quicksilver, the excess of the latter being squeezed out, and the stiff amalgam used warm. Inferior kinds are made with quicksilver and tin, or zinc. A popular nostrum of this kind is said to consist of 40 gr. of quicksilver and 20 of fine zinc filings, mixed at the time of using. Mr. EVANS states that pure tin, with a small portion of cadmium, and sufficient quicksilver, forms the most lasting and least objectionable amalgam. The following is the formula:—Melt 2 parts of tin with 1 of cadmium, run it into an ingot, and reduce it to filings. Form these into a fluid amalgam with mercury, and squeeze out the excess of mercury through leather. Work up the solid residue in the hand, and press it into the tooth. Or, melt some bees' wax in a pipkin over the fire and throw in 5 parts of cadmium, and, when melted, add 7 or 8 parts of tin in small pieces; pour the melted metals into an iron or wooden box, and shake them till cold, so as to obtain the alloy in a powder. This is mixed with 2½ or 3 times its weight of quicksilver in the palm of the hand, and used as above.

Another cement consists of about 73 parts of silver, 21 of tin, and 6 of zinc, amalgamated with quicksilver. An amalgam of copper is said to be sometimes used. But this class of stoppings is altogether disapproved of by other authorities. Pure leaf-gold seems the least objectionable.

11. MARMORATUM. Finely levigated glass, mixed with tin amalgam.

12. POUDRE METALLIQUE. The article sold under this name in Paris appears to be an amalgam of silver, mercury, and ammonium, with an excess of mercury, which is pressed out before using it.

13. FUSIBLE METAL. Melt together 8 parts of bismuth, 5 of lead, 3 of tin, and 1½ or 1·6 of quicksilver, with as little heat as possible.—CHAUDET.

PASTE FOR DESTROYING THE SENSIBILITY OF THE DENTAL PULP PREVIOUS TO STOPPING. Arsenious acid 20 grains, sulphate of morphia 20 grains, creasote q. s. [Unsafe; it is only inserted by way of warning against what may prove an unsuspected cause of mischief.]

PIVOTS FOR ARTIFICIAL TEETH. An alloy of platinum and silver.

SPRINGS FOR ARTIFICIAL TEETH. Equal parts of copper, silver, and palladium.—CHAUDET.

[For Cachou Aromatisé, and other compounds for sweetening the breath, see PERFUMERY.]

BEVERAGES,

DIETETIC ARTICLES AND CONDIMENTS.

BEVERAGES, AND POWDERS FOR PREPARING THEM.

We have placed here such beverages as are rather employed as a refreshing luxury than either medicinally or as regular articles of diet. Wines, spirits, &c., are necessarily excluded. The medicinal mineral waters will be found elsewhere.

Ginger Beer. 1. Infuse 3 oz. of bruised ginger in 4 gallons of boiling water till cold. Strain through tammy or flannel. Dissolve in the liquor 5 ℔ of loaf sugar, and add half a pint of solid yeast, and $2\frac{1}{2}$ oz. of cream of tartar. In cold weather it will be necessary to set the cask near the fire, so as to excite brisk fermentation. As soon as this subsides rack off the clear liquor, return it into the cask previously washed out, and allow it to work for a day or two longer. Then draw it off, and bottle. —Mr. Donovan.

2. Ginger sliced 1 oz., dried orange-peel $\frac{1}{2}$ oz.; tie them in a bag, and boil with 16 ℔ of water, and strain; add $\frac{3}{4}$ of an oz. of tartaric or citric acid, 25 drops of essence of lemon, and 24 oz. of loaf sugar. When sufficiently cool add 2 tablespoonfuls of fresh yeast; let it work for 12 hours, and bottle it.

3. Ginger sliced $\frac{3}{4}$ oz., essence of lemon (rubbed with sugar) $\frac{1}{2}$ dr., lump sugar 12 oz., boiling water 8 ℔; infuse till cold, and strain. Ferment as above, with 3 or 4 spoonfuls of yeast, and bottle.

4. Boil $2\frac{1}{2}$ oz. of bruised ginger and 3 ℔ of sugar in $3\frac{1}{2}$ gallons of water for 20 minutes; put into a large pan 1 oz. cream of tartar, and the juice and rind of 2 lemons; pour the boiling liquor over them, and stir the whole well together; when milk-warm add $\frac{1}{4}$ pint of good ale yeast, cover it, and let it work for 2 or 3 days, skimming it frequently; then strain it through a jelly-bag into a cask, add $\frac{1}{2}$ pint of brandy, bung down close, and in 2 or 3 weeks bottle it in the usual way.

5. Boil 22 ounces of bruised ginger in 3 gallons of water for $\frac{1}{2}$ an hour; add 20 ℔ of white sugar, 18 ounces of lemon juice, 1 ℔ of honey, and 15 gallons of water, and strain through a cloth. When cold add the white of one egg, and $\frac{1}{2}$ oz. of essence of lemon; after standing 4 days bottle, and lay the bottles in a cellar for 3 weeks.

6. Prepare a clear decoction or infusion of ginger with sugar and lemon as above; but instead of fermenting it with yeast, charge it strongly with carbonic acid gas by means of a machine.

7. *Imperial Pop.* Cream of tartar 3 oz., ginger 1 oz., white sugar 24 oz., lemon juice 1 oz., boiling water a gallon and half; when cool, strain, and ferment with 1 oz. of yeast, and bottle.

GIRAMBING, OR LIMONIATED GINGER BEER. 1. Boil $4\frac{1}{2}$ oz. of ginger with 11 quarts of water; beat up 4 eggs to a froth, and add them with 9 ℔ of sugar to the preceding. Take 9 lemons, peel them carefully, and add the rind and juice to the foregoing. Put the whole into a barrel, add 3 spoonfuls of yeast, bung down the barrel, and in about 12 days bottle it off. In 15 days it will be fit for drinking; but it improves by keeping.

2. To 10 gallons of water add $11\frac{1}{2}$ ℔ of loaf sugar, and the whites of ten eggs well beaten; boil till the scum rises, and add 6 oz. of bruised ginger; boil for 20 minutes, then pour the hot liquor on the rinds of 12 lemons thinly peeled; when cold put into a barrel the juice of 12 lemons, 1 oz., of isinglass, a gill of brandy, and a spoonful of yeast, and fill the barrel with the liquor. In a fortnight it will be ready to bottle.

GINGER BEER POWDERS. Fine powder of Jamaica ginger

4 or 5 drachms, bicarbonate of soda 3½ oz., refined sugar in powder 14 oz., essence of lemon 30 drops. Mix, and divide into 5 dozen powders. (Or 4 to 5 grains of ginger, 28 of bicarbonate of soda, 112 of sugar, and ½ drop of essence of lemon, in each powder.) In the other powder put 32 grains of tartaric acid; or 35 grains if a more decidedly acidulated beverage is required. Or from 30 to 33 grains of citric acid.

[Other formulæ are also in use. Dr. PEREIRA gives the following: Bicarbonate of soda 30 gr., white sugar 1 dr., powdered ginger 5 gr., in each blue paper: and 25 gr. of tartaric acid in each white paper. This is less agreeable, but perhaps more friendly to the stomach, than when the acid is in slight excess. The following is from the Pharmaceutical Journal:—Sugar 2 dr., sesquicarbonate of soda 2 scruples (misprinted 2 drachms in vol. 3,) ginger 4 or 5 gr., essence of lemon 1½ or 2 drops in each blue paper; with 35 gr. of tartaric acid.]

GINGER BEER POWDER, IN ONE BOTTLE. (The soda, acid, and sugar must be very carefully dried, separately, and at a temperature not exceeding 120.°) Fine powder of Jamaica ginger 4 or 5 dr., bicarbonate of soda 3½ oz., double refined sugar 14 oz., essence of lemon 30 drops, tartaric acid 4½ oz. The acid and soda should not be too finely powdered. Mix the powders, recently dried, in a warm mortar, and immediately put the mixture into dry bottles, and cork securely. A measure holding 3 drachms should accompany each bottle.

KING CUP; OR LEMON DRINK WITHOUT ACID. 1. Pour a quart of cold water on the thin peel of 1 or 2 lemons; let them infuse 6 or 8 hours; then strain.—Mr. BRANDE.

2. Pour a pint of boiling water on the outer rind of one lemon, a small piece of dried orange-peel, and a moderate-sized lump of sugar.

LEMONADE, ACIDULATED (NOT AERATED.) 1. Fresh lemon-juice 4 oz., fresh lemon-peel (thinly peeled) ½ oz., white sugar 4 oz., boiling water 3 pints. Strain when cold.—Mr. BRANDE.

2. *Imperial.* Cream of tartar 1½ drachm, a slice of thin lemon-peel, a lump of sugar; pour on them a quart

of boiling water. Strain when cold. To be taken as a cooling drink,

3. *Common.* Cut 2 lemons into slices, add 2 oz. of sugar, and pour on them a quart of boiling water. It is sometimes made with cold water.

4. *French.* Syrup of citric acid 2 oz., water a quart, spirit of lemon-peel a teaspoonful.

5. Juice and thin peel of 1 lemon, citric acid 1 drachm, sugar 3 oz., boiling water a quart. It may be varied by substituting for the sugar syrup of raspberries, or of other fruits.

AERATED OR EFFERVESCING LEMONADE. This may be made by putting into each bottle (soda-water bottle) 1 oz. or 1½ oz. of syrup of lemons, and filling it up with simple aerated water from the machine. [The syrup is made by dissolving 30 oz. of lump sugar in 16 oz. of fresh lemon juice, by a gentle heat. It may be aromatized by adding 30 or 40 drops of essence of lemon to the sugar; or by rubbing part of the sugar on the peel of 2 lemons; or by adding to the syrup an ounce of a strong tincture of fresh lemon peel; or of the distilled spirit of the same.]

EFFERVESCING LEMONADE, WITHOUT A MACHINE. Put into each bottle 2 dr. of sugar, 2 drops of essence of lemon, ½ dr. of bicarbonate of potash, and water to fill the bottle; then drop in 35 or 40 grains of citric or tartaric acid in crystals, and cork immediately, placing the bottles in a cool place, or preferably, in iced water. Mr. BARTLETT recommends 2 scruples of sesquicarbonate of soda, 2 dr. of sugar, 4 drops of essence of lemon, and half a pint of water; lastly, a dr. of tartaric acid in crystals. Care must be taken to avoid accidents from the bursting of the bottles. Another form is—Into a soda-water bottle nearly filled with water add 1 oz. of sugar, 2 drops of essence of lemon (dropped on the sugar,) 20 grains of bicarbonate of potash in crystals; and, lastly, 30 to 40 grains of citric acid, also in crystals. Cork immediately.

MILK LEMONADE. Dissolve 1½ ℔ of sugar in a quart of boiling water, add ¼ pint of fresh lemon juice, and the same of sherry; and, lastly, two-thirds of a pint of cold milk. Stir together, and strain.

DRY LEMONADE, OR ACIDULOUS LEMONADE POWDER. Citric acid ¾ oz., refined sugar 8 oz., essence of lemon 36 drops. Some recipes direct a larger quantity of acid, others a much larger proportion of sugar.

EFFERVESCING LEMONADE POWDERS. Bicarbonate of soda 3½ oz., refined sugar 14 oz., essence of lemon 60 drops. [Sometimes 12 or more grains of the powdered yellow rind of lemon peel are added to colour it.] Mix, and divide into 60 powders, or 140 gr. in each blue paper. In the white papers put from 30 to 32 gr. of citric acid, or from 32 to 35 gr. of tartaric acid. Or the mixed alkaline powder and the acid may be put into separate bottles, furnished with measures holding the proper quantity of each.

EFFERVESCING LEMONADE POWDERS, IN ONE BOTTLE. *Note.*—The powders must all be separately and carefully dried, at a moderate temperature, before mixing, and when mixed be carefully secured from the air.

1. Bicarbonate of soda 1 oz., refined sugar 3½ oz., tartaric acid 1¼ oz., essence of lemon 30 drops; mix, and put into well corked bottles.

2. Mix 3½ oz. of bicarbonate of soda, 14 oz. of double refined sugar, 60 drops of essence of lemon, and 4 oz. to 4½ oz. of tartaric acid.

3. *Lemon Kali. Acidulated Kali.* Sesquicarbonated soda 8 oz., tartaric acid 8 oz., refined sugar 16 oz., essence of lemon 100 drops; mix.—Pharmaceutical Journal.

ORANGEADE, OR SHERBET. 1. Juice of 4 oranges, thin peel of 1 orange, lump sugar 4 oz., boiling water 3 pints.

2. Juice and peel of 1 large orange, citric acid ½ dr., sugar 3 oz., boiling water a quart.

EFFERVESCING OR AERATED ORANGEADE, OR SHERBET.

1. Mix 1 ℔ of syrup of orange-peel, a gallon of water, and 1 oz. of citric acid, and charge it strongly with carbonic acid gas with a machine.

2. Syrup of orange juice ¾ oz., aerated water half a pint.

3. Simple syrup ½ fluid oz., tincture of orange-peel ½ dr., citric acid 1 scruple; fill the bottle with aerated water.

4. Put into a soda-water bottle ½ oz. to 1 oz. of syrup of orange peel, 30 gr. of bicarbonate of potash, 8 oz. of water, and lastly 40 gr. of citric acid in crystals, and cork immediately.

5. Put into each bottle 2 or 3 dr. of sugar, 2 drops of oil of orange-peel, 30 gr. of bicarbonate of potash, or 25 gr. of bicarbonate of soda; water to fill the bottle, and 40 gr. of citric acid, as before.

AERATED SHERBET OR ORANGEADE POWDERS. Powdered sugar 14½ oz., powdered orange-peel 12 gr., oil of orange-peel 60 drops, essence of cedrat 12 drops, bicarbonate of soda 3½ oz.; mix, and put 145 gr. in each blue paper. In the white paper put 32 gr. of tartaric (or rather 30 gr. of citric) acid. Or the alkaline and acid powders may be put into separate bottles, with a measure holding the proper proportion of each. The orange-peel may be omitted.

AERATED SHERBET POWDERS, IN ONE BOTTLE. Double refined sugar 14½ oz., [powdered orange-peel 12 gr.] bicarbonate of soda 3½ oz., essence of cedrat 12 drops, oil of orange-peel 60 drops, tartaric acid 4 oz. The powders must be carefully dried, mixed quickly, and afterwards kept dry and securely corked. A measure holding nearly 3 dr. of the powder should accompany each bottle.

ORANGEADE POWDER, NOT AERATED. Citric acid ½ oz., sugar 8 oz., oil of orange-peel 20 drops.

SODA POWDERS. The usual proportions are—30 or 32 gr. of bicarbonate of soda in each blue paper; and 25 or 26 gr. of tartaric acid in each white paper.

ACIDULATED EFFERVESCING POWDERS; for making effervescing drinks with concentrated syrups of lemon, ginger, &c. Put into separate papers, distinguished by their different colours, 20 gr. of bicarbonate of soda, and 28 gr. of citric or tartaric acid. One of each powder to be dissolved separately in one-third of a tumbler of water, and a teaspoonful of the syrup added to the acid solution, and the liquids mixed.

[The CONCENTRATED SYRUPS are thus made—

Concentrated Syrup of Ginger. Simple syrup 7½ fluid ounces, essence of ginger (1 part ginger to 4 of spirit) ½ oz.

Concentrated Syrup of Lemon-peel. Strong tincture of lemon-peel* 1 oz., simple syrup 7½ fluid ounces.

Concentrated Syrup of Orange-peel. Strong tincture of fresh orange-peel* ½ oz., simple syrup 7½ fluid ounces.

Syrup of raspberries, pine-apples, and other fruits may be used with the above powders in the same way.]

For Seidlitz and other Medicated Powders, see MINERAL WATERS and POWDERS, at the end of PATENT MEDICINES, &c.

SPRUCE BEER. Water 10 gallons, treacle, or lump sugar (according to the colour required) 6 ℔; essence of spruce 4 oz.; add yeast and ferment as for ginger beer.

SPRUCE BEER POWDERS. In each blue paper put 5 scruples of powdered sugar, 28 gr. of bicarbonate of soda, and 10 gr. essence of spruce. In each white paper 30 gr. of tartaric acid.

TREACLE BEER. 1. Brown sugar 1 ℔, treacle 1 ℔, bruised ginger 1 oz., hops ¼ oz.; boil for a few minutes in 3 quarts of water, strain, and add 5 quarts of cold water; add a spoonful of fresh yeast; let it work all night, and bottle it in the morning.

2. Treacle 14 ℔, hops 1½ ℔, water 36 gallons, yeast 1 ℔. Boil the hops with the water, add the treacle, and strain. Cool to 80°, and ferment with the yeast. In winter ½ oz. of Cayenne pods with the hops is an improvement.—FAMILY FRIEND.

CAPILLAIRE. To a pint of boiling water add 3 oz. of fine maidenhair; remove from the fire, cover, and set near the fire for 3 hours; strain, and add ¼ pint of orange-flower water. Boil a gallon of fine syrup till reduced to 7 pints, then add the infusion, and boil for 10 minutes; strain through a jelly-bag, and when quite cold, bottle the syrup. It is used to give a fine flavour to water.

* These tinctures are thus made:—Fresh lemon-peel, thin, and cut small, 4 oz.; rectified spirit 8 oz.; digest for some days, and strain. Fresh peel of Seville oranges 4 oz., spirit 16 oz.

LIMONIATED CAPILLAIRE. Refined sugar 24 oz., water 12 oz.; dissolve by a gentle heat; and add essence of lemon 30 drops, neroli 3 drops, citric acid 2 oz., orange-flower water 4 oz.

SYRUP OF PINE APPLE. Expressed juice of pine apple a pint; loaf sugar 2 ℔. Boil gently, and when cold filter.

SYRUP D'ORGEAT. See Syrupus Amygdalæ, Pocket Formulary. Another formula for this elegant syrup is the following:—Take 20 oz. of sweet and 8 of bitter almonds, 9 ℔ of white sugar, and 4 pints of water. Blanch the almonds, dry them well, beat them with a portion of the sugar, and gradually add two-thirds of the water; strain through linen, wash the almonds on the strainer with the rest of the water, and dissolve the sugar in the strained liquor by a gentle heat. Pour the syrup into an earthen vessel, remove the scum, and when nearly cold add 2 oz. of orange-flower water.

ACIDULATED RASPBERRY SYRUP. Put 6 ℔ of raspberries into a china or glass bowl, or an earthen pan not glazed with lead, with a quart of water in which has been dissolved 2½ oz. of tartaric (or preferably *citric*) acid, and let it remain 24 hours; then strain it, taking care not to bruise the fruit. To each pint of clear liquor add 1½ ℔ of pounded loaf sugar, and stir it with a silver spoon till dissolved; leave it for a few days, then bottle it close. A little of this syrup, or of either of the two following, with water, forms a refreshing drink in warm weather, and in some febrile disorders.

ACIDULATED STRAWBERRY SYRUP. As RASPBERRY SYRUP, using 2 oz. of citric acid, instead of 2½ oz. of tartaric acid.

RASPBERRY VINEGAR. Put a pint and a half of best wine vinegar to 3 ℔ of fruit in a glass or porcelain vessel; leave them together for a fortnight, then strain without pressure. Or put an equivalent quantity of strong acetic acid (4 oz. of the usual strength) to the fruit, in the same way. Or it may be made as directed above for ACIDULATED RASPBERRY SYRUP.

WHEY POWDER. Sugar of milk in fine powder 2 oz., powdered white sugar 8 oz., gum Arabic ½ oz.; mix.

An ounce dissolved in a quart of water as a substitute for whey.

WHEY may be made by adding a little infusion of rennet (prepared calf's stomach) to milk, and gently heating it till curdled. It is also made by heating a quart of milk nearly to boiling, and adding a little of either lemon juice, orange juice, solution of citric acid, vinegar, or white wine, or cream of tartar sufficient to turn it. It is then strained. If required *bright*, beat up the white of an egg with a portion of the whey, mix with the rest, boil for a moment, and run it through a jelly bag.

One or two recipes in Confectionary may be introduced here.

ORANGE MARMALADE. 1. Procure some large Seville oranges with clear skins, peel them, squeeze out the pulp and juice, taking care to remove all the pips. Boil the peel, divided into quarters till they are sufficiently tender; scrape clean all the inside from them, lay them in folds, and cut them into very thin slices about an inch long. Weigh your juice, pulp, and boiled peel, and add broken lump sugar equal in weight to the whole, and boil for half an hour, carefully removing the scum. Then put it into pots, and when quite cold cover them over.

2. Instead of using all Seville oranges, let only half or a third of them be bitter, and the rest common sweet oranges. Proceed in the same way. Some add honey.

CURRANT JELLY. Pick the currants, put them in an earthen jar, and place it in boiling water till the juice is extracted. Strain through a sieve without pressing them, and boil the juice in an enamelled saucepan with its weight of loaf sugar, removing the scum as it rises. When it will jelly on the back of a cold spoon, it is sufficiently done. A little of the jelly dissolved in warm water forms an agreeable beverage.

DIETETIC ARTICLES.

As the ingredients of some of the following compounds are usually sold by druggists, who may be expected to furnish information as to the manner of using them, and as they may all be regarded as auxiliaries to medical treatment, some notice of them here seems desirable, though it must necessarily be brief and incomplete.

ARROW-ROOT. [West India arrow-root is the fecula of the tubers of the Maranta arundinacea; East India arrow-root is obtained from the Curcuma angustifolia; South Sea or Tahiti arrow-root from the Tacca pinnatifida. They have all the same properties, and are used in the same manner.] Mix a dessert spoonful of arrow-root with sufficient cold water to form a soft paste; rub it till quite smooth, and add half a pint of boiling water, stirring it briskly. Boil it for a minute or two, and when removed from the fire add a table spoonful of sherry or other white wine (where wine is admissible,) with a little grated nutmeg or lemon-peel, and sugar to the taste. For young children milk should be used instead of water, and the wine omitted: it is also more nourishing in this form for those invalids with whom milk agrees.

TOUS LES MOIS. [The fecula of a species of Canna.] It is used in the same way as arrow-root; but rather less is required. It forms a more tenacious, but less transparent jelly.

SAGO. [The granulated fecula of the pith of one or more species of the Sago Palm.] Wash an ounce of pearl sago in cold water; then boil it very gently in a pint of fresh water, stirring it frequently till dissolved. It may be flavoured with wine, spices, and sugar, as directed for arrow-root. For children, and for consumptive and debilitated patients, it may be made with milk instead of water. The common sago, being in larger grains, requires more time to dissolve; and is usually steeped for some hours before boiling it.

TAPIOCA. [Obtained from the tuberous roots of the Cassava,

Janipha manihot. It is usually sold in small lumps formed by drying the fecula on hot plates.] It is used in the same way as sago; but requires to be previously steeped for some hours, or to be simmered for a longer time. It forms a clear jelly, which may be flavoured with wine, spices, and sugar, as directed for arrow-root; but is more nourishing when made with milk.

SAGO POSSET, for invalids. Macerate a table spoonful of sago in a pint of water for 2 hours on the hob of a stove, then boil for 15 minutes, assiduously stirring. Add sugar, with an aromatic, as ginger or nutmeg, and a table spoonful or more of white wine. If the wine be not permitted, flavour with lemon-juice.

SAGO OR TAPIOCA MILK, for invalids. Take an ounce of either of these feculæ, and soak it in a pint of cold water for an hour; then pour off this water, and, adding 1½ pint of good milk, boil slowly until well incorporated.—Dr. A. T. THOMSON.

TAPIOCA PUDDING, for invalids. Beat up ½ ounce of sugar with the yolks of 2 eggs, and stir the mixture into a pint of tapioca milk.—Dr. THOMSON.

Arrow-root milk and pudding may be made like the corresponding preparations of tapioca.

PANADA, for invalids. Place in a saucepan some very thin slices of bread crumb, and add rather more water than will cover them. Boil now until the bread becomes pulpy, strain off the superfluous water, and beat up the remainder into the consistence of gruel. Sweeten with white sugar, and add, if permitted, a little sherry wine.

BARLEY WATER. See DECOCTUM HORDEI, and DECOCTUM HORDEI COMPOSITUM. ROBINSON'S Patent Barley is a convenient preparation: printed directions accompany it.

ASSES' MILK, ARTIFICIAL. Eringo root, pearl barley, sago, rice, of each 1 oz. Wash them with cold water, then boil them with 3 pints of water to 1½ pint, and strain. Put a teaspoonful to a cup of boiling milk, and sweeten to the taste. [*Bonbons de lait d'ânesse* are made with sugar of milk, white sugar, gum, and starch or arrow-root.]

LINSEED TEA. Take 1½ oz. of clean linseed, and ½ an oz. of bruised liquorice root; put them into a warm teapot or jug, and pour on them 2 pints of boiling water; let them stand, covered, near the fire, for 3 or 4 hours, stirring them occasionally; then strain. To save time, the ingredients may be boiled for 15 or 20 minutes, instead of infusing them; but the tea so made is less agreeable.

ICELAND MOSS. Infuse an ounce of picked Iceland Moss for 15 minutes in half a pint of hot water; strain off the water, and boil the moss in a quart of fresh water till reduced to a pint and a half. Half an ounce of liquorice root may be added, towards the end of the boiling, if agreeable: or milk may be used instead of water.

JELLY OF ICELAND MOSS. See Gelatina Lichenis, Pocket Formulary. Another form is the following:—Infuse 2 ℔ of the moss for half an hour in sufficient boiling water to cover it; drain the moss, and boil it in 2½ gallons of water for an hour, and strain. Boil the moss with fresh water, adding an oz. of isinglass; strain; mix the product of the two boilings, and let it stand till clear. Evaporate the clear liquor to the consistence of a stiff jelly, adding, towards the end, 6 ℔ of fine lump sugar, 2 oz. of French brandy, and half an ounce of orange-flower water. It may be taken, almost at pleasure, dissolved in water or milk.

ICELAND MOSS CHOCOLATE. See Chocolata Lichenis, Pocket Formulary.

IRISH MOSS, OR CARRAGEEN. Steep a ¼ of an oz. of the moss in cold water for a few minutes; then withdraw it, shaking the water from each sprig, and boil it in a quart of milk till it attains the consistence of jelly, and sweeten to the taste. A decoction of the same quantity of moss in a quart of water is also used as a demulcent in coughs, &c. BLANC-MANGE may be made by washing ½ oz. of the moss as above, and boiling it in 1½ pint of new milk to such a consistence that it will retain its form when cold, sweetening and flavouring it to the taste. An agreeable jelly may be made by boiling it with water instead of milk, and adding lemon or orange juice or peel, wine, &c.

CEYLON MOSS. Boil ½ oz. of the prepared moss in a quart of water for 25 minutes; or till a spoonful taken out forms a firm jelly in 2 or 3 minutes: then flavour with wine, cinnamon, or with lemon or orange juice or peel; and sweeten to the taste. Boil for five minutes longer, and press through a jelly-bag, or doubled muslin. Pour it into earthen moulds, and leave it undisturbed till it has set. If the jelly is required *bright*, it must be clarified with white of egg, as directed for gelatine jelly. For BLANC-MANGE add 1 oz. of prepared moss to a quart of boiling water, and boil gently till reduced to a third; add the milk and flavouring ingredients, and pour into earthen moulds.

AUSTRALIAN MOSS. This has been introduced for the same uses as Irish and Ceylon mosses, but has not been very generally adopted. Soak ½ oz. of the moss in water for an hour or two, pour away the water, and boil the moss in a quart of fresh water till dissolved. Strain through a hair sieve, and sweeten and flavour to the taste.

SALEP. [The dried root of some species of orchis.] Boil ½ oz. of salep powder in a pint of water till dissolved; strain, and sweeten and flavour to the taste.

HARTSHORN JELLY. Boil 4 oz. of true hartshorn shavings (previously washed in warm water) in a quart of water till reduced to a pint; strain, and sweeten and flavour to the taste. For children and consumptive patients, the simple jelly may be mixed with milk and a little sugar. To make a bright jelly for the table, boil 4 oz. of washed hartshorn shavings in 1½ pint of water, till reduced to ¾ of a pint, and add 2 oz. of sugar, and a tablespoonful of lemon or orange juice. Strain with pressure; beat up the white of an egg with a little cold water, mix this thoroughly with the jelly, and evaporate the liquid till a little taken out solidifies on cooling. Add a little fresh lemon-peel, and strain through a jelly-bag.

GELATINE JELLY. Steep 1 oz. of NELSON'S or other purified gelatine in half a pint of cold water for ten minutes; then add the same quantity of boiling water, and stir till it is dissolved, applying heat if required: add the juice and peel of two lemons, sugar, and wine sufficient to make up the whole a pint and a half. If required bright, have ready the white and shell of an egg well beaten together, stir them briskly into the jelly, boil for 2 or 3 minutes without stirring, and pass through a jelly-bag. As a nourishing diet for children and invalids, a little of the gelatine simply dissolved in water may be mixed with milk, or the dry gelatine dissolved in milk by heat.

ISINGLASS JELLY. Isinglass is used in the same way as gelatine, but as it is not wholly soluble in water, it requires straining. To make a bright jelly, it requires more egg for its clarification than gelatine. A very pleasant jelly is made with the Acidulated Raspberry or Strawberry Syrup (page 280) thus:—Dissolve 1½ oz. of isinglass in a very little water, put this to a quart of the syrup, warm it and stir it well; then strain it into a mould. In warm weather put 2 oz. of isinglass.

ARROW ROOT BLANC-MANGE. Beat up 2 oz. of genuine arrow-root with a little cold milk to the consistence of cream; pour on it 1½ pint of boiling milk, stirring it all the time. Flavour and sweeten to the taste, boil for 10 minutes, stirring it constantly, pour it into moulds, and leave it until next day.

BLANC-MANGE. This may be made with either isinglass or gelatine. Boil ½ oz. in 16 fluid oz. (the old wine pint) of new milk; stir it constantly till it boils, let it simmer for a few minutes till the isinglass is dissolved; strain, add sugar to the taste, and a few drops of almond flavour, or other flavouring ingredients, and pour into moulds.

CHOCOLATE. This is prepared from the finest cacao nuts (seeds of Theobroma cacao) after roasting, winnowing, &c., by grinding them on a hot stone or plate, or beating them in a hot mortar, to a smooth paste. Sugar is generally added, and vanilla or other flavouring ingredient.

CHOCOLATES, Medicated. See Chocolata, Pocket Formulary.

WHITE CHOCOLATE. White sugar 3 ℔, rice flour 27½ oz., English or Indian arrow-root 8 oz., tincture of vanilla ½ oz., butter of cacao 8 oz., powdered gum Arabic 4 oz.; form a paste with boiling water, and put it into moulds.

COCOA. This should also be prepared from the seeds of Theobroma cacao; and the rock, roll, and flake cocoas, often consist of this alone. But most of the paste cocoa, and soluble cocoa powder, is mixed with saccharine and farinaceous matters. This is the case even with much of the *Homœopathic Cocoa*, which professes to be unadulterated. A common proportion for soluble cocoa appears to be two-thirds of pure cocoa, and one-third of sugar and farina; the latter being one or more of the following—Wheat flour, sago meal, potato flour, arrow-root, &c. The *Paste Cocoa* often contains only about half its weight of cocoa, the rest being sugar and water, with sometimes the addition of sago meal or other farina.

BROMA. This consists of about 8 ounces of pure cocoa, 3½ of sugar, and 4½ of sago meal, arrow-root, &c.

WACAKA DES INDES. Roasted cacao beans (chocolate) in powder 2 oz., sugar 6 oz., cinnamon ¼ oz., vanilla (powdered with part of the sugar) ½ dr., ambergris 3 gr., musk 1½ gr. Sometimes a drachm of prepared annatto is added, and the ambergris and musk omitted.

RACAHOUT DES ARABES. This is professedly a preparation of acorns (perhaps those of the Quercus ballotta, which are naturally sweet, or of other kinds deprived of their bitterness by being buried in the earth;) but it is imitated by the following:—1. Chocolate in powder 1 oz., rice flour 3 oz., sugar 9 oz., potato arrow-root 3 oz., vanilla (pulverized with part of the sugar) 1 dr. Mix.

2. Chocolate in powder 4 oz., salep 1 oz. (or powdered tragacanth 1 oz.,) potato arrow-root 5 oz., sugar (flavoured with vanilla) 8 oz.—CADET.

DICTAMIA. Sugar 7 oz., potato arrow-root 4 oz., flour of brent barley (triticum monococcum) 3 oz., Trinidad and Granada chocolate, each 1 oz., vanilla 15 gr.

PALAMOUD. Chocolate 1 oz., rice flour 4 oz., potato arrow-root 4 oz., red sanders in fine powder, 1 dr. Mix. [In the above by chocolate is meant the cacao beans roasted and pulverized without addition. Indian arrow-root or Tous les Mois may be substituted for the potato arrow-root.]

FERCULUM SAXONIA. Barley flour 21 oz., sugar 7 oz., cinnamon 1 dr. Mix, and bake them in an oven, enveloped in a paste of wheat flour, and placed in an earthen vessel. When sufficiently baked, remove the crust, and when the contents are cool, reduce them to powder. About ½ oz. to 1 oz. is boiled with broth, &c., as a nourishing diet. It is often medicated with the addition of sarsaparilla, bark, &c.

FARINACEOUS FOOD, &c. The following compounds are accompanied with full directions for use:—

BASTER'S *Soojee and Compound Farina.* Wheat flour, with sugar.

BRIGHT'S *Nutritious Farina.* The basis is said to be potato starch.

BRIGHT'S *Breakfast Powder.* A combination of chocolate with his nutritious farina.

BRADEN'S *Farinaceous Food.* Chiefly wheat flour carefully baked.

BULLOCK'S *Semola.* Wheat flour, from which a portion of the starch has been removed, so as to leave a definite proportion of gluten.

DENHAM'S *Farinaceous Food.* As BRADEN'S, with perhaps a mixture of barley flour.

GARDINER'S *Alimentary Preparation.* Very finely ground rice flour.

HARD'S *Farinaceous Food.* Carefully baked wheat flour.

HUNT'S *Breakfast Powder.* Rye, carefully roasted as coffee. [For Dandelion Coffee, see page 182.]

LEATH'S *Alimentary Farina.* Baked wheat flour, with sugar, potato flour, and a small quantity of Indian corn meal, and tapioca.

MAIDMAN'S *Nutritious Farina.* Potato flour, tinged with some pink colouring matter.

PALMER'S *Vitaroborant.* See ERVALENTA, below.

PLUMBE'S *Farinaceous Food.* South Sea arrow-root, combined with pea flour.

Prince of Wales's Food. Potato flour.

Semolina. A hard kind of wheat, containing much gluten, ground into coarse grains. But some articles sold under this name appear to be compounds of gluten, artificially granulated, resembling BULLOCK'S Semola.

ERVALENTA, REVALENTA ARABICA, LENTIL POWDER, &c. These consist chiefly either of the European or Egyptian lentil.

Ervalenta. WARTON'S consists of the French or German lentil, with either Indian corn, or, more probably, a species of corn called *Durra*, used by the Arabs. But Dr. SCHENK states that what is sold at Paris consists of the flour of French beans and Indian corn.

Revalenta Arabica. A mixture of the red (Egyptian or Arabian) lentil with barley flour. Some samples contain sugar, others salt, and a flavouring ingredient.

Lentil Powders. Some consist entirely of lentil flour (French or German,) or Egyptian, or both kinds mixed. Others contain barley flour in addition. NEVILL'S consists of 1 oz. of curry powder to 4 ℔ of lentil flour. The LANCET gives the following recipes for lentil powder:—1. Arabian lentil flour 2 ℔, barley flour 1 ℔, salt 3 ounces.

2. Pea flour 2 ℔, Indian corn flour 1 ℔, salt 3 oz.

GRUEL is made either from oatmeal, or from groats or grits (oats deprived of their cuticle) either whole or crushed (Embden groats.) Dr. THOMSON directs 3 oz. of groats, previously washed, to be boiled slowly in 4 pints of water, till reduced to 2 pints, then strained through a sieve. The Embden groats require less boiling. Dr. KITCHENER directs one or two tablespoonfuls of oatmeal (according as the gruel is preferred thin or thick) to be well mixed with 3 spoonfuls of cold water gradually added, a pint of boiling water poured on it, and the whole boiled for 5 minutes, constantly stirring it; it is then skimmed and strained through a hair sieve; a little butter is usually added, and sometimes milk, with salt, or otherwise sugar and spices to the taste. Thorough trituration of the oatmeal and cold water, and constant stirring of the gruel while on the fire, render long boiling unnecessary.

BOILED WHEAT. Steep the wheat in water for 10 or 12 hours, then boil it for half an hour. [As a substitute for vegetables, and to obviate constipation.—Mr. L. BULLOCK.]

BEEF TEA. Professor LIEBIG directs 1 ℔ of beef, free from fat, to be minced very small, mixed with an equal weight of cold water, and heated slowly to boiling; when it has boiled for a minute or two, strain through a cloth. It may be coloured with roasted onion or burnt sugar, and salted to the taste. Dr. SEYMOUR directs 2½ ℔ of lean beef cut small to be put into 3 pints of cold water, and simmered slowly, without boiling, till reduced to a pint and a half; then carefully strained.

EXTRACT OF MEAT. Cut the lean of fresh-killed meat very small, put it into eight times its weight of cold water, and heat it gradually to the boiling point. When it has boiled for a few minutes, strain it through a cloth, and evaporate the liquor gently by water-bath to a soft mass. 2 ℔ of meat yield 1 oz. of extract. Fat must be carefully excluded, or it will not keep.—LIEBIG.

TROPHAZOME. Mince 16 oz. of meat, free from fat, very fine, pour on it 8 oz. of cold or lukewarm water (not exceeding 100°;) mix well, and let it stand for an hour, stirring it 3 or 4 times. Press out the fluid (about 6 oz.;) mix 8 oz. more of water with the meat, stir it occasionally, and in half an hour strain with pressure. Repeat this with 8 oz. more water. Break up the pressed meat, and put into a small tin vessel; place this in a water-bath of cold water, heat gradually to the boiling point, and keep it boiling for 20 minutes. Mix the fluid which exudes with the others, add salt, spices, and other flavouring ingredients, and boil for 20 minutes in a covered vessel. It may be thickened with 1 oz. of semola.—Mr. BULLOCK.

BREAD, UNFERMENTED. Mix carefully ½ oz. of bicarbonate of soda and ¼ oz. of salt with 4 ℔ of flour; mix this with a quart (or rather 41 or 42 fluid oz.) of very cold water, previously mixed with ½ a fluid oz. and 20 minims of muriatic acid of 1·16 specific gravity, into a thin dough, with as little kneading as possible, and let it be *immediately* placed in the oven; it requires rather more time than fermented bread. By mixing 26 measures of the acid with 46 of water, a diluted acid is obtained, of which a fluid ounce and a half may be taken for every ½ oz. packet of soda.—Mr. DEANE.

A pamphlet on the subject directs for *Brown Bread*, 3 ℔ of wheatmeal and 10 dr. (Apoth. weight) of bicarbonate of soda to be well mixed, and made into dough, with 25 oz. of cold water, previously mixed with 12½ fluid dr. of muriatic acid.

The proportions used first by Dr. WHITING, and subsequently by Mr. DODSON, in the preparation of unfermented bread and biscuits, were—7 ℔ of wheaten flour, 350 to 500 gr. of carbonate of soda, 2¾ pints of water, with muriatic acid 420 to 560 gr., or as much as may be sufficient. The soda, dissolved in a small quantity of water, is first carefully kneaded with the dough, and the acid being afterwards rapidly mixed in, the bread is baked without delay.

A third formula is that of Mr. J. SAVORY, and is recommended as excellent by Dr. PEREIRA. Intimately mix with 1 ℔ of flour, sesquicarbonate of soda 40 gr., and powdered white sugar a teaspoonful, in a large basin with a wooden spoon. Then gradually add cold water about ½ pint, previously mixed with 50 drops of common muriatic acid, and stir constantly, so as to form very speedily an intimate mixture. Divide into 2 loaves, and put into a quick oven immediately.

Another form of unfermented bread is as follows:—mix 1 oz. of bicarbonate of soda, ¾ oz. of tartaric acid, and ¼ oz. of salt, with 7 ℔ (half a peck) of flour; mix the whole thoroughly, taking care that all the ingredients are perfectly dry; add, in 2 or 3 portions, 4 pints of cold water, and incorporate quickly; place it in tins, and send it to the oven immediately. If not baked in tins, less water must be used.

(Biscuits and cakes made without yeast, and containing no butter, are prescribed in some dyspeptic cases; of such the following are examples:—)

ABERNETHY BISCUITS. Make into a stiff biscuit paste, 1 quart of milk, 6 eggs, 8 oz. of loaf sugar, and ½ oz. of caraway seeds, with flour sufficient to bring the whole to the required consistence. Make the biscuits thin, dock them with holes to prevent them from swelling up, and bake in an oven at a moderate heat.

SPONGE BISCUITS. Beat the yolks of 12 eggs for ½ an hour, then put in 1½ ℔ of finely powdered sugar, and whisk it briskly until it rises in bubbles; beat the whites to a strong froth, and whisk them well with the sugar and yolks; then work in 14 oz. of flour, with the rinds of 2 lemons grated. Bake in tin moulds buttered, for 1 hour in a quick oven, sifting over them a little fine sugar.

RICE CAKE. Beat the yolks of 15 eggs for nearly half an hour with a whisk, mix well with them 10 oz. of finely sifted white sugar; put in ½ ℔ of ground rice, a little orange flower water or brandy, and the rinds of 2 lemons grated; then add the whites of 7 eggs, well beaten up, and stir the whole for ¼ of an hour; put into a hoop, and bake for ½ an hour in a quick oven.

MEAT BISCUITS. A thick extract of meat (made by boiling fresh-killed beef or other meat, and evaporating the strained liquid) is kneaded with wheaten flour, and the dough rolled out and divided into biscuits, which are dried or baked in an oven. They are kept in the form of biscuits, or coarsely ground: 1 ounce makes a pint of rich soup, which may be salted or flavoured to the taste.

GLUTEN BREAD (for diabetic patients.) It is sometimes made with the gluten of flour, a small portion only of the starch being retained. Dr. PERCY proposes the following method:—Take the matter left after removing the starch from 16 ℔ of rasped potatoes, ¾ ℔ of mutton suet, 12 eggs, ½ ℔ of butter, and ½ oz. of carbonate of soda; mix, and add 2 oz. of diluted hydrochloric acid; divide into 8 cakes, and bake immediately in a quick oven.

[Various alimentary preparations have lately been introduced, the basis of which is the gluten which remains in extracting the starch from wheat flour by the mechanical process. Mr. GENTILE'S *gluten flour* is a mixture of this with wheat flour. It contains 42 per cent. of gluten, and yields a nutritious and digestible *gluten biscuit*, *gluten bread*, and, with cocoa, *gluten chocolate*. Mr. BULLOCK'S *semola* and M. VERNON'S *granulated gluten* are of the same nature. 30 parts of wheat flour, 10 of fresh gluten, and 7 of water, form a paste resembling *Italian macaroni*, vermicelli, &c.]

BAKING POWDER. See page 172.

CUSTARD POWDER. Rub up together gum tragacanth 2 oz., potato starch 1 ℔, powdered turmeric 2½ dr., with oil of bitter almonds ½ dr., and essence of lemons 1 dr. Put up into 1-oz. packets. (From 1 pint of new milk take 2 tablespoonfuls to work up with the powder; boil the remaining milk with 2 ounces of lump sugar, and pour it, while boiling, into the basin, stirring quickly until thoroughly mixed. Bake as a custard.)—Mr. SCHOLEFIELD.

Without the colouring, this forms *Blanc-mange Powder.*

CONDIMENTS, AND VARIOUS CULINARY COMPOUNDS.

CURRY POWDER. The recipes for "true Indian Curry Powder" are numerous, and vary much in the number and proportion of the ingredients. The total quantity of powder in each of the following recipes being nearly equal, the relative proportion of the different colouring, heating, and flavouring ingredients, will at once be seen. Dr. KITCHENER complains that the proportion of cayenne is generally so large, that a proper quantity of the powder cannot be used to obtain the benefit of the other ingredients; and the Editor of the Pharmaceutical Journal justly observes that many recipes contain too large a proportion of turmeric. All the ingredients should be of fine quality and recently ground.

	1	2	3	4	5	6	7	8	9	10	11	12
Turmeric	9	6	6	8	9	9	9	4	6	6	7	8
Coriander seed	9	16	12	22	10	9	16	12	11	16	13	12
Mustard, *scorched.*	3	...	...	...	3	3	...	4	...	...	...	...
Cayenne.............	2¼	4	1½	1	1¼	¾	1½	2	1	2	1	1
Pepper, black or long............	6 bl.	3 bl.	8 long	2 bl.	3 bl.	3 bl.	2½ bl.	4 bl.	5 bl.	1¼ bl.	5 bl.	4 bl.
Pimento	...	...	...	...	...	...	...	...	2	¾	...	...
Cloves	1	...	...	...	½	...	...	...	½	¼	...	...
Cinnamon	2	...	...	...	...	¾	...	...	3	¾	...	...
Cardamom	2	3	...	...	1½	1½	...	...	...	...	...	2
Ginger	1	...	...	...	3	3	...	...	2	1½	...	4
Mace	1	...	...	...	...	...	¼	¼	...	½	...	...
Fenugrec	...	...	3	...	...	...	...	2	2	3½	3	...
Cummin	...	...	2	...	1	...	3	2	...	...	3	1

The addition of 1 oz. of garlic, or 2 oz. of shallots, to 2 ℔ of either of the above, will be approved by some palates. The *true* Indian curry is said to be thus made—coriander seed 6 dr., turmeric 5 scruples, fresh ginger 4½ dr., cummin seeds 18 gr., black pepper 54 gr., poppy seed 94 gr., garlic 2 heads, cinnamon a scruple, cardamom 5 seeds, 8 cloves, 1 or 2 chillies, half a cocoa-nut grated; all but the last to be ground on a stone.

BENGAL CHITNI. Chillies 1½ ℔, unripe mangoes (or apples) 1 ℔, red tamarinds 2 ℔, sugar candy 1 ℔, fresh ginger root 1½ ℔, garlic ¾ to 1½ ℔, sultana raisins 1½ ℔, fine salt 1 ℔, and 5 bottles of the best vinegar; soak the chillies for an hour in the vinegar, then grind all with a stone and muller to a paste.

ITALIAN TAMARA. Coriander seed, cloves, and cinnamon, of each 8 oz.; anise and fennel seeds, of each 4 oz.; mix.

MIXED SPICES, AND SAVOURY HERBS. 1. *Kidder's Sweet Spice.* Equal weights of cloves, mace, nutmegs, cinnamon, and sugar.

2. *Kidder's Savoury Spice.* Equal weights of salt, pepper, cloves, nutmegs, and mace.

3. *Ragout.* Salt 16 oz., pepper 8 oz., nutmeg, ginger, and allspice, each ¼ oz.; lemon-peel 8 oz., mustard flour 8 oz., cayenne 2 oz.; mix.

4. *Sausage.* Pepper 5 ℔, cloves 1½ ℔, nutmegs 1½ ℔, ginger 2½ ℔, aniseed ½ ℔, coriander seed ½ ℔; mix.

5. Dr. KITCHENER'S *Savoury Ragout.* Salt 2 oz., mustard, black pepper, and grated lemon-peel, of each 1 oz., allspice, ginger, and nutmeg, of each ½ oz., cayenne ¼ oz.

6. *Soup Herb and Savoury Powder.* Mix 3 parts of No. 7 with 1 part of No. 5.

7. Dr. KITCHENER'S *Soup Herb Powder, or Vegetable Relish.* Dried parsley, winter savoury, sweet marjoram, lemon thyme, of each 2 oz., dried lemon-peel, and sweet basil, of each 1 oz.; mix. They should be carefully dried in a Dutch oven, powdered, passed through a hair sieve, and kept in closely-covered bottles. For sauces, soups, &c.

8. *Pease Powder.* Pound together in a marble mortar

2 oz. each of dried mint and sage, $\frac{1}{4}$ oz. each of celery seed and black pepper, and rub them through a hair sieve.

HORSE RADISH POWDER. Take up the roots in November or December, dry them carefully with a gentle heat, and reduce to powder.

SOLUBLE CAYENNE. To 1 ℔ of the best cayenne pepper, add as much rectified spirit as will form it into a paste. Cover this up for 2 hours; then place it in a percolator, and gradually pour on it more spirit till a pint of liquid is procured. A little water cautiously poured on the pepper will displace most of the remaining spirit. Distil off most of the spirit for future use, and add to the residue 3 ℔ of fine salt, and evaporate the mixture to dryness by the heat of a water-bath. It is usually coloured, but it is better without it.

CULINARY ESSENCES, TINCTURES, &c.

ALMOND FLAVOUR. Essential oil of bitter almonds 1 part, rectified spirit 7 parts. Some put one part of oil to 15 of spirit: others, 1 part to 3. It should not be sold without a caution as to the quantity to be used; or rather, the oil should be first purified from its hydrocyanic acid, by mixing it with a solution of chloride of iron and cream of lime, with a little peroxide of mercury, and, after a few days' contact, carefully re-distilling the oil.

FLAVOURING ESSENCE. Purified oil of bitter almonds 8 drops, essence of lemon 12 drops, oil of cinnamon 8 drops, oil of nutmeg 4 drops, highly rectified spirit 1 oz. A few drops to be added to pudding, custards, &c.

LEMON FLAVOUR. Fresh lemon-peel, cut thin, 3 dr., essence of lemon 1 dr., alcohol 3 oz. [Another method is to rub a lump of sugar on clean dry lemons, till the yellow rind is taken up by the sugar; then scrape off the saturated part of the sugar, and keep it in a closely-covered pot for use.]

TINCTURE OF CINNAMON (KITCHENER'S.) Bruised cinnamon 3 oz., a bottle of Cognac brandy; digest for a fortnight, and strain. [Tincture of Allspice, Nutmeg, Cloves, in the same manner.]

ESSENCE OF CINNAMON. Bruised cinnamon 2 dr., oil of cinnamon 1 dr., highly rectified spirit 3 oz.; digest, and strain.

ESSENCE OF NUTMEG, MACE, CLOVES, ALLSPICE, &c. These are made from the spices and their essential oils, as ESSENCE OF CINNAMON.

ESSENCE OF CELERY. Celery seed ½ oz. to 1 oz., brandy 4 oz.; digest for 8 or 10 days, and filter.

ESSENCE OF CARAWAY. Bruised caraway seed 1 oz., rectified spirit 8 oz., oil of caraway ¼ oz., brown sugar ¼ oz., digest for 8 or 10 days and filter.

AROMATIC ESSENCE OF GINGER. Fresh grated ginger, 3 oz., fresh thin lemon peel 2 oz., brandy 1½ pint; macerate for 10 days.—Dr. KITCHENER.

ESSENCE OF PEAR, and ESSENCE OF PINE-APPLE. See Trade Chemicals.

ESSENCE OF CAYENNE (KITCHENER'S.) Put ½ oz. of cayenne pepper into half a pint of brandy; let it steep for a fortnight, then pour off the clear liquor. [A much stronger essence is sometimes kept, prepared by percolation, as directed for Soluble Cayenne.]

SPIRIT OF SAVOURY SPICES (KITCHENER'S.) Black pepper 1 oz., allspice ½ oz., nutmeg ¼ oz. (all pounded;) infuse in 16 fluid oz. of brandy for 10 days.

SPIRIT OF SOUP HERBS (KITCHENER'S.) Lemon thyme, winter savoury, sweet marjoram, sweet basil, each 1 oz., grated lemon-peel and shallots, each ½ oz., celery seed 1 dr.; infuse in a pint of brandy for 10 days.

SPIRIT OF SAVOURY SPICES. Infuse half the Savoury Ragout Powder (see MIXED SPICES, &c., No. 5, above) in a quart of brandy for 10 days.

KITCHENER'S SOUP HERB AND SAVOURY SPICE SPIRIT. A mixture of equal measures of the last two.

CULINARY VINEGARS, SAUCES, &c.

TARRAGON VINEGAR. Put fresh tarragon leaves into a stone jar, and pour on them a sufficient quantity of the best wine vinegar to cover them. Set the jar in a warm place for 14 days; then strain through a jelly bag. [In the same way may be made elder-flower, basil, green mint, and burnet-vinegars. Cress and celery vinegar are made with ½ oz. of the bruised seed to a quart of vinegar. Horse radish vinegar, with 3 oz. of the scraped root, 1 oz. of minced shallots, 1 dr. of cayenne, to a quart of vinegar. Garlic vinegar is made with 2 oz. of minced garlic to a quart of wine vinegar. Shallot vinegar in the same proportion. Chilli vinegar, with 50 English chillies, cut or bruised (or ¼ oz. cayenne pepper,) to a pint of the best vinegar; digest for 14 days.]

CAMP VINEGAR. Take 12 chopped anchovies, 2 cloves of garlic minced, 1 dr. of cayenne, 2 oz. of soy, 4 oz. of walnut catsup, and a pint of the best vinegar; digest for a month, and strain.

2. Vinegar a quart, walnut catsup a pint, mushroom catsup 3 tablespoonfuls, garlic 4 heads, cayenne ½ oz., soy 2 tablespoonfuls, port wine 2 glasses, 3 anchovies, and a tablespoonful of salt; put them into a bottle, shake daily for a month, and decant.

CURRY VINEGAR. Infuse 3 oz. of curry powder in a quart of vinegar, near the fire, for 3 days.

RASPBERRY VINEGAR. Macerate 2 ℔ of fresh raspberries with a pint of the best vinegar for 14 days and strain. Or to a quart of the juice add 2 oz. of strong acetic acid, or enough to render it sufficiently acid.

ESCHALOT WINE. Bruised shallots 3 oz., sherry wine a pint; infuse for 10 days. An ounce of scraped horse radish and a drachm of thin lemon-peel may be added. ["The most elegant preparation of the onion tribe."—Dr. KITCHENER.] Wines of several herbs may be made in the same proportion as the vinegars.

FRENCH MUSTARD. This is sold with a great variety of flavours. A good substitute may be made by mixing good flour of mustard with the liquor of walnut and other pickles; or with the flavoured vinegars, above. The following is one of the published recipes:—Salt 12 oz., scraped horse radish 8 oz., a clove of garlic, ½ oz. of sugar, a gallon of French vinegar (hot, but not boiling.) Macerate for 24 hours, and strain. Mix with flour of mustard, q. s.

MUSTARD FOR THE TABLE. Mix 8 spoonfuls of flour of mustard with 2 of salt, and 9 of water. Mix to a smooth paste, add 6 spoonfuls more of water, and mix.

ESSENCE OF ANCHOVIES. Beat 1 ℔ of Anchovies in a Wedgewood mortar, and put them into a pipkin with 4 oz. of vinegar; boil for a few minutes, and rub the pulp through a hair-sieve. Boil the bones in 1½ ℔ of water, strain, and add 2 oz. of salt, and 2 oz. of flour of starch, and the pulped anchovies; let it boil, and pass it through a hair-sieve. It is usually coloured with powdered bole, or with annatto. Gum tragacanth is sometimes used to stiffen it instead of flour. Another method is, to simmer anchovies in their own weight of water for 2 or 3 hours, removing any scum that may rise, strain with pressure through a strong canvas bag, and filter through flannel. This has the pure flavour of the fish; but a little cayenne and salt may be added, to preserve it.

ANCHOVY PASTE. Pound the fish in a mortar, and rub the pulp through a fine sieve. Put it into pots, and cover with clarified butter.

MUSHROOM CATSUP. Press the mushrooms in a tincture press, and boil the juice with ½ oz. black pepper-corns, 1 oz. pimento, ½ oz. of ginger, ¼ oz. cloves, 1½ oz. shallots, and 8 oz. of salt, to each gallon. Some add 4 oz. of brandy. Or sprinkle the mushrooms with salt (a pound to 2 pecks,) stir occasionally for 2 days, then squeeze them gently in a hair-sieve, and boil the liquor with pepper and other spices.

WALNUT CATSUP. 1. Mix 6 half sieves of green walnut-shells with 2 or 3 ℔ of salt in a wooden vessel: let them stand 6 days, beating them frequently till they become pulpy; then drain off the juice, and boil it up with 4 oz. of ginger and allspice, and 2 oz. of long pepper and cloves.

2. Juice of walnuts 1 gallon, anchovies 2 ℔, shallots

1 lb, cloves, mace, and black pepper, of each 1 oz., and a clove of garlic. Boil for a short time, and bottle it.

LEMON PICKLE. Slice 6 lemons, rub them with salt, lay them in a stone jar, with 2 oz. each of allspice and white pepper; add $\frac{1}{4}$ oz. each of mace, cloves, and cayenne, and 2 oz. each of horse radish and mustard seed: pour over them 2 quarts of hot distilled vinegar; and, after standing for a few days, strain. Some add garlic or shallots.

QUIN SAUCE. Mushroom catsup $\frac{1}{2}$ pint, walnut pickle $\frac{1}{4}$ pint, port wine $\frac{1}{4}$ pint, 6 anchovies, and 6 shallots (both pounded;) soy, a tablespoonful, cayenne $\frac{1}{2}$ dr.; simmer together gently for 10 minutes, strain, and bottle.

WATERLOO SAUCE. Vinegar 4 pints, port wine 1 pint, cayenne 1 oz., walnut catsup $\frac{1}{2}$ pint, mushroom catsup $\frac{1}{2}$ pint, essence of anchovies 4 oz., powdered cochineal 1 oz., garlic, 12 cloves.

EPICUREAN SAUCE. Indian soy 2 oz., walnut catsup, mushroom catsup, each 8 oz., port wine 2 oz., bruised white pepper $\frac{1}{2}$ oz., shallots 3 oz., cayenne $\frac{1}{4}$ oz., cloves $\frac{1}{2}$ oz. Macerate for 14 days in a warm place, strain, and add white wine vinegar to make up a pint.

SAUCE SUPERLATIVE (Dr. KITCHENER'S.) Port wine, and mushroom catsup, of each a pint; walnut or other pickle liquor $\frac{1}{2}$ pint, pounded anchovies 4 oz.; fresh lemon-peel cut thin, sliced shallots, and scraped horse radish, of each 1 oz.; allspice and black pepper, of each $\frac{1}{2}$ oz.; cayenne 1 dr.; curry powder 3 dr.; celery seed 1 dr.; put them into a wide-mouthed bottle, stop it close, shake daily for a fortnight, and strain: a $\frac{1}{4}$ pint of soy may be added.

[A variety of sauces may be made by mixing, in different proportions, the ingredients of the last 4 sauces.]

CASSAREEP. The expressed juice of the roots of the bitter cassava; used as a condiment in the West Indies.

SOY. Boil a gallon of the seeds of dolichos soja till soft, add a gallon of bruised wheat, keep them in a warm place for 24 hours; add a gallon of salt, and 2 gallons of water, and after keeping them bunged up in a stone jar for 2 or 3 months, press out the liquor.

PICKLES.

A few recipes are here given as illustration of the methods employed in preparing these condiments. For full particulars the reader is referred to the popular treatises on Cookery. The best vinegar (pickling, or No. 24 vinegar) should be employed. Some prefer the crystal or white vinegar (distilled vinegar, or rather pure diluted wood-vinegar) especially for white pickles; but the best wine vinegar is more agreeable. Stoneware jars, not glazed with lead, should be used to keep the pickles in; or otherwise green glass jars.

SPICED VINEGAR, FOR PICKLES GENERALLY. Bruise in a mortar 2 oz. of black pepper, 1 oz. of ginger, ½ oz. of allspice, and 1 oz. of salt. If a hotter pickle is desired, add ½ dr. of cayenne, or a few capsicums. For walnuts add also 1 oz. of shallots. Put these into a stone jar, with a quart of vinegar, and cover them with a bladder wetted with the pickle, and over this a piece of leather. Set the jar on a trivet near the fire for 3 days, shaking it 3 times a day, then pour it on the walnuts or other vegetables. For walnuts it is used hot, but for cabbage, &c., cold. But to save time, it is usual to simmer the vinegar gently with the spices; which is best done in an enamelled saucepan.

BEET ROOT. Boil the roots till 3 parts done (from 1½ to 2½ hours:) then take them out, peel them, and cut them in thin slices. Put them into a jar, and pour on them sufficient cold spiced vinegar (as above) to cover them.

CABBAGE, White. Cut it in thin slices, put them into an earthen pan, sprinkle them with salt, and let them lie for 2 days; then drain them, and spread them out before the fire for some hours; put them into a stone jar, and add sufficient white vinegar, or pale wine vinegar, to cover them, and a little mace and white pepper corns.

RED CABBAGE. Remove the outer leaves and stalks, and cut the cabbage in quarters, then shred them into a colander, and sprinkle them with salt; next day drain them, put them into a jar, and pour on them sufficient cold spiced vinegar to cover them. Others hang up the cabbage for a few days to dry, then shred the leaves, and put them in layers in a jar with a little salt, pepper, and ginger, and fill up with cold vinegar. Others use vinegar without spice.

CAULIFLOWER AND BROCOLI. These should be sliced, and salted for 2 or 3 days, then drained, and spread upon a dry cloth before the fire for 24 hours; then put into a jar, and covered with spiced vinegar. Dr. KITCHENER says, that if vegetables are put into cold salt and water (a $\frac{1}{4}$ ℔ of salt to a quart of water) and gradually heated to boiling, it answers the same purpose as letting them lie some days in salt.

CUCUMBERS. Gherkins. Small cucumbers, but not too young, are wiped clean with a dry cloth, put into a jar, and boiling vinegar, with a handful of salt, poured on them. Boil up the vinegar every 3 days, and pour it on them till they become green; then add ginger and pepper, and tie them up close for use. Or cover them with salt and water (as above) in a stone jar, cover this, and set them on the hearth before the fire for 2 or 3 days, till they turn yellow; then put away the water, and cover them with hot vinegar, set them near the fire, and keep them hot for 8 or 10 days, till they become green; then pour off the vinegar, cover them with hot spiced vinegar, and keep them close.

MANGOES. Large cucumbers, or small melons, are split so that a marrow-spoon may be introduced, and the seeds scooped out; they are then parboiled in brine strong enough to float an egg, dried on a cloth before the fire, filled with mustard seed and a clove of garlic, and then covered with spiced vinegar. True mangoes the same.

MUSHROOMS. Clean them with water and flannel, throw them into boiling salt and water in a stewpan, and let them boil for a few minutes. Drain them in a colander, and lay them on a linen cloth, covering them with another. Put them into bottles with a blade or two of mace, and fill up with white vinegar, pouring some melted mutton fat on the top, if intended to be kept long.

NASTURTIUMS, FRENCH BEANS, and other small green vegetables, are pickled in the same way as GHERKINS.

ONIONS. 1. Let them lie in strong salt and water for a fortnight; then take them out and peel them; put them in fresh salt and water for another fortnight; take them out, wash them clean, and let them lie in fresh water all night. Next day put them on a cloth to drain; then put them in a jar, and pour over them hot spiced vinegar. If you wish them of a nice colour, use white vinegar.

2. Peel small silver button onions, and throw them into a stewpan of boiling water; as soon as they look clear, take them out with a perforated spoon, and lay them on a folded cloth, covered with another, and when quite dry, put them into a jar, and cover them with hot spiced vinegar. When quite cold, bung them down, and cover with bladder wetted with pickle, and leather.

WALNUTS. Take 100 young walnuts, lay them in salt and water for 2 or 3 days, changing the water every day. (If required to be soon ready for use, pierce each walnut with a larding pin, that the pickle may penetrate.) Wipe them with a soft cloth, and lay them on a folded cloth for some hours. Then put them in a jar, and pour on them sufficient of the above spiced vinegar, hot, to cover them. Or they may be allowed to simmer gently in strong vinegar, then put into a jar with a handful of mustard seed, 1 oz. ginger, ¼ oz. of mace, 1 oz. of allspice, 2 heads of garlic, and two split nutmegs, and pour on them sufficient boiling vinegar to cover them. Dr. KITCHENER recommends the walnuts to be gently simmered with the brine, then laid on a cloth for a day or two, till they turn black, put into a jar, and hot spiced vinegar poured on them.

TOMATOES. As Gherkins. See CUCUMBERS.

PICCALILLI, INDIAN, OR MIXED PICKLE. 1. To each gallon of strong vinegar put 4 oz. of curry powder, 4 oz. of good flour of mustard, 3 oz. of bruised ginger, 2 oz. of turmeric, 8 oz. of skinned shallots, and 2 oz. of garlic (the last two slightly baked in a Dutch oven,) ¼ lb of salt and 2 drachms of cayenne-pepper. Digest these near the fire, as directed above for spiced vinegar. Put into a jar, gherkins, sliced cucumbers, sliced onions, button onions, cauliflower, celery, brocoli, French beans, nasturtiums, capsicums, large cucumbers, and small melons. All, except the capsicum, to be parboiled in salt and water, drained, and dried on a cloth before the fire. The melons and large cucumbers to be prepared as directed above for mangoes. Pour on them the above pickle.

2. Take 1 ℔ of ginger-root, and ½ ℔ of garlic (both previously salted and dried,) 2 gallons of vinegar, ½ oz. of turmeric, ¼ ℔ of long pepper. Digest together for 2 or 3 days near the fire in a stone jar; or gently simmer them in a pipkin or enamelled saucepan. Then put in the above vegetables, or almost any except red cabbage and walnuts, all previously salted and dried.

BRINE, OR PICKLE, FOR PORK, &c. Brown sugar, bay salt, common salt, of each 2 ℔; saltpetre ½ ℔, water a gallon. Boil gently, and remove the scum. Another meat pickle is made with 12 ℔ of salt, 2 ℔ of sugar or treacle, ½ ℔ of nitre, and sufficient water to dissolve it. To cure HAMS, mix 5 oz. of nitre with 8 oz. of coarse sugar; rub it on the ham, and in 24 hours rub in 2 ℔ of salt, and in a fortnight 2 ℔ more. The above is for a ham of 20 ℔; it should lie in the salt a month or 5 weeks.

WESTPHALIAN ESSENCE,—CAMBRIAN ESSENCE OF WOOD SMOKE. These appear to be crude pyroligneous acid, or wood vinegar, and are used to give to hams, &c. the smoked flavour. The following has been published as the recipe for Essence of Smoke, but we apprehend it is far from being correct:—Macerate for several weeks ½ dr. of Barbadoes tar, 1 dr. of liquid burnt sugar, 5 dr. each of port wine and vinegar, 2 dr. of salt, and 7 oz. of water.

LEMON JUICE, factitious. Dissolve 4 oz. of citric acid in 3 pints of water, with 8 drops of essence of lemon (rubbed with the acid, or dissolved in a little spirit or tincture of fresh lemon-peel.) After standing a few days filter it, and keep it in well-closed bottles.

ORANGE JUICE, factitious. Citric acid 1 oz., water 2 pints, oil of orange-peel 4 drops, tincture of orange-peel ½ oz. As the last.

TRADE CHEMICALS.

MISCELLANEOUS PREPARATIONS, & COMPOUNDS EMPLOYED IN THE ARTS, IN DOMESTIC ECONOMY, CHEMICAL RESEARCH AND AMUSEMENT, &c.

THIS division of the work comprises those chemical compounds which are employed for other purposes than those of medicine, and which have not been noticed in the former parts of this volume. It includes a variety of miscellaneous articles which are sometimes sold by the retail druggist, or the materials of which he is expected to furnish, or with the composition of which it is desirable he should be acquainted. The limits of the work do not admit of a minute description of the processes and manipulations employed in the manufacture of such chemicals as are only made on the large scale, and never by the retailer; nor of those chemical arts which have no immediate connexion with the trade.

ACETATES. Such as are employed in medicine will be found in the Pocket Formulary. The only Acetates requiring notice here are the following:—

ACETATE OF ALUMINA. This is made, for the use of dyers and calico printers, by decomposing acetate of lime with alum. It may be conveniently made by adding to a boiling solution of 5 parts of alum, a solution of 6 parts of sugar of lead. When the mixture is cold, the clear liquid is poured off; from which the dry salt may be obtained by careful evaporation. It contains, besides acetate of alumina, some sulphate of potash.

ACETATE OF IRON, OR IRON LIQUOR. Usually obtained, for the use of dyers, by digesting scraps of iron in re-distilled wood-vinegar. (See page 347.)

ACETATE OF LIME. Impure acetate (or pyrolignite) of lime, is made by neutralizing pyroligneous acid with cream of lime or chalk, and evaporating to dryness. By using pure acetic acid a purer acetate is obtained.

ACETATE OF SODA. By mixing the above impure acetate of lime, in solution, with a solution of sulphate of soda, filtering, and evaporating the clear liquid, an impure acetate of soda is obtained; which by repeated crystallization is rendered colourless, and fit for yielding pure concentrated acetic acid by distillation with sulphuric acid.

ACETIMETRY. The strength of vinegar is estimated for the duty by an instrument named an acetimeter, which determines the quantity of acetic acid present by the specific gravity of the vinegar after neutralization by slaked lime. Dr. URE'S plan is to add to a given weight of vinegar bicarbonate of potash till exactly neutralized; every 2 gr. of the bicarbonate indicate 1 gr. of real acetic acid. In this and the following operations it is convenient to use a tube graduated into 100 equal divisions, numbered from the top downward (See ALKALIMETRY, below.) The quantity of test solution used is then seen at once. In the present case the 200 grains of the alkaline carbonate being dissolved in sufficient water to fill the graduated portion of the measure, each of the divisions used in neutralizing 100 grains of vinegar is equivalent to one per cent. of absolute acetic acid.

ACID, ACETIC. See VINEGAR. For the methods of procuring the concentrated acetic acid, see Acidum Aceticum, Pocket Formulary. The process of the Edinburgh Pharmacopœia yields a stronger acid than that of the London Pharmacopœia. A strong acid, very suitable for making aromatic spirit of vinegar, is procured by distilling crystallized verdigris in an earthen retort coated with clay, into a series of 3 globes, connected by opposite tubulures, and kept constantly cool, the last being furnished with a WELTER'S safety tube. The acid which comes over is usually coloured, and requires to be rectified by a slow and careful redistillation in a glass retort. Acetic acid of moderate strength may be rendered stronger by redistilling it over acetate of potash, rejecting the first portions that come over, and taking care that the temperature does not rise above 572° F. By redistilling it, rejecting the first and last portions, glacial acetic acid is procured. The same acetate of potash may be used repeatedly. The process of the Dublin Pharmacopœia yields a good product of glacial acetic acid.

ACID, CHLORIC. Dissolve 7 parts of crystallized carbonate of soda, and 7½ of tartaric acid in 24 of boiling water; add to the boiling solution 6 parts of chlorate of potash in 16 of water, at 212°, agitating the mixture. When quite cold filter, and add a solution of 6 parts of oxalic acid in 18 of water, heated not above 134°. Agitate well, and place the vessel in a freezing mixture of muriatic acid and sulphate of magnesia, and filter. [Not absolutely pure, but sufficiently so for technical purposes. It may be obtained pure by decomposing chlorate of barytes by sulphuric acid.]

ACID, CHROMIC. It may be obtained pure by mixing bichromate of potash with nitrate of silver in solution, washing the precipitate, and decomposing it with an equivalent quantity of muriatic acid. In a few minutes the clear solution may be poured off. A cheaper method, where great purity is not required, is to add from 120 to 150 volumes of strong sulphuric acid to 100 volumes of a cold saturated solution of bichromate of potash. Dry the acid which separates on porous tiles. Or add 2 parts of concentrated sulphuric acid to 1 part of dry chromate of lead, leave the paste for 12 hours, then treat it with water; decant the clear red liquid, and evaporate it in a retort. Keep it boiling for some time, then allow it to cool. Most of the acid separates in crystals; more may be obtained by evaporating the solution till its density is 1·55.

ACID, CINNAMIC. It is most readily procured by distilling genuine balsam of tolu by a gentle heat. The white crystalline mass which condenses on the neck of the retort, is purified by pressing it between blotting paper, dissolving in boiling water, and crystallizing.

ACID, FLUORIC. The anhydrous acid is made by distilling powdered fluor spar with twice its weight of oil of vitriol, in a leaden, or better, a *silver* alembic, the pipe of which fits into a bottle of the same material, surrounded with ice. But as it is usually required in a diluted state, water equal in weight to the spar may be put into the receiver. Great care must be taken, as the acid, both in its gaseous and liquid form, is very destructive.

ACID, HIPPURIC. Mix the urine of the horse with milk of lime, boil for some minutes, and strain. Boil down the clear liquid to $\frac{1}{8}$ of its bulk, avoiding burning; add hydrochloric acid, press the impure acid, boil it with fresh milk of lime, and again precipitate with hydrochloric acid.

ACID, IODIC. Mr. A. CONNELL'S *Method.* Put 50 grains of iodine into a large tall flask; add 1 oz. of fuming nitric acid, boil, and as the iodine sublimes and condenses on the sides of the flask, continually wash it back again with the acid. Continue this until none of the iodine remains unchanged. Then pour the whole into a shallow evaporating dish, and evaporate to dryness. Redissolve, and again evaporate till all the nitrous acid is got rid of.

ACID, MURIATIC, OR HYDROCHLORIC. Commercial muriatic acid is largely produced by the action of sulphuric acid on common salt, in the manufacture of sulphate of soda for the purpose of making soda ash and washing soda by the decomposition of that salt. From the impurity of the ingredients it is apt to be contaminated with arsenic and sulphurous acid; as well as sulphuric acid, and iron. It may be purified from arsenic by redistilling it over strips of bright copper. Dr. GREGORY'S method of procuring *pure* muriatic acid is as follows:—Put into a matrass 6 parts, by weight, of purified salt, and 10 oz. of oil of vitriol previously diluted with 4 of water and cooled. Fix in the matrass a tube twice bent at right angles and having a bulb blown on the descending limb. Into a bottle surrounded with ice and water introduce distilled water equal in weight to the salt employed, and let the bent tube dip an eighth of an inch into the water. Apply a gentle heat of a sand-bath to the matrass as long as acid comes over. In about 2 hours the operation will be finished. The water is increased two-thirds in bulk, and converted into hydrochloric acid of 1·14 or 1·15 sp. gr. To procure it of 1·21 sp. gr. employ part of this acid during the first half of a similar operation, and it will speedily be saturated. See also Acidum Hydrochloricum purum, Pocket Formulary. Mr. PHILLIPS says a perfectly colourless acid may be obtained from the commercial sulphuric acid and common salt.

ACID, NITRIC, AND FUMING NITROUS ACID. Put into an iron or stoneware pot, nitre or nitrate of soda, add rather more than half its weight of strong sulphuric acid, and lute on a stone ware head. The vapour is conducted into a series of two-necked stoneware vessels containing each a sixth of their capacity of water. The acid is usually obtained of the density of about 1·45. It is coloured with nitrous acid gas, forming what is commonly but improperly termed *nitrous acid*. By gently heating the coloured acid in a retort, the nitrous acid is driven off, and the acid remains nearly colourless, usually of the density of 1·38 to 1·42. This is weaker than the Pharmacopœia directs, but sufficiently strong for most purposes. (See Acidum Nitricum, Pocket Formulary.) Its strength may be increased by mixing it with its volume of strong oil of vitriol, and slowly distilling off two-thirds of the nitric acid. This yields an acid of 1·5 sp. gr., such as is required for the preparation of gun-cotton, as well as in some pharmaceutical processes.

ACID, NITROMURIATIC. *Aqua Regia.* This is used in the arts, chiefly as a solvent for gold. By the mutual action of nitric and muriatic acids a compound of chlorine, nitrogen, and oxygen, is formed. The best proportions and strength of the acids are variously stated. Colourless nitric acid must be used. Mr. ELKINGTON employs 21 parts of nitric acid, sp. gr. 1·45; 17 parts of muriatic acid, 1·15 sp. gr.; and 14 parts of water. This dissolves 5 parts of gold. For the nitro-muriatic acid employed by dyers as a solvent for tin, see DYES, &c., below.

ACID, OXALIC. Digest by the aid of heat 1 part of treacle, or of potato starch, in 5 parts of nitric acid, sp. gr. 1·42, diluted with 10 parts of water, as long as gaseous products are evolved. By evaporation the acid is obtained in crystals, and must be re-crystallized till sufficiently pure. Mr. LEWIS THOMSON directs 28 oz. of sugar, 184 oz. of nitric acid of 1·245 sp. gr., to be digested at 125° F. It yields 30 or 31 oz. of acid. M. SCHLESINGER directs 4 parts of dry sugar, and 33 of nitric acid of 1·38 sp. gr. to be boiled to one-sixth of the original volume, and allowed to crystallize. This is the best method of operating on a small scale, when the amount of product is not the principal object.

ACID, PHOSPHORIC. See Pocket Formulary. *Dry* phosphoric acid is thus obtained.—On a flat plate place a large bell glass, and under it a small porcelain cup or crucible. Introduce into the latter a piece of phosphorus, dried with blotting paper, and set it on fire by a heated wire. Let the bell glass be raised on one side to admit sufficient air to maintain combustion; and as the phosphorus is consumed, introduce successive pieces, taking care that the glass does not become too hot. When the quantity of acid is considerable, knock it from the plate with an iron spoon, and put it into stoppered bottles. Several glasses may be used at once. It is used as a desiccating body, having the strongest attraction for water of any known substance. Also in making a stopping for teeth—see TEETH CEMENTS.

ACID, PYROGALLIC. Heat powdered nutgalls in a dish covered with thin filtering paper pasted to its edges, and surmounted with a bell-formed receiver, kept cool. A solution of the condensed acid, decolorized by animal charcoal, and mixed with spirit, is used to stain the hair (and skin) brown.

ACID, SULPHURIC. This is only made on a large scale; but the commercial acid requires purification for many chemical as well as pharmaceutical purposes, as it is usually contaminated with tin and lead, and frequently with arsenic, or selenium, and compounds of nitrogen. The purification of oil of vitriol by distillation is attended with some difficulty. No luting must be employed; and to prevent the violent jumpings which attend the ebullition, strips of platina, or fragments of rock crystal, should be introduced into the retort. The receiver should be large, and the whole defended from currents of cold air. The first portions which come over should be rejected till the indigo test proves it to be free from nitric acid. By boiling a portion of the acid with a few drops of solution of sulphate of indigo, the latter is discoloured if nitric acid is present. The Edinburgh Pharmacopœia directs the nitrous acid to be got rid of by heating 8 fluid ounces of commercial oil of vitriol to near the boiling point with from 10 to 15 gr. of sugar. When sulphuric acid is diluted with water, the *metallic* impurities may be removed by a little solution of sulphuret of barium, and allowing the precipitates to subside, when the pure diluted acid may be decanted for use.

DRY OR ANHYDROUS SULPHURIC ACID. Into a retort, placed in a freezing mixture, and having a receiver attached, put some dry phosphoric acid (see above,) and add $\frac{3}{4}$ths of its weight of strong sulphuric acid. Remove the retort from the freezing mixture, and place the receiver attached to it there; a gentle heat being now applied to the retort, the anhydrous acid is obtained in silky crystals.

ACID, SULPHUROUS. For the mode of obtaining an aqueous solution of this acid, see Acidum Sulphurosum, Pocket Formulary. The following are cheaper methods of obtaining it for bleaching purposes, &c. BERTHIER directs a mixture of 100 parts black oxide of manganese, and 12 or 14 of sulphur, to be heated in a glass retort, and the gas received into water kept very cold. Mr. REDWOOD directs $\frac{1}{2}$ oz. of powdered charcoal to be acted on by 4 fluid oz. of oil of vitriol. Treacle is sometimes used instead of charcoal; as also is linseed oil.

ACID, TANNIC. *Tannin.* Place coarsely-powdered Aleppo galls in a damp cellar for 3 or 4 days, then mix them with sufficient sulphuric ether to form a soft paste.

Place this in a close vessel for 24 hours, then wrap it in linen ticking, and submit it to the action of a powerful press. Scrape off the tannin from the surface of the ticking, remove the *cake* from within it, rub this into powder, form it into a paste with a mixture of 100 parts of ether and 6 of water, well shaken together before pouring it on the galls, and proceed as before. Let the syrupy liquid thus obtained be thinly spread on plates, and dried at 113° Fahrenheit.

ACIDS, MIXED, FOR GALVANIC BATTERIES. 1. For troughs, for general purposes, medical galvanism, &c.: Nitric acid 1 fluid oz., sulphuric acid 1½ fluid oz., water 4 pints.

2. Dr. FARADAY. Oil of vitriol 2 fluid oz., nitric acid 1 fluid oz., water 5 pints. It should be tried by dipping into it a piece of sheet zinc. A continuous succession of *small* bubbles should be produced.

3. For Mr. SMEE's Battery. One measure of sulphuric acid to 7 of water. The intensity of its action is increased by the addition of a few drops of nitric acid, but this tends to destroy the plates. In electro-metallurgy the water should only contain a sixteenth of sulphuric acid.

4. For Mr. GROVE's Battery. For the outer vessel, 1 part sulphuric acid to 7 of water: for the inner, concentrated nitric acid.

5. For DANIELL's Battery. For the porous tube containing the zinc, 1 part of sulphuric acid with ten of water. For the outer cylinder, a saturated solution of sulphate of copper, with a tenth part of sulphuric acid.

6. Nitro-sulphuric acid, for Dr. T. WRIGHT's Batteries: Nitric acid 1 part, sulphuric acid 5 parts. The zinc plate is immersed in a solution of muriate of ammonia or of salt, the platinized zinc in the above acid. The platinizing requires to be repeated every time the plate is washed.

ACIDIMETRY. Acids generally are estimated by the quantity of alkalies or carbonated alkalies required to neutralize them. Weigh 100 gr. of the acid and dilute it with a few times its weight of water. Then add sufficient dry or crystallized carbonate of soda, or carbonate of potash, to exactly neutralize the acid. The Alkalimeter tube may be used for the solution of the alkali. By a reference to the table of chemical equivalents, the quantity of real acid of any kind represented by the quantity of alkali required to neutralize it may be estimated.

ACIDULATED KALI. See BEVERAGES.

ALBUMINOUS SIZE. Beat up the white of an egg with twice its bulk of cold water, until well incorporated. Used as a varnish for leather binding and kid shoes; also to size drawing paper.

ALCOHOL. There is, perhaps, no better method of obtaining absolute alcohol than that of the Edinburgh Pharmacopœia. See Alcohol, Pocket Formulary.

ALKALIMETRY. The quantity of real alkali contained in the commercial alkalies (common soda, soda ash, potashes, pearlash, salt of tartar, &c.,) is ascertained by the quantity of an acid solution of known strength required to neutralize it. For this purpose a tube, termed an ALKALIMETER, is used, which will hold 1000 grains of water. The tube may be three-fourths of an inch internal diameter, and 9½ inches in length; or five-eighth inches diameter and 14 inches in height; and should be graduated into 100 equal divisions numbered from the top downwards. The quantity of test acid used is then at once seen. This consists of sulphuric acid diluted with water so that each measure (10 grains) is equivalent to one grain of pure soda. To use it, dissolve 100 grains of the impure soda in 3 ounces of hot water, filter, and wash the filter. Then add to the solution the test acid until the litmus or cabbage paper ceases to show an alkaline reaction. The same acid will serve for potash, if the number be multiplied by 3 and divided by 4.—PARNELL. There are several other methods of performing the process.

ALLOYS AND AMALGAMS. A few only of these metallic compounds require notice here:—

Fusible Metal. 1. Tin 8 parts, lead 4, bismuth 3; melt together, removing the scum. Used as a metal-bath.

2. DARCET'S, for the same purpose: Bismuth 8 parts, lead 5, tin 3.

3. Lead 3 parts, tin 2, bismuth 5. This melts at 197° Fahrenheit.

4. For anatomical injections: Melt together with a gentle heat 174 parts of tin, 312 of lead, 514 of bismuth, with a little charcoal: remove from the fire, and add 100 parts of mercury, previously heated. It is fluid at 173°; solid at 140° Fahrenheit.

Bronze. 1. For medals and small castings: Copper 95, tin 4.

2. Copper 89, tin 8, zinc 3.

3. *Ancient.* Copper 100, tin 7, lead 7.

4. KELLY'S. Copper 91, zinc 6, tin 2, lead 1.

5. For gilding: Copper 14, zinc 6, tin 4.

6. *Bell-metal.* Copper 78, tin 22.

German Silver. 1. Copper 40½, nickel 31½, zinc 25½, iron 2½.

2. Pure copper 55, nickel 23, zinc 17, iron 3, tin 2.

Gold, Factitious. Platina 7, copper 16, zinc 1; fuse together. See AURUM MUSIVUM.

Common Gold. Copper 16, silver 1, gold 2.

Or-molu. Copper 45 to 48, zinc 52 to 55.

Solders. 1. For Gold: Pure gold 12 parts, silver 2, copper 4.

2. *Soft Solder.* Tin 2 parts, lead 1.

3. For brass: Brass 2 parts, zinc 1.

Alloys for Electrotype. Clichée Moulds. Bismuth 8 parts, tin 4, lead 5, regulus of antimony 1; melt repeatedly together, and pour out in drops, till perfectly mixed.

Amalgam for Electrical Machines. 1. Fuse 1 oz. of zinc with ½ oz. tin, at as low a temperature as possible; then add 1½ oz. of quicksilver, previously made hot; mix, pour out, and when cold reduce it to powder, and triturate it with sufficient quicksilver to bring it to a proper consistence.

2. Zinc 1 part, tin 1, quicksilver 2; melt together.

3. Zinc 2, tin 1, mercury 5.

4. LA BEAUME'S. Pour into a chalked wooden box 6 oz. of quicksilver; put into an iron ladle ½ oz. bees'-wax, with 2 oz. purified zinc, and 1 oz. of grain tin; set it over a brisk fire, and when the metals are melted, pour

them into the box, avoiding the dross. When cold, reduce it to powder, and mix it with lard. Keep it in a box, covered with tallow, and spread it on leather for use.

Liquid Amalgam, for Silvering Globes, &c. Pure lead 1 oz., grain tin 1 oz.; melt in a clean ladle, and immediately add 1 oz. of bismuth. Skim off the dross, remove the ladle from the fire, and, before the metal sets, add 10 oz. of quicksilver. Stir together, avoiding the fumes.

Amalgam for Varnishing Figures. Melt 2 oz. of tin with ½ oz. of bismuth, and add ½ oz. of quicksilver. When cold, grind it with white of egg, and apply to the figure.

ALUM. It is prepared by lixiviating calcined aluminous schist, and concentrating the solution to 1·4 or 1·5 density, and adding the requisite quantity of muriate of potash, soap-boilers' ash, or kelp, to supply the alkali. By recrystallization it is obtained colourless. In some manufactories sulphate of ammonia, from gas liquor, is added to the lixivium, instead of muriate of potash. Roman or cubic alum is crystallized from a solution, the temperature of which is not allowed to exceed 104° F. It differs from common alum in containing a larger quantity of base, a portion of which separates if the solution be heated to 120°. Another kind of alum, sometimes used as a mordant, consists almost entirely of sulphate of alumina, and is probably made by boiling fine clay, free from iron, with sulphuric acid, and cooling the solution so as to obtain a solid mass. See DYES, &c.

AMADOU. Prepared from Boletus igniarius, B. fomentarius, and some other allied species of fungi. The fungus is cut into thin slices, the hard external parts removed, and the rest beaten with a mallet till soft. This forms *surgeon's agaric*. If intended for *German tinder*, it is soaked in a solution of nitre, and sometimes sprinkled with gunpowder, and carefully dried.

AMALGAMS. See ALLOYS, above.

AMMONIA, SULPHATE AND CARBONATE OF. An impure sulphate of ammonia, suitable for agricultural purposes, is obtained by neutralizing the ammoniacal liquor of gas works, with sulphuric acid. By recrystallization it may be obtained in a state of greater purity. The carbonate (hydrated sesquicarbonate) is obtained by mixing either this sulphate, or sal ammoniac, with chalk, and subliming it in iron retorts into leaden receivers. It is further purified by resubliming it with a gentle heat. A sketch of the apparatus employed will be found in Dr. PEREIRA'S "Elements," Vol. I.

ANATOMICAL INJECTIONS. 1. Tallow, resin, and wax, equal parts; melt over a slow fire; and add red lead or vermilion sufficient to colour. For coarse preparations.

2. A strong solution of isinglass, coloured as required. For delicate preparations.

3. AMALGAM INJECTION. Melt together 1 oz. each of bismuth, lead, and zinc, and, when melted, add 2 oz. of quicksilver. Also for delicate parts.

ANATOMICAL SUBJECTS, AND ANIMAL SUBSTANCES, TO PRESERVE. 1. M. GANNAL'S *Solution*. Common salt 2 ℔, alum 2 ℔, nitre 1 ℔, water 4 gallons. M. GANNAL injects into the carotid artery a solution of sulphate of alumina, of density 1.286. From 5 to 7 pints are required in summer, but less will suffice in winter.

2. Dr. BABINGTON injects pyroxylic spirit into the aorta, and a little into the cavity of the peritoneum and the rectum.

3. Mr. GOADBY, for insects, and for preparations of their organs. Bay salt 4 oz., alum 2 oz., corrosive sublimate from 2 to 4 grains, water 1 to 2 quarts. The weaker proportions should always be employed in the first instance. Let the insect, or its organs, be covered with the fluid, which should be changed frequently.

4. *For Mollusca*. Bay salt ½ oz.; arsenic ½ dr., sublimate 2 gr., water a quart; dissolve.

5. Mr. PIGNE, for preserving pathological specimens. Creasote 3 to 6 drops, water a pint.

6. Dr. STAPLETON, for pathological specimens. In a quart of saturated solution of alum, dissolve ½ dr. of nitre. A recent preparation immersed in this liquid becomes discoloured; but within a few days the colour returns. It is then put up in a saturated and filtered solution of alum. M. REBOULET proposes: Water 16 parts, chloride of lime 4, alum 2, nitre 1.

7. Chloride of tin 4 (or corrosive sublimate 5) parts, in 100 of water, with 2 of muriatic acid.—Mr. COOLEY.

8. *For preserving Animals.* Alum 32 oz., nux vomica 3 oz., water 5 pints; boil to 4½ pints. When cold, filter, or decant. This serves for injection. The residue, mixed with yolk of egg, is used for anointing the interior of the skin, and fleshy parts left in skinning animals.

9. *For preserving Feathers.* Strychnine 16 gr., rectified spirit a pint (dangerous.) See STUFFING BIRDS, &c.

ANNOTTO, PURIFIED. To a boiling solution of pearlash add as much annotto as it will dissolve. When cold, decant the clear solution, and neutralize with diluted sulphuric acid, avoiding any excess. Wash the precipitate with a little cold water, and dry it.

ANNOTTO, SOLUTION OF. Boil equal weights of annotto and pearlash with water, and dilute to the required colour.

ANTI-ATTRITION, AND AXLE GREASE. 1. One part of fine black-lead, ground perfectly smooth, with 4 parts of lard. Some recipes add a little camphor.

2. BOOTH'S AXLE GREASE. (Expired Patent.) Dissolve ½ ℔ common soda in 1 gallon of water, add 3 ℔ of tallow, and 6 ℔ palm oil, (or 10 ℔ palm oil only ;) heat them together to 200 or 210° F.; mix, and keep the mixture constantly stirred till the composition is cooled down to 60 or 70°. A thinner composition is made with ½ ℔ of soda, a gallon of water, a gallon of rape-oil, and ¼ ℔ of tallow or palm oil. [See also Lubricating Compounds.]

ANTI-FERMENT. Sulphite of lime; or equal parts of sulphite of lime and ground black mustard seed. Used to check the fermentation of cyder, &c.

AQUA FORTIS. Double aqua fortis is nitric acid of 1.36 specific gravity; single aqua fortis about 1·22.—Dr. PEREIRA. A compound acid was formerly used under this name by dyers, and for cleaning brass, consisting of strong spirit of nitre 20 ℔, oil of vitriol 7 ℔, water 30 ℔.—ELABORATORY LAID OPEN.

AQUA REGIA. See NITROMURIATIC ACID, above.

ARABINE. Gum Arabic dissolved in water, and precipitated by alcohol.

ARGENTUM MUSIVUM. Fuse ½ oz. each of grain tin and bismuth in a crucible, and add ½ oz. of mercury.

ARBOR DIANÆ. See TREES, Metallic.

AROMATIC PASTILS. See PERFUMERY.

AURUM MUSIVUM. Mosaic gold, or bisulphuret of tin. See Stanni Sulphuretum, Pocket Formulary. 1. Dr. URE directs 12 oz. of tin to be melted, and 3 oz. of mercury added. This amalgam is triturated with 7 oz. of sulphur, and three of sal ammoniac, and the powder put into a matrass, which is bedded deep in sand, and kept for several hours at a gentle heat. The heat is then raised, and continued for several hours, taking care not to raise it so high as to blacken the mass.

2. Melt together in a crucible, over a clear fire, equal parts of sulphur and the white oxide of tin; keep it continually stirred with a glass rod, until the compound appears as a yellow flaky powder. (This is used as a cheap bronze powder, &c.)

BALDWIN'S PHOSPHORUS. Heat nitrate of lime till it melts; keep it fused for 10 minutes, and pour it into a heated iron ladle. When cool, break it into pieces and keep it in a closely-stoppered bottle. After exposure to the sun's rays, it emits a white light in the dark.

BALLS FOR HORSES. See Veterinary Formulary.

BALLS, ASH. The ashes of fern, or other kinds of wood ashes, made into balls.

BALLS, HEEL. 1. Melt together 4 oz. of mutton suet, 1 oz. of bees'-wax, 1 oz. of sweet oil, ½ oz. oil of turpentine, and stir in 1 oz. of powdered gum Arabic, and ½ oz. of fine lamp-black.

2. Bees'-wax 8 oz., tallow 1 oz., powdered gum 1 oz., lamp-black q. s. These are used not merely by the shoemaker, but to copy inscriptions, raised patterns, &c., by rubbing the ball on paper laid over the article to be copied. ULLATHORNE'S Balls answer the purpose very well. For copying ancient monumental brasses, a similar compound, coloured with bronze-powder instead of lamp-black, is sometimes employed.

BALLS FOR SCOURING—BREECHES BALLS, CLOTHES BALLS.

1. Bath-brick 4 parts, pipe-clay 8 parts, pumice 1, soft-soap 1; ochre, umber, or other colour to bring it to the desired shade, q. s.; ox-gall to form a paste. Make it into balls, and dry them.

2. Pipe-clay 4 oz., fuller's-earth ½ oz., whiting ½ oz.,

white pepper ¼ oz., ox-gall sufficient to form it into a paste.

3. Pipe-clay 3 oz., white pepper 1 dr., starch 1 dr., orris powder 1½ dr. It may be kept in powder, or formed into balls, as above.

BALLS, BLACKING. See BLACKING, below.

BALLS, FURNITURE. See FURNITURE PASTE.

BARIUM, PEROXIDE OF. Heat pure barytes to low redness in a platinum crucible; then gradually add chlorate of potash in the proportion of 1 part of the latter to 4 of the former. Cold water removes the chloride of potassium, and the peroxide remains as a hydrate.

BARYTES, CHLORATE. See CHLORATE OF BARYTES.

BEETLE POISON. Put a drachm of phosphorus in a flask with 2 oz. of water; plunge the flask into hot water, and when the phosphorus is melted, pour the contents into a mortar with 2 or 3 oz. of lard. Triturate briskly, adding water, and ½ ℔ of flour, with 1 or 2 oz. of brown sugar.—PHARMACEUTICAL JOURNAL. Plaster of Paris, with oatmeal, is said to destroy cockroaches.

BEETLE WAFERS. These are made with flour, sugar, and red lead, heated in wafer irons.

BENZOLE. A volatile liquid, procured by distilling light coal naphtha at a temperature not exceeding 200° F., by the method patented by Mr. MANSFIELD. It is a solvent for gutta percha; and also, with heat and long digestion, of India rubber.

BEVERAGES, AND POWDERS FOR PREPARING THEM. See above, page 273.

BIRD LIME. Boil the middle bark of the holly 7 or 8 hours in water; drain it, and lay it in heaps in the ground, covered with stones, for 2 or 3 weeks, till reduced to a mucilage. Beat this in a mortar, wash it in rain-water, and knead it till free from extraneous matters. Put it into earthen pots, and in 4 or 5 days it will be fit for use. An inferior kind is made by boiling linseed oil for some hours, until it becomes a viscid paste.

BISULPHURET OF CARBON. This is used in the arts, as a solvent for India rubber, gutta percha, &c. To procure it, MULDER recommends the following process as the most convenient. Provide an iron bottle (a quicksilver bottle answers very well,) and make a second opening into it. To one opening adapt a copper tube bent twice at right angles; and to the other a straight tube dipping into the bottle. Having nearly filled the bottle with pieces of charcoal (recently heated to redness,) and having screwed on the bent and straight tubes, place the bottle in a furnace, closing the mouth of the latter with a stone or clay cover in two pieces, hollowed in the centre so as to fit the upper part of the bottle, and defend it from the action of the fire. Connect the curved tube with a WOOLFE'S bottle half filled with water, and placed in a freezing mixture; and when the iron bottle is sufficiently heated, introduce by the straight tube fragments of sulphur, and immediately close the mouth of the tube with a plug. The bisulphuret, as it comes over, falls to the bottom of the water. Separate it from the water, and distil over dry muriate of lime.

BLACKING, LIQUID, FOR SHOES, &c. [*Note.*—By ivory-black, *bone*-black, which is usually sold under this name, is intended. True ivory-black has a more intense colour, but is too dear for general use.] 1. Ivory-black 3 oz. treacle 2 oz., sweet oil ½ oz.; mix to form a paste; add gradually ½ oz. of oil of vitriol, and then half a pint of vinegar, and 1¾ pint of water, or sour beer. Some prefer mixing the oil of vitriol, with the sweet oil.

2. Ivory-black 2 ℔, treacle 2 ℔, sweet oil ½ ℔; mix and add ¾ ℔ oil of vitriol, and beer or vinegar to make up a gallon.

3. Ivory-black 3 ℔, treacle 4 ℔, vinegar a pint, oil of vitriol 8 oz., water a gallon.

4. Ivory-black 2 ℔, neat's-foot oil 4 oz.; mix, and add 3 quarts of sour beer, or vinegar, and a spoonful of any kind of spirits; stir till smooth, and add 2 oz. of oil of vitriol, and sprinkle on it ½ drachm of powdered rosin. Then boil together 3 pints of sour ale with a little logwood, and ¼ oz. of Prussian blue, 3 oz. of honey, and 8 oz. of treacle. Mix, but do not bottle it for 2 or 3 days.

5. Ivory-black 8 oz., brown sugar or treacle 8 oz., sweet oil 1 oz., oil of vitriol ½ oz., vinegar 2 quarts.

Mix the oil with the treacle, then add the oil of vitriol and vinegar, and lastly, the ivory black.

BLACKING FOR DRESS BOOTS. 1. Gum 8 oz., treacle 2 oz., ink a pint, vinegar 2 oz., spirit of wine 2 oz. Dissolve the gum and treacle in the ink and vinegar, strain, and add the spirit.

2. To the above add 1 oz. of sweet oil, and ¼ oz. lamp-black. [These are applied with a sponge, and allowed to dry out of the dust. They will not bear the wet.]

3. Beat together the whites of 2 eggs, a tablespoonful of spirit of wine, a lump of sugar, and a little finely-powdered ivory-black to thicken.

BLACKING, WITHOUT POLISHING. Treacle 4 oz., lamp-black ½ oz., yeast a tablespoonful, 2 eggs, olive oil a teaspoonful, oil of turpentine a teaspoonful. Mix well. To be applied with a sponge, without brushing.

BLACKING, INDIA RUBBER (PATENT.) Ivory-black 60 ℔, treacle 45 ℔, vinegar (No. 24) 20 gallons, powdered gum 1 ℔, India rubber oil 9 ℔. (The latter is made by dissolving by heat 18 oz. of India rubber in 9 ℔ of rape oil.) Grind the whole smooth in a paint mill, then add, by small quantities at a time, 12 ℔ of oil of vitriol, stirring it strongly for half an hour a day for a fortnight.

BLACKING, PASTE. 1. These may be made with the ingredients of liquid blacking, using sufficient vinegar in which a little gum has been dissolved, to form a paste. Make it into cakes, and dry it.

2. *German Blacking.* Powdered bone-black is mixed with half its weight of molasses and one-eighth of its weight of olive-oil; and to this is added afterwards one-eighth of its weight of hydrochloric acid, and one-fourth of its weight of strong sulphuric acid. The whole is to be then mixed up with water into a sort of unctuous paste.—LIEBIG.

BAILEY'S *Blacking Balls.* Bruised gum tragacanth 1 oz., water 4 oz.; mix, and add 2 oz. of neat's-foot oil, 2 oz. of fine ivory-black, 2 oz. of Prussian blue, 4 oz. of sugar-candy; mix, and evaporate to a proper consistence.

For HEEL BALLS, see BALLS, above.

BLACKING FOR HARNESS. 1. Isinglass or gelatine ½ oz.,

powdered indigo ¼ oz., soft soap 4 oz., logwood 4 oz., glue 5 oz. Boil together in 2 pints of vinegar till the glue is dissolved; then strain through a cloth, and bottle for use. This appears an unchemical composition; but is inserted (as are many similar ones) because it is in actual use. The next is of a different character.

2. Melt 8 oz. of bees'-wax in an earthen pipkin, and stir into it 2 oz. of ivory-black, 1 oz. of Prussian blue ground in oil, 1 oz. of oil of turpentine, and ¼ oz. of copal varnish. Make it into balls. To be applied with a brush, and polished with an old handkerchief.

3. Treacle ½ ℔, lamp black 1 oz., yeast a spoonful, sugar-candy, olive oil, gum tragacanth, isinglass, each 1 oz., a cow's gall. Mix all together with 2 pints of stale beer, and let it stand before the fire for an hour.

BLACK REVIVER. 1. Bruised nutgalls 1 ℔, logwood 1 ℔, water 5 quarts; boil to 4 quarts, and add sulphate of iron 4 oz.; dissolve, and strain. When cold, add 8 oz. of ox gall.

2. Galls 3 oz., logwood 1 oz., copperas, iron filings, and sumach, of each 1 oz., vinegar 2 pints.—GRAY'S SUPPLEMENT.

BLACK JAPAN. True asphaltum 1½ oz., boiled linseed oil 4 pints, burnt umber 4 oz. Heat together till the whole is incorporated, remove from the fire, and when sufficiently cool, add as much oil of turpentine as will bring it to a proper consistence.

BLEACHING LIQUID. Solutions of chloride of lime, and chloride of soda, are sold for this purpose, with directions for use. The following is also used;—Mix 3 ℔ of common salt and 1 ℔ of black oxide of manganese with as much water as will form a paste. Put the mixture into a retort, and add 2 ℔ of oil of vitriol previously diluted with 4 ℔ of water. Pass the gas into a solution of 1 ℔ of common pearlash, or 11 oz. of caustic potash, in 6 ℔ of water. The retort may be placed, after a short period, in hot water, to extricate the remaining gas. In bleaching cotton by chloride of lime, 1 ℔ is dissolved in 3 gallons of water for each pound of cloth; it is afterwards passed through diluted muriatic or sulphuric acid (1 part of acid to 30 of water,) and then washed.

BLIGHTS, REMEDIES FOR.

Apple-tree Canker. Having brushed off the white down, and the red stain underneath it, anoint the places with a mixture of train oil and Scotch snuff.

White blight of Apple tree. Apply a decoction of fox-glove mixed with fresh cow-dung into a paste.

Fly in Turnips. Steep the seed before sowing in train oil; or distribute slaked lime over the field as soon as the plants have appeared; or contrive, if possible, to fumigate the field with brimstone.

Mildew of Wheat. 1. To prevent it. Dissolve in 3½ gallons of cold water 3¼ oz. of sulphate of copper; for every 3 bushels of sowing grain. Throw this quantity of wheat into another vessel, and pour over it the prepared liquid, until it rises 5 or 6 inches above the corn. Stir thoroughly, and remove all the grains that swim. Throw the mixture into a basket, so as to drain off the liquid; wash it well in soft water, and dry before sowing.

2. To remove it. A solution of 1 ℔ of salt to the gallon of water, sprinkled with a flat brush over the growing corn.

Smut in Wheat. To prevent it. Boil 3 gallons of water, and slake in it about 36 ℔ of quick lime; add 3 gallons more of cold water, and pour the hot mixture on 4½ bushels of the grain placed in a tub, stirring incessantly. Turn over the mixture now and then for 24 hours. Allow the liquid to drain off, and sow the limed wheat as soon as it is sufficiently dry.

Blight in Vines. A solution of pentesulphuret of calcium is to be painted over the branches and twigs until they acquire a continuous coating of sulphur mixed with carbonate of lime.

For lice, aphides, and red spiders. See WASHES FOR VERMIN.

BLUE FOR LINEN. The ordinary kinds of cake blue consist of indigo and starch. Liefchild's patent blue is thus made:—Mix 4 parts of Chinese blue, 1 of Turnbull's, and 1 of oxalic acid; gradually add boiling water until the whole is dissolved, and lastly 4 parts of sulphate of indigo. The latter is made with 1 part of indigo, and 4 of sulphuric acid, neutralized with carbonate of ammonia.

BONES, SULPHATED. To a bushel of ground bones add from 10 to 14 ℔ of oil of vitriol, previously mixed with half its bulk of water. [It is sometimes mixed with an equal weight of salt and a sufficient quantity of bran. Turnip seed may be mixed with this compound, and sown together.]

BOOT-TOP LIQUID. 1. Solution of muriate of tin 3 dr.; French chalk, or Venetian talc, in powder, 1 oz.; salt of sorrel ½ oz.; flake white 1 oz., burnt alum ½ oz., powdered cuttle-fish bone 1 oz., white arsenic 1 oz., boiling water a quart. Probably sulphate of barytes might be substituted for arsenic, the use of which it is desirable to discourage.

2. Sour milk 3 pints, cream of tartar 2 oz., oxalic acid 1 oz., alum 1 oz.—Mr. REDWOOD.

3. Wash the tops with soap and water, and scrape them with the back of a knife. Then apply the following with a hare foot brush.—Oxalic acid 1 oz., water a pint. Use the back of a knife as before; then polish with the following:—Powdered gum Arabic ½ oz., red spirits of lavender 2 oz., powdered turmeric ½ oz.; pencil this over the top, let it half dry, then polish by rubbing it, one way only, with a flannel till it shines.

4. Sour milk 3 pints, butter of antimony 2 oz., cream of tartar 2 oz., citric acid, alum, burnt alum, of each 1 oz.—GRAY'S SUPPLEMENT.

5. *White Top.* One ounce each of magnesia, alum, cream of tartar, and oxalic acid; ¼ oz. salt of sorrel, and ¼ oz. of sugar of lead; dissolve in a quart of water, and apply with a sponge.

6. *Brown Top.* Oxalic acid, alum, annotto, of each 1 oz.; isinglass ½ oz.; sugar of lead ½ oz.; salt of sorrel ¼ oz; boil together in a quart of water for 10 minutes. Apply with a sponge.

BOOK-BINDERS' STAINS, FOR LEATHER. *Black.* A solution of 1 part of sulphate of iron in 6 of water. *Blue.* A solution of indigo. (See CHEMIC BLUE.) *Brown.* A solution of pearlash, or of common soda.

BOOT POWDER. Finely-powdered French chalk, or Venetian talc.

BREAD, UNFERMENTED. See DIETETIC ARTICLES, p. 290.

BRONZE POWDER. The best methods of preparing these powders are probably kept secret. The following are some of the published recipes:—

1. Gold leaf, or alloys of gold, reduced to powder by grinding them with sulphate of potash, or with honey, and washing away the extraneous matter with hot water, and drying the metallic powder.

2. Dutch metal, and other similar alloys, treated in the same way.

3. Verdigris 4 oz., tutty 2 oz., sublimate 1 dr., borax 1 dr., nitre 1 dr.; mix them into a paste with oil, and fuse the mixture in a crucible. This has failed in some hands—perhaps from the tutty being factitious.

4. Mix together 100 parts of sulphate of copper, and 50 of crystallized carbonate of soda; apply heat till they unite. Powder the mass when cold, and add 15 parts of copper filings; mix well, and keep it at a white heat for 20 minutes. Wash and dry the product.

See also AURUM MUSIVUM, and ARGENTUM MUSIVUM, above.

BRONZING LIQUIDS, FOR BRONZING COPPER MEDALS, FIGURES, INSTRUMENTS, &c. 1. Sal ammoniac 1 dr., oxalic acid 15 gr., vinegar a pint: after well cleaning the article to be bronzed, warm it gently, and brush it over with the liquid, using only a small quantity at a time. When rubbed dry, repeat the application till the desired tint is obtained. [For copper medals, electrotype casts, &c.]

Bronze for Plaster Figures. Dissolve palm soap in water, and add a mixed solution of sulphate of copper and sulphate of iron until no further precipitate occurs. Dry the precipitate, and mix it with oil of turpentine, or linseed oil. Sulphate of copper alone produces too bright a green. Palmite of iron is yellow. These may be precipitated separately, and mixed to the desired shade after being triturated with the oil. 10 ounces of soap will require 3 ounces of sulphate of copper.

3. Sal ammoniac 1 oz., cream of tartar 3 oz., salt 6

oz.; dissolve in a pint of hot water, add 2 oz. of nitre, and 2 oz. of nitrate of copper dissolved in ½ pint of water.

4. Salt of sorrel 1 oz., sal ammoniac 2 oz., white vinegar 14 oz. [To give an antique appearance to bronze figures, &c.]

5. A diluted solution of muriate of platina. [For copper binding screws, and other small articles.]

6. A weak solution of hydro-sulphuret of ammonia, or of sulphuret of potassium. [For electrotype medals.]

7. Immediately on removing the electrotype cast from the solution, brush it over with good black lead; then heat it moderately, and brush it over with a painting brush, the slightest moisture being used.

8. Boil 2 oz. of carbonate of ammonia and 1 oz. of acetate of copper, in ½ pint of vinegar, until nearly all the vinegar is evaporated. Pour into this a solution of 62 grains of sal ammoniac, and 15½ grains of oxalic acid, in ½ pint of vinegar; boil the whole, and filter. Apply it to the medal (which should be perfectly bright, and previously warmed) with a camel hair pencil for half a minute; then pour boiling water on it, wipe it with soft cotton very slightly moistened with linseed oil, and rub it with clean cotton. *For electrotype copper medals.* [They may also be bronzed by applying oxide of iron (jeweller's rouge, or crocus) in the same manner as directed above, for plumbago; or a mixture of these may be used.]

9. *Tin Castings.* Wash them over, after being well cleaned and wiped, with a solution of 1 part of sulphate of iron, and 1 of sulphate of copper, in 20 parts of water: afterwards with a solution of 4 parts of verdigris in 11 of distilled vinegar; leave for an hour to dry, then polish with a soft brush and colcothar.

BRONZING BALL. See BALL (HEEL.)

BROSSE DE CORAIL. The roots of lucerne (medicago sativa) cleaned, dried, and hammered at the end. Used as a tooth-brush.

BROWNING, OR BRONZING LIQUIDS, FOR GUN BARRELS.

1. Aquafortis ½ oz., sweet spirit of nitre ½ oz., spirit

of wine 1 oz., sulphate of copper 2 oz., water 30 oz., tincture of muriate of iron 1 oz.: mix.

2. Sulphate of copper 1 oz., sweet spirit of nitre 1 oz., water a pint; mix. In a few days it will be fit for use.

3. Sweet spirit of nitre 3 oz., gum benzoin 1½ oz., tincture of muriate of iron ½ oz., sulphate of copper 2 dr., spirit of wine ½ oz.; mix, and add 2 ℔ of soft water.

4. Tincture of muriate of iron ½ oz., spirit of nitric ether ½ oz., sulphate of copper 2 scruples, rain water ½ pint. The above are applied with a sponge, after cleaning the barrel with lime and water. When dry, they are polished with a stiff brush, or iron scratch brush.

BRUNSWICK BLACK. Melt asphaltum, and add to it half its weight of boiled linseed oil; mix, and when sufficiently cool, add enough oil of turpentine to bring it to the proper consistence.

BUG POISON. 1. Spirit of wine 8 oz., spirit of turpentine 8 oz., camphor ½ oz.: mix.

2. Distilled vinegar, or diluted wood vinegar a pint; camphor ½ oz.; dissolve.

3. Corrosive sublimate 3 oz., muriatic acid 3 oz., oil of turpentine 12 oz., water 6 pints. Or, 1 oz. of sublimate, 2 oz. of muriatic acid, a pint of oil of turpentine, and a pint decoction of tobacco.

4. Strong mercurial ointment 1 oz., soft-soap 1 oz., oil of turpentine a pint.

5. White arsenic 2 oz., lard 13 oz., corrosive sublimate ¼ oz., Venetian red ¼ oz.

6. Scotch snuff mixed with soft-soap.

7. *For Floors.* Corrosive sublimate 1 ℔, sal ammoniac 1 ℔, hot water 8 gallons. [It is said that if a branch of narrow leaved dittany or pepperwort (lepidium ruderale) be suspended in a room, all the bugs will settle in it, and may be taken. Fumigating the rooms with sulphur is a troublesome and disagreeable process, and not always successful.]

BURNETT'S (Sir W.) DISINFECTING FLUID. See DISINFECTING COMPOUNDS.

BUTTER, TO PRESERVE. Powder finely, and mix together, 2 parts of the best salt, 1 of loaf sugar, and 1 of nitre.

To each pound of butter, well cleansed from the milk, add 1 oz. of this compound. It should not be used under a month. [Butter that has an unpleasant flavour, is said to be improved by the addition of 2½ dr. of bi-carbonate of soda to 3 ℔ of butter. A turnipy flavour may be prevented by only feeding the cows with turnips immediately after milking them.]

BUTTER OF ANTIMONY. The liquid chloride of antimony, commercially known by this name, is usually made by dissolving crude or roasted black antimony in muriatic acid, with the addition of a little nitric acid. It usually contains pernitrate of iron.

BUTYRIC ETHER. Saponify butter with a strong solution of potash, dissolve the soap in the smallest quantity of alcohol by the aid of heat, add a mixture of alcohol and sulphuric acid till the solution is acid, and distil as long as the product has a fruity odour. Redistil the product from chloride of calcium. It is sold as essence of pine apple.

CAMPHINE. Highly rectified oil of turpentine. ENGLISH'S patent camphine is made by passing the vapour of oil of turpentine through caustic solutions of potash, soda, or lime; or through sulphuric acid.

CAMPHOR, ARTIFICIAL. This is formed by passing muriatic acid gas into oil of turpentine.

CAMPHOR BALLS, See SKIN COSMETICS, after PERFUMERY.

CANDIES. These belong rather to the confectioner than the druggist. The green stalks of angelica, the peels of orange, lemon, and citron, green roots of ginger, &c., are first boiled in water till soft, then in syrup till they are transparent, and dried in a stove, at a heat not exceeding 104° F. Candied horehound is made by boiling lump sugar with a little strong decoction or infusion of dried horehound, till a portion taken out and cooled becomes solid. It is then poured on to a slab, or into paper or tin moulds dusted with powdered sugar.

CANTON'S PHOSPHORUS. Put calcined oyster shells in layers, alternately with sulphur, and heat strongly in a covered crucible for an hour.

CAOUTCHOUC, SOLVENTS FOR. See SOLVENTS.

CAPSULES, GELATINOUS. These are used to contain copaiva and other nauseous liquids which do not dissolve gelatine, so that they may be swallowed without inconvenience. They are made by "dipping the bulbous extremity of an iron rod into a concentrated solution of gelatine. When the rod is withdrawn, it is to be rotated, in order to diffuse the gelatine equally over the bulb." When sufficiently hardened, they are removed, placed on pins to dry, and when dry filled with the balsam or oil, and the orifice closed with liquid gelatine. They are usually of an olive form, and contain 10 gr. of balsam in each. See Dr. PEREIRA'S "Elements," article COPAIVA. M. GIRAUD recommends the following composition for capsules:—Transparent gelatine 12 parts, syrup of gum 2 parts, syrup 2 parts, water 10 parts. Melt it in a water-bath, remove the scum, and dip the mould, previously oiled, into the compound.

CARBON. See CHARCOAL.

CARBONIC ACID. See GASES.

CARMINE. See PIGMENTS.

CASE HARDENING POWDER. This is merely ferroprussiate of potash, dried, and finely powdered. By sprinkling it on iron heated to bright redness, the metal becomes case-hardened, or superficially converted into steel. The iron should be plunged into cold water as soon as the powder has acted on it. The following compound is used for the same purpose:—Sal ammoniac 2 oz., burnt bone dust 2 oz., HENWOOD'S composition ½ oz. Used as the former.

CASSOLETTES. See PERFUMERY.

CAYENNE, SOLUBLE. See CONDIMENTS, p. 295.

CEMENTS AND LUTES, VARIOUS.

Shell-lac Cement. Fine orange shell-lac, bruised, 4 oz., highly rectified spirit 3 oz. Digest in a warm place, frequently shaking, till the shell-lac is dissolved. Rectified wood naphtha may be substituted for spirit of wine, where the smell is not objectionable. A most useful cement for securely joining almost any material. See LIQUID GLUE.

Shell-lac Cement, without Spirit. Boil 1 oz. of borax in 16 oz. water, add 2 oz. powdered shell-lac, and boil in a covered vessel till the lac is dissolved. Cheaper than the above, and for many purposes answers very well. Both are useful in fixing paper labels to tin, and to glass when exposed to damp.

Armenian Cement for Glass, China, &c. 1. KELLER'S. Soak 2 dr. of cut isinglass in 2 oz. of water for 24 hours; boil to 1 oz., add 1 oz. spirit of wine, and strain through linen. Mix this, while hot, with a solution of 1 dr. of mastic in 1 oz. of rectified spirit, and triturate with ½ dr. powdered gum ammoniac, till perfectly homogeneous.

2. Dr. URE'S *Diamond Cement.* Isinglass 1 oz., distilled water 6 oz., boil to 3 oz., and add 1½ oz., of rectified spirit. Boil for a minute or two, strain, and add while hot, first ½ oz. of a milky emulsion of ammoniac, and then 5 dr. of tincture of mastic. [There are various kinds of this cement sold, and some of the improvements introduced by peculiar makers have not been made public.]

Cement used in the East for uniting jewels, glass, and metals. Dissolve 5 or 6 pieces of gum mastic, each about the size of a large pea, in just as much spirit as will render it liquid. Soften some isinglass by steeping it in water; having dried it, dissolve as much of it in good brandy as will make a two ounce phial of strong glue, to which must be added two small bits of gum ammoniacum, rubbing until they are dissolved. Mix the two solutions; keep in a close phial; and when it is to be used, set the phial in boiling water.—Mr. ETON.

HŒNLE'S *Cement for Glass or Earthenware.* Shell-lac 2 parts, Venice turpentine 1 part, fuse together, and form into sticks.

Cheese Cement, for Earthenware, &c. Mix together white of egg beaten to a froth, quick lime, and grated cheese, and beat them to a paste.

Curd Cement. Add ½ pint of vinegar to ½ pint of skimmed milk; mix the curd with the whites of 5 eggs well beaten, and sufficient powdered quick lime to form a paste. It resists water, and a moderate degree of heat.

Glass Flux, for mending broken China, &c. Mix 3 parts of red lead, 2 of fine white sand, and 3 of crystallized boracic acid; fuse the mixture, levigate it, and apply it with thin mucilage of tragacanth. Heat the repaired article gently so as partially to fuse the cement.

Cement for joining Spar and Marble Ornaments, &c. Melt together 8 parts of resin, 1 of wax, and stir in 4 parts, or as much as may be required, of Paris plaster. The pieces to be made hot.

HENSLER'S *Cement.* Grind 3 parts of litharge, 2 of recently burnt lime, and 1 of white bole, with linseed oil varnish. [Very tenacious, but long in drying.]

SINGER'S *Cement for Electrical Machines and Galvanic Troughs.* Melt together 5 ℔ of rosin and 1 ℔ of bees'-wax, and stir in 1 ℔ of red ochre (highly dried, and still warm,) and 4 oz. of Paris plaster, continuing the heat a little above 212°, and stirring constantly till all frothing ceases. Or (for troughs,) Rosin 6 ℔, dried red ochre, 1 ℔, calcined plaster of Paris ½ ℔, linseed oil ¼ ℔.

Botany Bay Cement. Botany Bay gum, melted and mixed with an equal quantity of brick dust.

Cap Cement. As SINGER'S; but 1 ℔ of dried Venetian red may be substituted for the red ochre and Paris plaster.

Bottle Cement. Rosin 15 parts, tallow 4 (or wax 3) parts, highly dried red ochre 5 parts, or ivory black q. s. The common kinds of sealing wax are also used.

Turner's Cement. Bees'-wax 1 oz., rosin ½ oz., pitch ½ oz. Melt, and stir in fine brickdust q. s.

Coppersmith's Cement. Powdered quicklime, mixed with bullock's blood, and applied immediately.

Engineer's Cement. Equal weights of red and white lead, with drying oil, spread on tow or canvass. For metallic joints, or to unite large stones, in cisterns, &c.

Cement for Steam Pipes. Good linseed oil varnish ground with equal weights of white lead, oxide of manganese, and pipe clay.

Iron Cement, for closing the joints of iron pipes. Iron borings, coarsely powdered, 5 ℔, powdered sal ammoniac 2 oz., sulphur 1 oz., water sufficient to moisten it. It quickly hardens; but if time can be allowed, it sets more firmly without the sulphur. It must be used as soon as mixed, and rammed tightly into the joints.

GAD'S *Hydraulic Cement.* Powdered clay 3 ℔, oxide of iron 1 ℔, boiled oil to form a stiff paste.

Cements for Masonry of Chambers for Chlorine, &c. Equal parts of pitch, rosin, and plaster of Paris.

Roman Cement. A mixture of clay, lime, and oxide of iron, separately calcined, and finely powdered. It must be kept in close vessels, and mixed with water when used.

Marine Cement. See GLUE MARINE.

MAISSIAT'S *Cement, as an air-tight covering for bottles, &c.* Melt India-rubber (to which 15 per cent. of wax or tallow may be added,) and gradually add finely-powdered quick lime till a change of odour shows that combination has taken place, and a proper consistence is obtained.

Cement for attaching Metal Letters to Plate Glass. Copal varnish 15 parts, drying oil 5 parts, turpentine 3 parts, oil of turpentine 2 parts, liquefied glue 5 parts; melted in a water-bath, and 10 parts of slaked lime added.

Japanese Cement. Mix rice flour intimately with cold water, and boil gently.

French Cement. Mix thick mucilage of gum Arabic with powdered starch.

Common Paste. To a dessert-spoonful of flour add gradually half a pint of cold water, and mix till quite smooth; add a pinch of powdered alum, (some add also as much powdered rosin as will lie on a sixpence,) and boil for a few moments, stirring constantly. The addition of a little brown sugar, and a few grains of corrosive sublimate, is said to preserve it for years.

Soft Cement. Melt yellow wax with half its weight of common turpentine, and stir in a little Venetian red, previously well dried, and finely powdered. [As a temporary stopping for joints and openings in glass and other apparatus, where the heat and pressure are not great.] See the next.

Lutes or Cements for closing the Joints of Apparatus. 1. Mix Paris plaster with water to a soft paste, and apply it immediately. It bears nearly a red heat. It may be rendered impervious by rubbing it over with wax and oil.

2. Slaked lime, made into a paste with white of egg, or a solution of gelatine.

3. *Fat Lute.* Finely powdered clay moistened with water, and beaten up with boiled linseed oil. Roll it into cylinders, and press it on the joints of the vessels, which must be perfectly dry. It is rendered more secure by binding it with strips of linen moistened with white of egg.

4. Linseed meal beaten to a paste with water.

5. Slips of moistened bladder, smeared with white of egg.

Luting for Acids. Dissolve 1 part of India rubber in 2 parts of linseed oil, by heat, and work it into a stiff paste with 3 parts, or as much as sufficient, of white clay.

Lutes for Coating Retorts. 1. Dissolve 1 oz. of borax in ½ pint of water, and add slaked lime to form a thin paste. Brush this over the retort, and let it dry gradually. Then apply a coating of slaked lime and linseed oil well beaten together. Let it dry for a day or two before use, and fill up any cracks which may appear with lime and linseed oil.

2. For bearing a stronger heat: Stourbridge clay, mixed with a little sand to prevent it splitting off: a little cut tow, or horse-dung, or asbestos, is usually added, to increase its coherence. It should be well beaten to a stiff paste, and rolled out before application. The glass should be first rubbed over with a little of the lute mixed with water, then placed in the centre of the paste, rolled out to about ¼ or ⅓ of an inch thickness, and the edges of the latter raised and moulded to the glass, taking care to press out all the air.

MOHR'S *Lute.* Mix equal parts of brick-dust and litharge, and beat them into a paste with linseed oil. Apply this with a stiff brush, and dust it over with coarse sand: dry it in a warm place.

For cements for plugging teeth, see TEETH COSMETICS, page 270.

CHARCOAL. Wood charcoal is made by burning wood with only a partial access of air. For chemical purposes, that made in iron cylinders, in the manufacture of wood vinegar, is preferred.

CHARCOAL, ANIMAL. The most common form is that of

bone black (commonly called ivory black,) made by distilling bones, from which the grease has been removed by boiling, in iron or earthen retorts, the ammoniacal liquor, &c., being collected in proper receivers. The residue is bone black. When used for the purpose of decolorization, further treatment is required: either the bone earth may be entirely removed by muriatic acid, as directed in the Pharmacopœia; or more commonly, in the refining of sugar, and for other manufacturing purposes, this is only partially effected, in some such way as the following:—Mix 8 ℔ of the bone black, coarsely powdered, with sufficient water to form a paste, and add 1 ℔ of muriatic acid. In an hour, pour boiling water on the mass, let it settle, pour off the liquid, add more water, and repeat this till the water comes off free from taste. Drain and press the black in a cloth, and dry it. Its power is increased by mixing it with a little potash, heating it to dull redness in a covered crucible, and again washing it.

Chameleon Mineral. Mix equal weights of black oxide of manganese and pure potash, and heat them in a crucible. Keep the compound in closely-stopped bottles. A solution of it in water passes through various shades of colour from green to red.

Chemique, or Chemic Blue—Sulphate of Indigo. To 7 or 8 parts of oil of vitriol, in a glass or earthen vessel, placed in cold water, add gradually 1 part of fine indigo in powder, stirring the mixture at each addition with a glass rod, or piece of tobacco-pipe. Cover the vessel for 24 hours, then dilute with an equal weight of water. Sometimes it is sold without diluting. The German fuming acid answers best, 4 or 5 parts of it being sufficient for 1 of indigo. For dyeing silk, &c., carbonate of potash, soda, or ammonia, is added, to neutralize the acid, taking care not to add it in excess.

Chlorate of Barytes. Saturate solution of chloric acid, prepared as directed page 306, with fresh precipitated carbonate of barytes, filter, and crystallize.

Chlorate of Potash. Slake 7 oz. of quicklime, add it to a pint of solution of caustic potash of 1·110 sp. gr.;

heat the mixture slightly, and pass through it a rapid current of chlorine gas until no more is absorbed. Evaporate nearly to dryness, re-dissolve in boiling water, filter, and evaporate the filtered solution, and the washings of the filter, for crystallization.—Mr. CALVERT. Or dissolve chloride of lime in water, add solution of muriate of potash, and boil to dryness. Dissolve the mass in hot water, and filter if necessary: on cooling, a large quantity of chlorate of potash is deposited.—LIEBIG. For another process, see Potassæ Chloras, P. F.

CHLORIDE OF LIME, OR CHLORINATED LIME. *Bleaching Powder.* Chlorine gas (slowly evolved from a mixture of 10 parts of common salt and 10 to 14 parts of oxide of manganese, placed in an alembic of lead, and heated by steam, and with 12 to 14 parts of oil of vitriol previously diluted with a fourth of its weight of water, added) is conveyed into a chamber where sifted slake lime is thinly spread on shelves. It is so cheaply made by the large manufacturers for bleaching purposes, that it is seldom prepared by druggists. The liquid chloride of lime may be made either by triturating the dry chloride with a little cold water till perfectly smooth, then adding more water, and filtering the solution; or by passing chlorine gas into a mixture of lime and water. The DUB. PHARM. directs a solution of 1035 sp. gr. The Paris Codex directs 1 part of dry bleaching powder to be diffused in 45 of water. SOUBEIRAN directs 1 part to 50; but prefers passing the gas from 1 part of oxide of manganese and 4 of muriatic acid, into a mixture of 1 part of lime and 50 of water.

CHLORIDE OR HYPOCHLORITE OF POTASH. *Eau de Javelle.* Pass chlorine gas, as above, into a solution of 1 ℔ of carbonate of potash in a gallon of water. Or mix 8 oz. of dry chloride of lime with 6 pints of water; and dissolve 16 oz. of carbonate of potash in a quart of water. Mix the liquids, and filter.

CHLORIDE OF SODA, OR CHLORINATED SODA. See Soda Chlorinata, and Liquor Sodæ Chlorinatæ, in the Pocket Formulary. A more ready way of preparing it, for other purposes than dispensing prescriptions, is the following:—

Diffuse 1 ℔ of chloride of lime in 30 ℔ of water. Dissolve 2 ℔ of crystallized carbonate of soda in 15 ℔ of water. Mix the solutions, let the mixture settle, pour off the clear liquid, and filter it. See P. F., 5th ed., p. 513.

CHLORINE. See GASES.

CHLOROFORM. Into a copper still placed in a water-bath put 7 gallons of water; heat to 100° F.; add 10 ℔ of lime slaked in a solution of 20 ℔ of chloride of lime. Add 3 ℔ of rectified spirit; mix them well, lute on the head immediately, and raise the heat rapidly to 212°. When the extremity of the neck of the still becomes hot, damp the fire, and the distillation will continue regularly. When it ceases, add to what remains in the still 17½ pints of water, raise the heat to 100°, add 8 ℔ of lime, and 20 ℔ of chloride of lime, stir carefully, add the distilled liquor from which the chloroform has been separated, with 1¾ pint of spirit; stir, and proceed as before. If the still is large enough, this may be repeated 3 or 4 times, with a constantly increasing product. The chloroform sinks to the bottom of the distilled liquid, and may be rectified by distilling it with oil of vitriol. Its density should not be less than 1·496: LIEBIG says 1·480, but at that density it is not pure. Chloroform may be obtained by a similar process from rectified wood naphtha (pyroxylic spirit,) but it is then contaminated with an empyreumatic oil, lighter than water, which cannot be entirely separated from it. It is therefore unfit for inhalation; but when rectified over sulphuric acid and chloride of calcium, may be used as a solvent. The process recommended by Dr. SIMPSON is that of DUMAS:—Chloride of lime in powder 4 ℔, water 12 ℔, rectified spirit 12 oz. Mix in a capacious still, and distil as long as a dense liquid, which sinks to the bottom of the water which comes over with it, is produced. It is rectified as the last. For other methods, see Pocket Formulary.

CHOCOLATE. See Chocolata, Pocket Formulary.

CHROMATE OF POTASH. Mix 4 parts of chrome ore (chromate of iron) with 2 of pearlash and 1 of nitre, and heat the mixture in a reverberatory furnace for several hours.

Lixiviate, and crystallize. The chromate is converted into bichromate by adding sulphuric acid, or rather acetic acid, to the solution.

CHROMATE OF LEAD. See PIGMENTS.

CHROME OXIDE. Mix bichromate of potash with half its weight of muriate of ammonia; heat the mixture to redness, and wash the mass with plenty of boiling water. Dry the residue.

CHROMIC ACID. See ACID, CHROMIC.

CLOTHES, POWDER TO KEEP AWAY MOTHS FROM. Mix powdered pipe-clay 1½ ℔, white pepper and starch, each 1 oz., root of Florentine iris 1½ oz., with spirits of wine 2 oz. To be dusted over the clothes when laid by.

COLLODION. Mix in a glass, stoneware, or porcelain vessel, 30 parts of strong sulphuric acid and 20 of powdered nitre; place the vessel in cold water; add 1 part of carded cotton-wool, and open and stir it in the acid mixture by means of 2 glass or porcelain rods, or stems of tobacco pipes, for 2 or 3 minutes. Then remove the cotton into a large quantity of cold water, press it, and wash it in a stream of water, opening it with the fingers, till the water passes through it free from acidity. Squeeze it strongly in a dry cloth, and then open it, and dry it gradually in a warm situation, free from danger. One part of this prepared cotton, with 16 of rectified ether, and 1 of alcohol, agitated together, soon forms a gelatinous solution. See Pocket Formulary, for its medical preparations.

COLLODION for photographic purposes. Mr. COLLINS. Put into a large tumbler ½ oz. of strong nitric acid (sp. gr. 1·50,) and add ½ oz. of oil of vitriol. Weigh out 30 grains of cotton-wool (or of paper made from linen rags,) and with two glass rods stir it well into the acid, that the cotton may become quickly saturated. It must not be allowed to become soft and gummy. From 15 to 20 seconds is generally sufficient for this immersion. The cotton is next removed by the glass rods, and plunged into a basin of cold water, placed under a running tap,—the cotton being worked about in this until it ceases to redden a piece of blue litmus paper. Remove it, express the water, first by wringing in a clean cloth, then between folds of blotting paper. Hang up to dry. Take nine fluid ounces of rectified ether, and dissolve in it 15 grains of this dry prepared cotton. Add 1 oz. of alcohol, cork the bottle tightly, and allow it to stand until any flocculent matter has subsided. Finally, decant into a stoppered bottle for use. (To prepare this collodion for forming a sensitive surface on glass, on which, if poured in a thin layer, it now leaves only a transparent coating by the evaporation of the ether and spirit, it must first be *iodized.* To a saturated solution of iodide of potassium in alcohol, as much iodide of silver is to be added by degrees as the liquid will dissolve—a process which must be performed by candle-light. To every ounce of collodion, made as above, add 20 drops of this iodide mixture, and keep it now carefully from the light.) See PHOTOGRAPHY.

COLLODION, ELASTIC (for surgical purposes.) Mix together, in a stoneware or porcelain pot, sulphuric acid (of sp. gr. 1·847) 300 parts, very dry nitrate of potash 200 parts; and add carded cotton 10 parts. Leave in contact for 12 minutes; withdraw the cotton, wash it in cold water to remove the acid which it retains, and, after 2 or 3 rinsings, immerse it again in a solution of 30 parts of subcarbonate of potash in 1000 of water; plunge it again into simple water, agitating well; and lastly, dry at a temperature of 77° to 86° Fahr. The product is xyloidine. Place now 8 parts of this xyloidine, with 125 parts of sulphuric ether, in a wide-mouthed flask, and add 8 parts of alcohol (sp. gr. ·825.) Agitate. Make next a mixture of Venice turpentine 2 parts, castor oil 2 parts, white wax 2 parts, sulphuric ether 6 parts. Heat together the first three substances, add the ether, and mix all with the solution of xyloidine.—M. LAURAS.

COLOURS, VARIOUS. The principal dry colours will be found under PIGMENTS. Other colours are noticed below.

COLOURS FOR DRUGGISTS' SHOW BOTTLES. In making these, distilled water should be used, and rather more of the colour than will fill the carboys made, to avoid the necessity of adding water to fill up after filtration, as this sometimes renders them turbid. The carboys should be perfectly clean, and also dry, or otherwise rinsed out with a portion of the filtered liquid.

1. *Blues.* Sulphate of copper 4 to 8 oz., water a gallon, oil of vitriol 1 oz.

2. *Royal Blue.* Sulphate of copper 8 oz., water a gallon; dissolve, and add water of ammonia till the full colour is developed; then water to make up 2 gallons.

3. *Finest Royal Blue.* Nitrate of copper 3 oz., water sufficient to dissolve it; add water of ammonia as long as the colour becomes deeper, then water to make up 2 gallons.

4. *Paler.* Crystallized acetate of copper ½ oz., muriatic acid 1½ oz., water of ammonia q. s., water to make up 2 gallons.

5. *Light Blue.* Crystallized acetate of copper a scruple, water of ammonia 2 oz., water 2 gallons.

Green. 1. An infusion of saffron added to the above blues.

2. Sulphate of copper 4 oz., bichromate of potash ½ dr., water q. s.

3. By adding to the above deep or light blues a small quantity of chromate or bichromate of potash till the desired tint is produced, various shades of green may be obtained.

4. Sulphate of copper, with muriate of soda, or muriate of iron.

5. *Emerald Green.* Nitrate of copper 3 oz., muriatic acid 4 oz., nitric acid 4 oz., water 2 gallons.

6. *Very Fine Emerald.* Nickel 3 oz., muriatic acid 4 oz., nitrous acid 2 oz.; digest for 24 hours, add 2 gallons of water, and filter.

Red. 1. Dried rose petals 8 oz., boiling water a gallon; digest for 12 hours, strain; digest the roses with more water, and strain; mix the infusions, add a pint of diluted sulphuric acid, and filter.

2. Cochineal ½ oz., boiling water a gallon; digest, strain, add ½ oz. of sulphuric acid, and water to make up 2 gallons.

3. *Crimson.* Iodine, and iodide of potassium, of each 2 dr.; triturate with a dr. of water, and add 3 gallons of water, and 4 oz. of muriatic acid.

4. *For External Lamps.* Camphine, strongly coloured with alkanet root.

Pink. 1. Infuse ½ oz. of good madder in a quart of boiling distilled water; when cold, add 1 oz. of strong ammonia, and filter into 2 gallons of distilled water.

2. Dissolve muriate or nitrate of cobalt in water, and add sufficient carbonate of ammonia to re-dissolve the precipitate first thrown down; then water q. s.

Purple. To the last add sufficient of the blue No. 3, to give the desired shade.

Lilac. Smalts 4 oz., nitric acid 4 oz.; let it stand 24 hours, add 2 gallons of water, 1 oz. of alum, and 4 oz. of water of ammonia. Or rather as the purple.

Yellow. 1. Chromate or bichromate of potash, with water q. s.

2. Bichromate of potash 2 dr., hot water 4 oz.; dissolve, and add 4 oz. sulphuric acid, and 2 gallons of water.

3. Bichromate of potash, nitrate of potash, and water.

Amber. 1. Deep chrome yellow 3 oz., pearlash 9 oz., water 2 gallons; boil gently for half an hour, take it off to cool, and add 6 oz. muriatic acid, and water to the desired colour.

2. Dragon's blood, digested with sulphuric acid, and diluted with water to the desired shade.

Olive. Sulphate of iron 3 oz., sulphuric acid 3 oz., water 2 gallons; dissolve, and add the green No. 5, q. s. to brighten the colour.

LIQUID COLOURS FOR MAPS, &c. See INKS, DYES, CHEMIQUE BLUE, LAKE LIQUOR, &c. Gamboge and some of the cake colours, mixed with water, are also used.

COLOURS FOR CONFECTIONERS. Many fatal accidents occur from confectionary being coloured with poisonous pigments. The following may be safely used:—Cochineal and its preparations, sap green, vegetable lakes, Prussian blue; a mixture of a yellow lake and Prussian blue for green.

COLOURING FOR BRANDY, &c. Sugar melted in a ladle till it is brown, and then dissolved in water, or lime water.

COLOURS FOR LIQUEURS. Pink is given by cochineal;

yellow by saffron or safflower; violet by litmus; blue, by sulphate of indigo, saturated with chalk; green, by the last with tincture of saffron, or by sap green.

COLOURS FOR LEATHER. See BOOKBINDERS' COLOURS.

COLOURS, IMPROVED VEHICLES FOR. 1. One measure of saturated solution of borax, with 4 of linseed oil. The pigment may be ground with the oil or the mixture.

2. A solution of shell-lac with borax, as in making COATHUPE'S Ink. See INK.

3. Water colours, mixed with gelatine, and afterwards fixed by washing with a solution of alum.

4. Curd of milk, washed and pressed, then dried on fine net, and when required for use, mixed with water and the colouring matter.

COPPER, OXIDE OF. The *black* oxide is made by calcining the nitrate; or by adding caustic potash to sulphate of copper, in solution, and washing and drying the precipitate. The red oxide may be made as directed for Bronze Powder, No. 4, or in the moist way thus:—Pour a solution of 27 parts of sugar in 60 of water, over 9 parts of hydrated oxide of copper, weighed in its compressed but still moist state. A solution of 18 parts of caustic potash in 60 of water is added, and the whole agitated together without heat, and filtered. The clear liquid heated in a water-bath, and continually stirred, deposits the red oxide, and the liquid becomes colourless.

NITRATE OF COPPER. Dissolve copper in nitric acid to saturation, evaporate to dryness, re-dissolve, filter, and evaporate, so that the salt may crystallize. Or add a solution of sulphate of copper to a solution of nitrate of lead, so long as sulphate of lead is precipitated; filter, evaporate, and crystallize. For the other salts of copper, see CUPRUM, Pocket Formulary.

COTTON POWDER. See GUN COTTON.

DEPILATORIES. See HAIR COSMETICS, page 258.

DEXTRINE, OR STARCH GUM. Heat 4 gallons of water in a water-bath to between 77° and 86° Fahrenheit; stir in 1½ or 2 ℔ finely ground malt; raise the temperature to 140°, add 10 ℔ of potato or other starch; mix all thoroughly, raise the heat to 158°, and keep it between that and 167° for 20 or 30 minutes. When the liquid becomes thin, instantly raise the heat to the boiling point, to prevent the formation of sugar. Strain the liquor and evaporate it to dryness, as the dextrine will not keep long in a liquid form. Another method is to boil solution of starch with a few drops of sulphuric acid, filter the solution, and add alcohol to throw down the dextrine. See GUM [BRITISH] for another form of dextrine.

DEXTRINE VARNISH. Dextrine 2 parts, water 6 parts, rectified spirit 1 part.—BARON DE SYLVESTRE.

DIASTASE. Macerate ground malt in cold water; strain with pressure, heat the clear solution in a water-bath, to 158° Fahrenheit to coagulate the albumen; filter again, and add rectified spirit as long as diastase falls. If required very pure, re-dissolve it in water, and again precipitate with spirit. Dry it at a low temperature. Well malted barley contains about 1 per cent. of pure diastase; one part of which is capable of converting 2000 parts of starch into dextrine or sugar.

DIETETIC ARTICLES. For these see another division of the work.

DISINFECTING AND DEODORIZING COMPOUNDS. 1. SIR WM. BURNETT'S *Patent Solution.* It is made by dissolving zinc in commercial muriatic acid to saturation.

2. ELLERMAN'S *Deodorizing Fluid.* This consists chiefly of perchlorides and chlorides of iron and manganese.

3. LEDOYEN'S *Solution.* This is a solution of nitrate of lead, and contains about 20 oz. of the salt in a gallon. The specific gravity should be 1·40. A similar compound may be made by mixing 13½ oz. of litharge with 6 pints of water, and adding 12 oz. of nitric acid at 1·38 specific gravity (or 8 oz. at 1·50;) and digesting at a gentle heat till the solution is complete.

4. SIRET'S *Compound.* Sulphate of iron 20 ℔, sulphate of zinc 3½ ℔, wood or peat charcoal 1 ℔, sulphate of lime 26½ ℔: mix, and form into balls. To be placed in cesspools, &c., to deodorize them. M. SIRET has subsequently modified this compound, thus—Sulphate

of iron 100 parts, sulphate of zinc 50, tan or oak-bark powder 40, tar 5, and oil 5 parts.

5. COLLINS' *Disinfecting Powder.* Mix 2 parts of dry chloride of lime with one of burnt alum. To be set in shallow dishes in rooms, &c., with or without the addition of water. [See also CHLORIDE OF LIME, and CHLORIDE OF SODA. Peat charcoal also possesses powerful deodorizing properties.]

DUBBING, CURRIERS'. Made by boiling cuttings of sheep-skins in common cod oil.

DRYERS FOR PAINTERS. White copperas 1 ℔, sugar of lead 1 ℔, white lead 2 ℔; ground with boiled oil.

DRYING AND BOILED OIL. Linseed oil is mixed with powdered litharge, and heated till it becomes thick. A *pale* drying oil is obtained by mixing with linseed oil sufficient dry sulphate of lead to form a milky liquid, and shaking it repeatedly for some days, letting it stand exposed to the light. When it has become quite clear, it may be poured off from the dregs. The sulphate of lead, when washed from the mucilage, may be again used for the same purpose. LIEBIG directs 1 ℔ of acetate of lead to be dissolved in half a gallon of rain water, and 1 ℔ of finely-powdered litharge added: the mixture is either boiled, or exposed for a long time to a moderate heat, and frequently stirred, till no more particles of litharge can be seen. A white deposit is formed, which may be left in the liquid, or separated by filtration; 20 ℔ of linseed oil, in which 1 ℔ of levigated litharge has been diffused, are gradually added to the lead solution, previously diluted with an equal bulk of water, and the mixture frequently stirred. It is then left to clear itself in a warm place; but to obtain it bright it must be filtered through coarse paper or cotton. It may be bleached by exposure to the sun. The lead solution which subsides from the mixture may be filtered and used again, after dissolving in it 1 ℔ of litharge as before. The oxide of lead contained in the oil may be removed from it by agitating it with diluted sulphuric acid, and letting it stand to settle. See also OILS (Clarified Linseed Oil.)

DUPUYTREN'S POMMADE. See HAIR COSMETICS, after PERFUMERY.

DYES AND COMPOUNDS USED IN DYEING. A few of the principal colouring matters and mordants may here be noticed; for further information, the reader is referred to "Dr. Ure's Dictionary of the Arts," "Parnell's Applied Chemistry," "Berthollet on Dyeing," &c.

Blue Dyes. The most important of these is indigo. Being insoluble in water, it is prepared for use by sulphate of iron and alkalies or lime, by fermentation and alkalies, and by solution in sulphuric acid.

1. Triturate 1 ℔ of indigo with water and a little caustic potash; then add 3 ℔ of lime, and afterwards 2½ ℔ of sulphate of iron in solution, stirring them well together. The solution contains *disoxygenized indigo*, which is soluble in lime and alkalies. The cotton, linen, &c., to be dyed is repeatedly dipped in the solution, and afterwards rinsed in water soured with muriatic acid.

2. To 45 or 50 gallons of water, heated to 122° F., add 12 oz. of indigo, 8 oz. of madder, 8 oz. of bran, and 24 oz. of potash. In 36 hours introduce 12 oz. more of potash, and the same in 12 hours after. In 72 hours, add a little lime to check the fermentation. Wool, silk, linen, and cotton may be dyed in this bath. Another form of this dye is—indigo 2 parts, common soda 5 parts, lime 2 parts, clarified honey 1 part, water as much as may be sufficient. Keep it warm in an earthen jar till the indigo is dissolved.

3. A solution of indigo in sulphuric acid (see CHEMIC BLUE) is used as a dye, but a purer tone of colour is obtained by the following method:—The sulphate of indigo, mixed with water, is heated in a copper kettle; wool is immersed in it, and the whole is allowed to cool for 24 hours. The wool is then taken out, washed till the water comes off colourless and free from acid; it is then boiled in water containing about 2 per cent. of pearlash, or other alkaline carbonate, for a quarter of an hour. The quantity of pearlash should be equal to one-third the weight of the indigo.

Logwood, with verdigris, or sulphate of copper, gives a

blue dye, bordering on violet: with alum and tartar, a violet.

Prussian Blue is sometimes used in dyeing, after being triturated and digested for 24 hours with its weight of muriatic acid. A blue is also given by immersing silk, &c., in a solution of peracetate of iron, then in a solution of prussiate of potash, and afterwards rinsing it in acidulated water. Boiling water is sufficient to discolour articles thus dyed.

Red Dyes. The various shades of red are given by madder, cochineal, lac dye, safflower, &c.; fixed by aluminous or tin mordants. Less permanent dyes are produced by Brazil wood, peach wood, and archil. Some of these require peculiar treatment. Safflower contains a yellow as well as a red colouring matter. The first, being soluble in cold water, is extracted by putting the safflower in a bag, and kneading it under water. The safflower, thus deprived of the yellow matter, yields its red colour to alkaline liquids; at the time of using which, lemon juice or some other acid is added sufficient to saturate the alkali. Pink saucers are made by adding lemon juice to an alkaline infusion of washed safflower, and allowing the colouring matter to deposit. Madder also contains a dun colouring matter which deteriorates the red unless previously removed. This may be partially effected by washing it in cold water: another mode is to treat the madder with its own weight of sulphuric acid, which carbonizes the other matters, but leaves the red colour uninjured. As madder gives out but little of its red colouring matter to water, the decoction is not strained off, but the madder left in the bath. With acetate of iron, madder yields a purple tint. Lac dye, as imported from India, requires acids for its solution. See Lac Solvent, below.

Yellow Dyes. These are given by French berries, quercitron bark, turmeric, weld, yellow wood, &c. Also by some mineral colours, as the following:—The material to be dyed is first padded in a solution of bichromate of potash (8 oz. to a gallon of water,) then in a solution of acetate or nitrate of lead. Cotton is dyed yellow by alternate dippings in iron liquor and lime water, or solution of pearlash. A yellow colour is given to silk by passing it through a mixture of equal measures of nitric acid (sp. gr. 1·288) and water, heated to 95° or 100° Fahrenheit, and from thence into a stream of water, or a mixture of chalk and water. This is termed mandarining.

Nankeen Dye is made by boiling annatto with an equal weight of pearlash in sufficient water. Orange is given by annatto; or by a mixture of red and yellow dyes; or by the successive application of acetate of alumina, a bath of quercitron, and the madder-bath.

Greens are given to woollens by first dyeing them blue, immersing the article in acetate of alumina, drying it, and finally immersing it in a quercitron-bath. For silks, the order is reversed.

Browns are given by catechu, by walnut-peels with alum, by redwood and copperas, by madder and black dye, &c.

Drabs are given by fustic with iron liquor.

Blacks. These are given by salts of iron, with galls, sumach, and logwood. The best black cloths are previously dyed blue with indigo.

By the mixture of various dyes, every variety of shade is produced: and often several tints from one colouring matter by the use of different mordants.

Mordants are earthy and metallic compounds, the base of which unites both with the fibres of the material to be dyed and the colouring matter, thus rendering the dyes fixed. In *calico printing*, the mordants are formed into a paste with some gum or other thickening material, and printed with wooden blocks on the cloth; which, after being dried, &c., is passed through the liquid dyes. The colouring matter combines with the parts so printed, but is easily discharged from the other parts.

The principal Mordants are the following:—

Alum Mordants. 1. Alum with one-fourth its weight of tartar.

2. Acetate of Alumina. (See page 304.) This is

commonly prepared in solution for the purpose: 100 parts of alum in solution, with 150 parts of pyrolignite of lime of 20° B. density, is sometimes employed.

3. A solution of alum, with crystallized carbonate of soda, in the proportion of 1 oz. to each pound of alum.

4. HAUSMANN'S. This consists of a solution of alum with sufficient strong solution of caustic potash to re-dissolve the precipitated alumina; to which mixture a portion of linseed oil is added.

5. To 50 gallons of boiling water add 100 lb of alum; dissolve, and add slowly 10 lb of crystallized carbonate of soda. When the effervescence is over add 75 lb of sugar of lead.

Tin Mordants. 1. *Protochloride of Tin.* To strong muriatic acid add gradually small pieces of grain tin till no more is dissolved. It may be obtained in crystals by evaporation. In re-dissolving them, it is necessary to add to the water a few drops of muriatic acid.

2. *Nitro-muriate, or Perchloride of Tin.* Mix 1 measure of nitric acid with 4 of muriatic acid, and add tin in small quantities as long as any is dissolved. Or mix 4 oz. of muriatic with 1 of nitric acid, and 1 of water; dissolve in it, by small portions at a time, 2 drachms of grain tin.

3. Aqua fortis (or equal parts of nitric acid and water) 8 parts, sal ammoniac 1 part; mix, and add gradually 1 part, or as much as it will dissolve, of grain tin.

4. Dr. BANCROFT'S *Murio-sulphate of Tin.* Digest 2 parts of tin with 3 of strong muriatic acid for an hour. Add very cautiously 1½ part of oil of vitriol. Keep up the heat as long as hydrogen is evolved: on cooling, it crystallizes. Dissolve this salt in water, so as to form a solution containing one part of tin in 8.

5. *New Tin Crystals.* Add 3 lb of sal ammoniac to a gallon of solution of tin; evaporate, and crystallize.

6. *Mordant for Lac Dye.* Mix 27 lb of muriatic acid with 1½ lb of nitric acid (sp. gr. 1·19,) put it into a stone bottle, and add tin in small bits till 4 lb are dissolved.

Lac Spirit, used as a *Solvent* for lac dye, in preference to muriatic acid alone, is thus made:—Add gradually 3 ℔ of tin to 60 ℔ of muriatic acid. Digest ¾ ℔ of this solvent on each pound of the dye for 6 hours. Plum or puce spirit, peach spirit, and grain or scarlet spirit, are names given by dyers to different solutions of tin employed in dyeing these colours. For scarlet, the nitro-muriatic solutions (Nos. 2 and 3, above) are used.

Iron Liquor. Scraps of iron are placed in casks or other vessels, and covered with rectified raw pyroligneous acid. There are usually a series of vessels, through which the solution is successively passed till it is fully saturated.

To produce good and permanent dyes, several successive processes are required, which cannot be described here. In domestic dyeing, for trifling articles, the dye and mordant are often boiled together, and the silk, &c. immersed in the liquid. The following are some examples:—*Crimson.*—Boil 1 oz. Brazil-wood with 1 dr. of alum and ½ dr. of cream of tartar in a quart of water. *Purple, or Lilac.*—Archil 1 oz. (or cudbear 1 oz.,) pearlash 1 dr., hot water a quart. *Rose, or Flesh-colour.*—Pink saucers, with a little lemon-juice will be found convenient. *Violet.*—Boil 4 oz. of logwood, with 1 oz. alum and ¼ oz. of tartar, in a quart of water. *Blue.*—Add to the water as much sulphate of indigo (chemic blue) as will give it the required colour. Or one of the other solutions of indigo (above) may be used. *Yellow.*—Boil 2 oz. of turmeric, or 4 oz. quercitron, or a drachm of saffron, with ½ oz. of alum, in a quart of water. *Green.*—Add to the yellow dye sufficient chemic blue to render it green. *Rose-red,* for silk.—Put your silk into a hot solution of alum and tartar; then into a hot decoction of madder. *Scarlet,* for silk.—Dye it yellow with saffron and alum; then put it into a decoction of cochineal and madder. *Black.*—Boil 1 oz. of logwood, ¼ oz. sumach, and 1 dr. of copperas, in 4 pints of water. *Buff.*—Boil 1 oz. of fustic, 1 dr. of alum, in 4 pints of water.]

EAU DE JAVELLE. See CHLORIDE OF POTASH.

EGGS, TO PRESERVE. JAYNE'S Liquid (expired patent) is thus made:—Take a bushel of lime, 2 ℔ of salt, ½ ℔ of cream of tartar, and water sufficient to form a solution strong enough to float an egg. In this liquid, it is stated, eggs may be preserved for two years.

ELAINE. See OLEINE.

ELECTRIC TISSUE. Steep linen or cotton in a mixture of strong sulphuric acid, and 3 of pure nitric acid, for an hour. Squeeze out the acid, wash with water until no sensible acidity remains, plunge it in a weak alkaline solution, then in water, and dry. By friction it yields a large quantity of resinous electricity.

ELECTROTYPE MOULDS. These are sometimes made with fusible metals; sometimes with non-metallic compounds, having their surface covered with a conducting substance. The *fusible metal* is composed of 8 parts of bismuth, 3 of tin, and 5 of lead. The French Clichée moulds consist of 8 parts of bismuth, 4 of tin, 5 of lead, and 1 of antimony. These are repeatedly melted together till perfectly mixed; and after being poured out on a suitable surface, are well stirred, and the medal forcibly pressed on the compound at the moment it is about to become solid. *Composition Moulds* are made with 8 oz. of spermaceti, 1¾ oz. of white wax, and the same of strained mutton suet. These are melted together, and a little fine plumbago or flake-white stirred in. To copy plaster casts, the cast is set in a plate of hot water, with its face above the water, till it has absorbed water; it is then surrounded with a ring of cardboard, and the melted composition poured on it. The composition mould requires to be brushed over with finely-powdered genuine black lead.

ELECTROTYPE MOULDS. *Elastic.* To 12 parts of carefully-melted glue, add 3 parts of treacle, and incorporate them perfectly. [For copying medals where the figures are in high relief.] *Gutta-Percha Moulds* are made by softening a piece of gutta percha by warm water (150° to 160°,) and pressing the medal into it by a screw. See SOLUTIONS.

ENGRAVINGS, PROCESS FOR CLEANING. Put the engraving on a smooth board, and cover it thinly with common salt, finely powdered; pour and squeeze lemon-juice upon this salt, so as to dissolve a considerable portion of it. Now elevate one end of the board, that it may form an angle of about 45° with the horizon. Pour lastly on the engraving boiling water from a tea-kettle, until the salt and lemon-juice be all washed off; the engraving will then appear perfectly clean, and free from stains. It must be dried gradually, on the same board, or on some smooth surface.—FRANCIS.

ENGRAVING MIXTURE, FOR WRITING ON STEEL. Sulphate of copper 1 oz., sal ammoniac ½ oz. Pulverize separately, adding a little vermilion to colour it, and mix with 1½ oz. of vinegar. Rub the steel with soft soap, and write with a clean hard pen, without a slit, dipped in the mixture.

ESSENCE OF JARGONELLE PEAR. Acetate of Amylene is sold under this name. It is made by distilling a mixture of one part of oil of grain, 2 of acetate of potash, and 1 of oil of vitriol. Wash the distilled liquid with alkaline water, agitate with dry chloride of calcium, and redistil it from litharge.

ESSENCE OF PINE APPLE. See BUTYRIC ETHER.

ESSENCE OF BUGS. Oxalate of Amylene has been so termed. It is made by heating oil of grain with excess of oxalic acid and distilling the oily liquid which separates at 500°.

[For PERFUMED ESSENCES, see PERFUMERY. For CULINARY ESSENCES, see page 295.]

ETCHING FLUIDS. *For Lithography.* Dissolve 3 oz. of fused chloride of calcium in 9½ oz. of water, add to the solution 2 oz. of gum Arabic, and 1 oz. of pure hydrochloric acid.—CHEVALLIER.

For Copper. 1. Aqua fortis 2 oz., water 5 oz.; mix.

2. Iodine 2 parts, iodide of potassium 5 parts, water 5 to 8 parts.

3. CALLOT'S *Eau Forte, for Fine Touches.* Dissolve 4 parts each of verdigris, alum, sea-salt, and sal ammoniac, in 8 parts of vinegar; add 16 parts of water, boil for a minute, and let it cool.

For Steel. 1. Iodine 1 oz., iron filings ½ drachm, water 4 ounces; digest till the iron is dissolved.

2. Pyroligneous acid 4 parts, by measure, alcohol 1 part; mix, and add 1 part of double aqua fortis (sp. gr. 1·28.) Apply it from 1½ to 15 minutes.

3. Mix 10 parts of pure hydrochloric acid, 70 of distilled water, and a solution of 2 parts of chlorate of potash in 20 of water. Dilute before using with from 100 to 200 parts of water.

See PHOTO-LITHOGRAPHY, and PHOTOGRAPHIC ETCHING ON STEEL.

ETCHING VARNISHES. 1. White wax 2 oz., asphaltum 2 oz.; melt the wax in a clean pipkin, add the asphaltum in powder, and boil to a proper consistence. Pour it into warm water, and form it into balls, which must be kneaded and put into taffeta for use.

2. White wax 2 oz., Burgundy pitch and black pitch each ½ oz.; melt together, and add by degrees 2 oz. of asphaltum in powder, and boil till a drop cooled on a plate becomes brittle.

3. Equal quantities of linseed oil and mastic, melted together.

FILTERING POWDER. Fullers' earth washed, dried, and coarsely powdered; mixed with prepared bone black (see CHARCOAL, ANIMAL) coarsely powdered.

FININGS, FOR GIN. Subcarbonate of potash 4 oz., roche alum 8 oz. Brewers' Finings consist of isinglass dissolved in stale beer.

FIRES, TO EXTINGUISH. DR. CLANNY'S *Solution* consists of 5 ounces of sal ammoniac to a gallon of water. The compound used in Phillips's Fire Annihilator is said to consist of dried prussiate of potash, sugar, and chlorate of potash.

FIRES, COLOURED. The ingredients for these compounds must be dry, not too finely powdered, and mixed very uniformly. The nitrate of strontian requires to be gently heated in an iron pan till it falls to powder. The chlorate of potash must be pulverized separately, and mixed very lightly with the other powders; the whole must then be passed through a sieve once or twice.

White Fires. 1. Nitre 30, sulphur 10, black antimony 5; mix.

2. Nitre 48, sulphur 13¼, black antimony 5 parts; mix.

3. Nitre 12, sulphur 16, black antimony 4, charcoal ¼, white arsenic ¼; mix.

4. Nitre 46½, sulphur 23, meal powder 12½, zinc filings 18.

5. For stars: Nitre 57, sulphur 28, zinc filings 15.

Blue and Purple Fires. 1. Chlorate of potash 9, dried verdigris 2, sulphur 1 oz.; mix.

2. Nitre 12, sulphur 16, black antimony 4, charcoal ¼ oz., orpiment ¼.

3. Chlorate of potash 9, sulphur 12, refiner's blue verditer 3 oz.; mix.

4. *Purple.* Chlorate of potash 5, nitrate of strontian 16, realgar 1, sulphur 2, lamp black 1; mix.

5. Nitre 5, sulphur 2, metallic antimony 1; mix.

6. *Purple.* Chlorate of potash 2 oz., sulphur 1 dr., oxide of copper 1 oz.; mix.

7. *Violet.* Chlorate of potash 1 dr., pure copper ½ dr., sulphur a scruple, charcoal 16 gr.; mix.

Yellow Fires. 1. Nitre 3 oz., meal powder 3 oz., flowers of sulphur 3 oz., dried salt 2 oz.; mix.

2. Nitrate of soda 6, sulphur 1, lamp black 1; mix.

Red Fires. 1. Chlorate of potash 10, nitrate of strontian 80, sulphur 26, charcoal 6; mix.

2. Chlorate of potash 3, nitrate of strontian 24, sulphur 7, lamp-black 1, sulphuret of antimony 2. [Half the lamp-black or charcoal only may be added at first; and if on trial it does not burn freely, add more.]

3. Chlorate of potash 1, nitrate of strontian 5, sulphur 1, black sulphuret of antimony 1; mix.

4. Chlorate of potash 2½, nitrate of strontian 20, sulphur 6½, sulphuret of antimony 2, charcoal ½; mix.

5. Chlorate of potash 5, nitrate of strontian 28, sulphur 13, sulphuret of antimony 4, lamp-black 1.

6. Chlorate of potash 35, nitrate of strontian 360, sulphur 93, sulphuret of antimony 60, charcoal 10.

7. Nitrate of strontian 72, sulphur 20, coal dust 2, gunpowder 6; mix.

8. 40 parts of nitrate of strontian, 13 of sulphur, 2 of lime-tree charcoal. Mix, and add by mixing with a horn spatula, 5 parts of dry and finely-powdered chlorate of potash.

Lilac Fire. Chlorate of potash 49, sulphur 25, dry chalk 20, black oxide of copper 6 parts. For pans.

Green Fires. 1. Sulphur $10\frac{1}{2}$, nitrate of barytes $62\frac{1}{2}$, chlorate of potash $23\frac{1}{2}$, sulphuret of arsenic $1\frac{3}{4}$, charcoal or lamp-black $1\frac{3}{4}$; mix.

2. Sulphur 13, nitrate of barytes 77, chlorate of potash 5, metallic arsenic 2, charcoal 3; mix.

3. Nitrate of barytes 20, sulphur $1\frac{1}{2}$, sulphuret of antimony $\frac{1}{2}$, chlorate of potash 10, charcoal $\frac{1}{4}$; mix.

4. Nitrate of barytes $10\frac{1}{2}$ dr., sulphur 2 dr., chlorate of potash 162 gr., lamp-black 26 gr.; mix.

5. Dry nitrate of barytes 12 parts, sulphur 4, dry and finely-powdered chlorate of potash 5 parts. The chlorate to be mixed by a horn spatula.

COLOURED FLAMES. The flame of alcohol may be coloured by mixing certain salts with the spirit. A green colour is given by muriate of copper, or boracic acid; red by nitrate of strontian, nitrate of iron, or nitrate of lime; yellow by nitrate of soda, &c.

FIRE-PROOFING. *For Paper*, see PAPER. For dresses, &c. A strong solution of sulphate of ammonia.

FLINTS, LIQUOR OF. Soluble glass. Mix 70 parts of pearlash, 54 of washing soda, and 152 of silicious sand, and fuse the mixture in a crucible. It is soluble in water, and the filtered solution evaporated to dryness leaves a transparent glass. It has been proposed to render wood, muslins, &c., incombustible by means of the solution. Dr. TURNER directs 3 parts of carbonate of potash, and 1 of silica. See SOLUBLE GLASS.

FLY POISON. A common poison for flies consists of white arsenic, or King's yellow, with sugar, &c., but the use of such compounds may lead to fatal accidents. A sweetened infusion of quassia answers the same purpose, and is free from danger. Pepper, with milk, is also used; and also some adhesive compounds by which they are fatally entangled.

FLOWERS, COMPOUND FOR PROMOTING THE BLOWING OF. Sulphate of ammonia 4 oz., nitre 2 oz., sugar 1 oz., hot water a pint. Keep it in a well-corked bottle. For hyacinth glasses add 8 or 10 drops of the liquid to the water, changing the water every 10 or 12 days. For flowering plants in pots, add a few drops to the water employed to moisten them.

FLUXES. In a general sense these are substances which promote the fusion of minerals, but particularly which cleanse a reduced metal, by assisting its separation from its impurities. They also serve to defend it from the action of the air, and some of them assist in the reduction of oxides.

Black Flux. Into an earthen crucible, heated sufficiently hot to cause feeble combustion, but not to fuse the flux, throw successive portions of a mixture of 1 part of nitre, and 2 of crude (or cream of) tartar. Keep the flux in a close bottle.

White Flux. Into a large earthen crucible, heated to redness, throw successive portions of a mixture of 2 parts of nitre and 1 of tartar. Keep it as the last.

Crude Flux, is the mixture of nitre and tartar, before deflagration.

Dr. CHRISTISON'S *Flux for reducing arsenic.* Mix crystallized carbonate of soda with $\frac{1}{8}$ of charcoal, and heat gradually to redness.

FRESENIUS'S *Flux,* for reducing sulphuret of arsenic. Dry carbonate of potash 3 parts, cyanide of potassium 1 part.

Cornish Flux. Cream of tartar 10 parts, nitre $3\frac{1}{2}$, borax 3.

MORVEAU'S *Flux.* Pulverized glass (free from lead) 8 parts, calcined borax $\frac{1}{2}$ part, charcoal $\frac{1}{2}$ part.

Mr. TAYLOR'S *Flux.* Saturate a solution of tartaric acid with carbonate of soda, evaporate to dryness, and calcine in a covered platinum crucible.

Sal enixum (the acid sulphate of potash left in distilling nitric acid,) sandiver or glass-gall, fluor spar, limestone, &c., are also used as Fluxes.

FREEZING MIXTURES. The salts should be in a crystallized state, with as much water in them as possible without being damp. They should be coarsely pulverized at the time of using, and put into the water contained in a basin or other suitable vessel. The water to be frozen should be enclosed in a thin vessel, and immersed in the freezing mixture. To obtain extreme degrees of cold, the ingredients and vessels employed should be previously cooled by one of the freezing mixtures.

1. Sal ammoniac 5 oz., nitre 5 oz., water 16 oz.

2. Mix 4 oz. of nitrate of ammonia, 4 of crystallized carbonate of soda, and 4 of water. In 3 hours 10 oz. of water may be frozen.

3. Nitrate of ammonia and muriate of ammonia in equal proportions, water q. s.

4. Nitrate of ammonia 5 parts, nitrate of potash 5, sulphate of soda 8, water 16 parts.

5. Phosphate of soda 9 parts, diluted nitric acid 4 parts.

6. Sulphate of soda 8 parts, muriatic acid 5 parts.

7. Sulphate of soda 6 parts, nitrate of ammonia 5 parts, diluted nitric acid 4 parts.

8. Mix 1 part by weight of powdered sal ammoniac, with 2 of powdered nitre. Reduce common washing soda to powder. Keep these powders in well-closed bottles, and when required for use, take equal measures of each, and add an equal bulk of water, or sufficient to dissolve the salts.

9. Muriate of ammonia 11 dr., nitre 10 dr., sulphate of soda 2 oz. Powder separately, and mix in a tin vessel with 5 oz. of water.

With Ice.

1. Snow or pounded ice 2 parts, muriate of soda 1 part.

2. Snow 2 parts, cryst. muriate of lime 3 parts.

3. Snow 8 parts, muriatic acid 5 parts.

4. Snow or pounded ice 12 parts, muriate of soda 5 parts, nitrate of ammonia 5.

5. Snow 7 parts, diluted nitric acid 4 parts.

6. Snow 3 parts, diluted sulphuric acid 2 parts.

French Polish. This is an alcoholic solution of shell-lac; some of the softer resinous gums are usually added, but too much of them renders the polish less durable. Highly rectified spirit, not less than 60 over proof, should be used. Rectified wood naphtha is sometimes substituted, to which the unpleasant smell is the only objection.

1. Orange shell-lac 22 oz., rectified spirit 4 pints; dissolve.

2. Shell-lac 3 oz., gum sandarac ½ oz., rectified spirit a pint.

3. Shell-lac 4 oz., gum thus ½ oz., rectified spirit a pint; dissolve, and add almond or poppy oil 2 oz.

4. Shell-lac 5 oz., seed-lac 1 oz., gum juniper ½ oz., mastic 1 oz., rectified spirit a pint.

5. Shell-lac 3 oz., seed-lac 3 oz., gum juniper 1½ oz., mastic 1 oz., rectified spirit a quart.

6. Shell-lac 5 oz., oxalic acid ½ oz., rectified spirit a pint; dissolve, and add linseed oil 4 oz.

7. Shell-lac 5 oz., gum benzoin 5 oz., oxalic acid 10 dr., rectified spirit a quart; dissolve, and add ½ pint of linseed oil.

8. Shell-lac 8 oz., gum elemi 1½ oz., rectified spirit 4 pints.

9. Shell-lac 10 oz., seed-lac 6 oz., gum thus 3 oz., sandarac 6 oz., copal varnish 6 oz., rectified naphtha 8 pints. Or dissolve 8 oz. each of seed-lac, gum thus, and sandarac, separately in a pint of naphtha; and 1 ℔ of shell-lac in 8 pints of naphtha. Then mix 6 oz. of copal varnish, 12 oz. of the solution of seed-lac, 6 oz. of the solution of frankincense, and 12 of the solution of sandarac, and 5¾ ℔ of the solution of shell-lac. Let the copal varnish be put into the tincture of shell-lac, and well shaken, and the other ingredients added. A correspondent informs me that this polish cannot be excelled.

10. Copal ¼ oz., gum Arabic ¼ oz., shell-lac 1 oz. Pulverize, mix, and sift the powders, and dissolve in a pint of spirit.

11. Shell-lac 5 oz., rectified naphtha a pint.

French polish is sometimes coloured with dragon's blood, turmeric root, &c. The general directions for preparing the polish are to put the gums with the spirit in a tin bottle, and set it on the hob, or in water, so as to keep it at a gentle heat, shaking it frequently. The cork should be loosened a little before shaking it, taking care that there is no flame near to kindle the vapour. When the gums are dissolved, let it settle for a few hours, and pour off the solution from the dregs. The method of using it is to have a roll of list, over the end of which five or six folds of linen rag are placed. The polish is applied to the linen with a sponge, and a little linseed oil is dropped on the centre of it.

FULMINATING COMPOUNDS. *Fulminating Powder.* Mix together in a warm mortar 3 parts of pulverized nitre, 2 of dry subcarbonate of potash, and 1 of sulphur. A small quantity heated on an iron shovel or ladle till it fuses, suddenly explodes with great violence. It should be used with great caution. Another kind of fulminating or detonating powder is made by mixing 3 gr. of chlorate of potash with 1 of sulphur; by strongly triturating it with strong pressure in a marble mortar, a succession of sharp explosions is produced. The same mixture, or 6 gr. of chlorate of potash, 1 of sulphur, and 4 of charcoal, struck with a hammer on an anvil, gives a loud report.

Chloride of nitrogen and *iodide of nitrogen* cannot be meddled with without extreme danger. *Fulminating gold*, and the *fulminating silver* prepared with ammonia, are also dangerous compounds, even in minute quantities. As they serve no practical use, the mode of preparing them is omitted.

Fulminating mercury (HOWARD'S, as improved by Dr. URE.) Dissolve by a gentle heat 1 oz. of quicksilver in 7½ fluid oz. (or 10 oz. by weight) of nitric acid, of 1·4 specific gravity, in a glass retort, the beak of which is loosely inserted into a large balloon, or bottle. When the mercury is dissolved, the solution, at the temperature of 130° Fahrenheit, should be slowly poured through a funnel into 10 fluid oz. of alcohol of ·830 specific gravity, contained in a vessel that will hold 6 times the quantity of ingredients. When the action ceases, pour the contents of the matrass on a double filter in a glass funnel; wash out any powder that may remain in the matrass with a little cold water, and throw this also on the filter; and wash the fulminate with more water till it passes free from acid. When sufficiently drained, lift the filter out of the funnel, and lay it open on a copper or earthen plate, and dry the fulminate at 212°, or under, by hot water or steam. Its manufacture requires great caution; some valuable lives have been sacrificed in its preparation.

Fulminating Silver (BRUGNATELLI'S.) On 100 gr. of pulverized nitrate of silver, in an open glass vessel, pour first an oz. of alcohol, and then as much strong nitrous acid. The mixture boils, and gives out ethereal vapours. When all the powdered nitrate has taken the form of white clouds, cold distilled water must be added to suspend ebullition, otherwise the fulminate will be dissolved. Collect the powder on a filter, and dry it at a low temperature. Dr. TURNER directs one part of silver to be dissolved in 10 of nitric acid, at a gentle heat, 20 parts of rectified spirit to be added, and the mixture warmed. When it begins to boil, set it aside to cool, collect and wash the crystals on a filter, and carefully dry them. This is more violent and dangerous than fulminating mercury.

FUMIGATIONS. See Fumigatio, Pocket Formulary, for their medicinal uses. Though not strictly belonging to this place, it may be useful to give a few directions for the management of these important agents, as disinfectants and purifiers.

Chlorine Fumigation. This is probably the most effective in destroying noxious effluvia and putrid odours, and in checking the spread of contagious diseases. But as the gas is itself deleterious, except in a very diluted state, it must be used with caution in occupied apartments. To disinfect rooms from which the occupants have been removed, mix common salt and black oxide of manganese in equal quantities. Mix also in an earthen basin equal weights of oil of vitriol and water, and when it has cooled, put it into a bottle for use. Into a China or earthen basin put from 1 to 3 oz. of the powder, according to the size of the room, and pour over it twice or thrice as much of the mixed acid. Place it in the apartment, and close the doors and windows for a few hours; the doors and windows are then thrown open till the smell of chlorine disappears. Dr. A. T. THOMSON directs a mixture of 1 oz. of salt and ½ oz. of oxide of manganese to be put into a China cup, and 6 fluid drachms of oil of vitriol poured on it, the cup being placed in a pipkin of hot sand. Instead of the above ingredients, some chloride of lime may be placed in a large jar or basin, and a mixture of acetic acid and water poured on it. When used in or near the apartments of the sick, great care must be taken that the chlorine is so diluted with air that it shall occasion no annoyance to the invalid. Some contrivances have been adopted to render the extrication of chlorine gradual and continued. SMITH'S Chlorine Fumigator, and the more simple one of Messrs. HEATHFIELD & BURGESS, are very convenient. Another method is proposed by Mr. SCANLAN, in the Pharmaceutical Journal, vol. vii. page 343. By such contrivances, chlorine may with care be safely employed in houses occupied by the sick (in the passages, stairs, &c.) to prevent the spread of infectious fevers; but chloride of lime, simply mixed with water, in the proportion of not more than an oz. to a quart, is usually sufficient to purify the chamber of the sick. It should be occasionally sprinkled on the floor, and also placed about the room in shallow dishes, or a linen cloth moistened with it, suspended on a line. The same method may be pursued in all places where unpleasant smells prevail.

Nitric Fumigation. Put into a China cup equal measures of sulphuric acid and water, and add to it, from time to time, small quantities of powdered nitre; or put 2 or 3 drachms of powdered nitre into a cup, and pour over it about an equal quantity of oil of vitriol. Stir it with a piece of glass, or tobacco pipe, and remove it from time to time to different parts of the apartment. For large rooms, 2 or 3 cups may be required. It is often recommended to apply heat; but Dr. BATEMAN, of the Fever Hospital, found this unnecessary and objectionable, especially in the apartments of the sick. No metallic or wooden stirrers, or vessels, must be used.

Muriatic Fumigation. This is now almost disused, being less efficacious than the preceding. It is obtained by putting a few drachms of common salt into a cup, and pouring on it an equal quantity of oil of vitriol. The vapours are very injurious to the lungs.

Acetic Fumigation. The vapour of vinegar, and especially of strong acetic acid, is employed as a disinfectant, but its efficacy is now considered to be very limited. It may be used by keeping the vinegar boiling over a lamp. A coarser method sometimes used is to plunge a red-hot poker into a cup of vinegar. Aromatic vinegar, merely held to the nose, may afford some slight protection to those who attend upon the sick.

Sulphur Fumigation. The fumes of burning sulphur may possibly have some effect in decomposing miasmata and noxious effluvia; but as they have no advantage over chlorine, and are very disagreeable, and otherwise objectionable, they are not likely to be employed. Formerly the following powder was burnt to destroy contagious miasmata. Flowers of sulphur, nitre, and powdered myrrh, of each 1 oz.

Tar Fumigation. The vapour of boiling tar has been used as a disinfectant, as well as a palliative in some affections of the respiratory organs. The usual plan is to keep the tar boiling over a lamp. See Fumigatio Picea, Pocket Formulary.

Benzoin, styrax, and other odoriferous gums, cascarilla bark, coffee berries, and the compounds termed aromatic pastiles, are burnt as purifiers and disinfectants. But little confidence is now placed in them as prophylactics against infection. The same may be said of camphor and tobacco. They should not be depended on to the exclusion of more efficient means, nor be made a substitute for free ventilation, and the removal of all sources of noxious effluvia, when practicable.

FUMIGATING PASTILES. See PERFUMERY.

FURNITURE CREAM. 1. Soft water a gallon, soap 4 oz., bees'-wax in shavings 1 ℔; boil together, and add 2 oz. of pearlash. To be diluted with water, laid on with a paint brush, and polished off with a hard brush or cloth.

2. Wax 3 oz., pearlash 2 oz., water 6 oz.; heat them together, and add 4 oz. of boiled oil, and 5 oz. spirit of turpentine.

3. The same is sometimes given to a mixture of 1 oz. of white or yellow wax, with 4 of oil of turpentine.

FURNITURE PASTE. 1. Melt 1 ℔ of bees'-wax with ¼ pint of linseed oil, and add ½ oz. of alkanet root; keep it at a moderate heat till sufficiently coloured; then remove from the fire, add ¼ pint of oil of turpentine, strain through muslin, and put it into small gallipots to cool.

2. Scrape 4 oz. of wax, and put it into a pipkin with

as much oil of turpentine as will cover it, and ¼ oz. of powdered resin; melt with a gentle heat, and stir in sufficient Indian red to colour it.

3. Equal weights of bees'-wax, spirit of turpentine, and linseed oil.

FURNITURE OIL. 1. Linseed oil a pint, alkanet ½ oz.; digest in a warm place till coloured, and strain.

2. The same with ¼ pint of oil of turpentine.

3. Linseed oil a pint, alkanet root 1 oz., rose pink 1 oz.; let them stand in an earthen vessel all night.

4. A quart of linseed oil, 6 oz. of distilled vinegar, 3 oz. of spirit of turpentine, 1 oz. of muriatic acid, and 2 oz. spirit of wine.

5. Linseed oil 8 oz., vinegar 4 oz., oil of turpentine, mucilage, rectified spirit, each ½ oz.; butter of antimony ¼ oz.; muriatic acid 1 oz.; mix.

6. Linseed oil 16 oz., black rosin 4 oz., vinegar 4 oz., rectified spirit 3 oz., butter of antimony 1 oz., spirit of salts 2 oz.; melt the rosin, add the oil, take it off the fire, and stir in the vinegar; let it boil for a few minutes, stirring it; when cool put it into a bottle, add the other ingredients, shaking altogether. [The last two are especially used for reviving French polish.]

7. Linseed oil a pint, oil of turpentine ½ pint, rectified spirit 4 oz., powdered rosin 1½ oz., rose pink ½ oz.; mix.

8. Linseed oil 14 oz., vinegar 1½ oz., muriatic acid ½ oz.; mix.

FUSIBLE METAL. See ALLOYS.

GALL, CLARIFIED. Ox-gall is prepared for the use of artists in the following manner:—To a pint of fresh ox-gall, boiled and skimmed, add 1 oz. finely-powdered alum; leave it on the fire till the alum is dissolved, then let it cool, put it into a bottle, and cork it loosely. Treat another pint in the same way with 1 oz. of salt instead of alum. After standing more than 3 months, carefully decant from each bottle the clear portion, and mix them together. The colouring matter is precipitated, and a clear colourless liquid is obtained by filtration. It is used for mixing artists' colour, and to prepare ivory, oiled paper, &c., to receive the colours. Also for taking out grease spots.

GALVANIC BATTERIES, SOLUTIONS FOR. See page 311.

GANNAL'S SOLUTION. See page 315.

GANTEINE. (A composition for cleaning kid gloves; sometimes improperly termed *Saponine.*) Dissolve 3 oz. of soap by heat in 2 oz. of water, and when nearly cold add 2 oz. of eau de Javelle, and 1 dr. of water of ammonia; form a paste, which is to be rubbed over the glove with flannel till sufficiently clean.

GARANCINE. Madder (sometimes the spent madder of the dyer's bath) is mixed with its weight of oil of vitriol, added very gradually, so as to avoid overheating. The acid is then washed out.

GARROT'S COVERING FOR PILLS. Soak 1 oz. of purified gelatine in 2 or 3 dr. of water; keep it liquefied in a salt-water bath. The pills are stuck on long pins, and dipped in the solution; when cold the pins are withdrawn, after being heated by a small flame, which melts the gelatine and closes the hole.

GASES. These are generated in gas bottles fitted, by grinding, with an S-formed tube; or in flasks to which a bent tube is adapted by means of a cork; in a common retort; or sometimes in iron bottles with a metal tube. They are usually collected in vessels filled with water placed with their open end in a vessel of water. *Pepy's Gas Holder* is very useful for receiving, retaining, and transferring gases. The *pneumatic trough* consists of a vessel for holding water with a shelf for sustaining the jars or bottles that are to be filled; these are filled by sinking them under water, and are then lifted on the shelf, above which the water rises, with their open end downwards. The beak of the retort, or bent tubes, are so placed that the gas issuing from them rises through the water into the vessel; and takes the place of the water in them. Some gases being very easily absorbed by water, are collected over mercury. Sometimes they are collected in dry bottles. For light gases, as ammonia, place a bottle in a vertical position with its mouth downward over the tube from which the gas issues, which should touch the bottom of the bottle. When the bottle is filled with gas, and this escapes from the mouth, quietly withdraw the tube and close the bottle, still inverted, with a greased stopper. For gases heavier than air, as chlorine, or carbonic acid, the bottle must be placed with its mouth uppermost, and the tube delivering the gas must descend to the bottom of the bottle. When full of the gas, close it with the greased stopper. The tube connected with a flask in which a gas is generated should have a ball blown in it, into which asbestos may be introduced to arrest any particles thrown up by effervescence.

The following are the processes for procuring the principal gases:—

Ammoniacal Gas. This is obtained by mixing equal weights of slaked lime (previously cooled) and powdered sal ammoniac, and heating the mixture in a retort or flask. As water rapidly absorbs the gas, it must be collected over mercury, or in a dry bottle as described above.

Carbonic Acid Gas. This is obtained by acting on marble or chalk, or carbonate of soda or potash, by a diluted acid. For exact experiments it must be collected over mercury; otherwise it may be collected in a bottle (as above.) Mr. BENSON states that a saturated solution of sulphate of magnesia may be used in collecting this gas, instead of mercury.

Carbonic Oxide is obtained by acting on binoxalate of potash with 6 times its weight of oil of vitriol at a gentle heat: or by strongly heating, in an iron bottle or gun barrel, equal weights of chalk and iron filings. The gas must be passed through water containing lime or caustic potash to absorb the carbonic acid gas.

Chlorine. This gas may be obtained from oxide of manganese, common salt, and sulphuric acid, as directed in making chloride of lime (p. 333.) Or from muriatic acid and oxide of manganese (see Chlorinium, Pocket Formulary.) But more conveniently, on the small scale, by dissolving common salt in water, adding a sixth of its weight of nitric acid, and as much oxide of manganese. Apply a gentle heat, and the gas is abundantly produced without violent action. (Chemist, vol. i.)

Hydrochloric Acid Gas. It may be obtained by heating

together in a flask equal weights of salt and oil of vitriol; or simply by heating strong muriatic acid. It must be collected over mercury; or otherwise conducted to the bottom of a dry bottle, as described above.

Hydrogen Gas is readily procured by pouring on fragments of zinc, in a glass bottle, or flask with a bent tube, or retort, some diluted sulphuric acid (1 measure of strong acid to 5 of water.) It may be collected over water. If zinc be not at hand, fine iron wire, or the turnings or filings of iron, may be substituted for it. To procure gas of great purity, distilled zinc must be used.

Carburetted Hydrogen Gas. Light carburetted hydrogen is readily obtained by stirring the mud of stagnant pools. Heavy carburetted hydrogen is prepared by heating 1 part of alcohol with 6 or 7 of oil of vitriol, and conducting the mixed masses through milk of lime, which retains the sulphurous acid; and afterwards through oil of vitriol, which absorbs water, ether, and alcohol. Coal gas is a mixture of these gases, with other hydrocarbons, &c.

Phosphuretted Hydrogen. The spontaneously inflammable variety of this gas is made by boiling phosphorus with solution of potash in a small retort, the beak of which is kept under water: as each bubble of gas rises from the water, it inflames, and forms a ring of white smoke, which dilates as it ascends. The spontaneous inflammability of the gas when mixed with atmospheric air or oxygen, renders caution necessary in its preparation. The other varieties of phosphuretted hydrogen have no special interest or application.

Sulphuretted Hydrogen. Mix together 2 parts of iron filings, with 1 of sulphur, into a thin pap with water, and heat it gently in an iron vessel. Combination takes place with the evolution of heat. Cover it till cold. On this compound, contained in a gas bottle, or other suitable apparatus, pour sulphuric acid previously diluted with 7 parts of water. If more acid be afterwards required, dilute the strong acid with only 4 of water. It is absorbed by water.

Nitrogen, or Azote. Atmospheric air may be made to yield an unlimited supply of nitrogen, by exposing it to the action of substances which combine with its oxygen. By burning phosphorus in a large bell glass standing in water, and allowing it to stand over the water a few hours, nearly pure nitrogen is obtained, and may be further purified by agitating it with solution of pure potash. CORENWINDER procures it from his solution of nitrate of potash (which see) by mixing one measure of it with three of concentrated solution of sal ammoniac, and heating the mixture in a flask. The gas contains a little ammonia, from which it may be freed by passing it through diluted sulphuric acid.

Protoxide of Nitrogen. Nitrous Oxide of DAVY. It is most conveniently made by heating nitrate of ammonia (formed by neutralizing pure nitric acid, diluted with 3 parts of water, with carbonate of ammonia, and boiling the solution till a drop let fall on a cold plate solidifies, adding a little ammonia towards the end, to ensure neutrality) in a retort, at a heat not exceeding 500° Fahrenheit, till it is nearly all decomposed. It may be collected over warm water.

Oxygen Gas. Mix chlorate of potash with a third of its bulk of black oxide of manganese; put the mixture into a gas-bottle, or clean flask, to which a bent tube is fitted by a cork, and apply a gentle heat. The gas, which comes over freely, may be collected over water.

Ozone Gas. This is supposed to be oxygen in an allotropic and more active state. It is formed by putting into a wide bottle pieces of clean phosphorus with a little water, so that the phosphorus shall be partly in the water and partly uncovered. Close the bottle for some hours, when the air it contains will manifest the odour and effects of ozone.

Sulphurous Acid Gas. It is procured in a nearly pure state by heating 2 parts of quicksilver with 3 of oil of vitriol, and collecting the gas over mercury. By passing the gas through a tube surrounded with a freezing mixture, it is condensed into a liquid. For ordinary purposes, the gas may be obtained as directed under ACID, SULPHUROUS.

GELATINE, PURIFIED. *Grenetine.* It is made by various processes from gelatinous animal matters. NELSON'S

Patent Gelatine is made from cuttings of the hides of beasts, and skins of calves. These, freed from hair, flesh, fat, &c., are washed and scored, then macerated for 10 days in a ley of caustic soda, and afterwards placed in covered vessels at a temperature of 60° to 70° until they become tender: then washed from the alkali, exposed to the vapour of burning sulphur until they become sensibly acid, dissolved in earthen vessels heated to 150°, strained, put into settling vessels heated to 100° or 120° for nine hours, the clear liquor drawn off, and poured on the cooling slabs to the depth of ½ an inch. When cold, the jelly is cut in pieces, washed till free from acid, redissolved at 85°, poured on slabs, cut up, and dried on nets.

Bone Gelatine. The bones are boiled to remove the fat, then digested in diluted muriatic acid till the earthy matter of the bone is dissolved. The gelatine, which retains the form of the bone, is washed in a stream of water, plunged in hot water, and again in cold, to remove all remains of acid, and sometimes put into a solution of carbonate of soda. When well washed, it is dried on open baskets or nets. By steeping the raw gelatine in cold water, dissolving it in boiling water, evaporating the jelly, and cutting it into tablets, it may be dried and preserved in that form.

GERMAN PASTE, for feeding insectivorous singing birds. Blanched sweet almonds, 1 ℔, pea meal 2 ℔, butter 3 oz., saffron a few grains, honey q. s. Form the whole into a paste, and granulate it by pressing it through a colander. Some add the yolks of 2 eggs.

GILDING. Leaf gold is affixed to various surfaces, properly prepared by gold size, or other adhesive medium. Metallic surfaces are coated with gold by means of amalgam of gold and mercury, applied with a wire brush, wet with an acid solution of mercury, made by dissolving 10 parts of mercury in 11 of nitric acid, by a gentle heat, and adding 2½ parts of water. The article thus coated is heated over charcoal till the mercury is dissipated, and afterwards burnished. To give it a redder colour, it is covered with gilders' wax, (a compound of verdigris, ochre, alum, and yellow wax;) again exposed to heat, and afterwards washed and cleaned by a scratch brush and vinegar. An inferior kind of gilding is effected by dissolving gold, with a fifth of its weight of copper, in ultromuriatic acid, dipping rags in the solution, drying and burning them, and rubbing the ashes on the metallic surface with a cork dipped in salt and water.

GILDING, by immersion. Dissolve teroxide or terchloride of gold in a solution of pyrophosphate of soda, and dip the article to be gilt in it.

Electro-Gilding, by Elkington's patent process, is thus performed:—A solution of 5 oz. of gold (see ACID, NITRO-MURIATIC, p. 308) is prepared, and boiled till it ceases to give out yellow vapours: the clear solution is mixed with 4 gallons of water, 20 ℔ of bicarbonate of potash added, and the whole boiled for 2 hours. The articles, properly cleaned, are suspended on wires, and moved about in the liquid from a few seconds to a minute, then washed, dried, and coloured in the usual way.

The solution used in gilding with the voltaic apparatus is made by dissolving ¼ oz. of oxide of gold, with 2 oz. of cyanide of potassium, in a pint of distilled water.

GINGER BEER. See BEVERAGES.

GINGER BREAD, PURGATIVE. See page 187.

GLASS OF BORAX. Calcine borax with a strong heat till the water of crystallization is expelled, and the salt fuses into a clear glass.

GLASS, SOLUBLE. Mix 10 parts of carbonate of potash, 15 of quartz (or of sand free from iron and alumina,) and 1 part of charcoal. Fuse together. The mass is soluble in 4 or 5 parts of water; and the filtered solution evaporated to dryness yields a transparent glass, permanent in the air.—FUCHS.

GLASS. The different kinds of common glass consist essentially of silica with soda or potash; most of the white kinds also contain oxide of lead. Crown glass and green bottle glass contain a portion of lime. Green glass and some kinds of foreign white glass, are free from lead, and should therefore be selected for chemical uses.

To mark on Glass. Glass may be written on, for temporary purposes by French chalk; pencils of this substance will be found convenient. Glass may be written on with ink if the surface is clean and dry, and the pen held nearly perpendicular. The shell-lac ink (see INK) is the best for labels, as it resists damp, &c. *To scratch glass*, a scratching diamond is used; or a piece of flint, or crystal of quartz, or the point of a small 3 square file. *To engrave on glass*, fluoric acid is used, either in the liquid state, or in vapour. The glass must be warmed, and coated with wax, or engravers' cement, and the writing or design traced through the wax with a bradawl, or other pointed instrument. The liquid fluoric acid is poured on it, and left to act on the uncovered portions of the glass; or the fluor spar may be powdered and made into a paste with oil of vitriol, and laid over the prepared surface, and covered with lead foil or tea-lead: or bruised fluor spar is put in a Wedgewood evaporating basin, with sufficient oil of vitriol to form a thin paste, and the prepared glass laid over the basin, so that the vapours may act on the portions from which the wax has been removed. *To cut glass* (beside the usual method of dividing cut glass by a glazier's diamond,) the following means may be used:—To divide glass tubes or rods, form a deep mark round them with the edge of a sharp 3-square file, then with a hand placed on either side of the mark, break the rod with a slightly stretching as well as bending motion. A diamond or sharp flint may be substituted for a file. Flasks, globes, and retorts, may be divided by means of iron rings, having a stem fixed in a wooden handle. Make the ring red-hot, and apply it to the flask, &c. If the vessel does not break where it came in contact with the ring, wet the part, and it will generally separate. Another method is to twist together 2 or 3 threads of cotton, such as is used for wicks, moisten them with spirit of wine, and encircle the flask with them; then, holding the flask horizontally, set fire to the wick, and turn the flask with the fingers, so as to keep the flame in the direction of the thread. If the separation does not take place the first time, the process may be repeated after the glass has cooled. By these means a common oil flask may be divided into an evaporating dish and a funnel. By means of a stout iron rod, fixed in a wooden handle, and terminating in a blunt point, and heated to redness, broken retorts, globes, and flasks may be converted into useful evaporating dishes, &c. If any crack exists, it may easily be led in any direction, as it will follow the motion of the heated iron. If no crack exists, one must be produced by applying the point of the heated rod to any convenient spot on the edge of the broken glass, touching it afterwards with a moistened finger, if necessary. The edges of glass thus divided are rendered less apt to break by heating them in the flame of a blow-pipe, or grinding them smooth with emery on a flat stone. See FARADAY'S Manipulations.

Glass, to Silver. The term *silvering* is applied to the process of coating the surface of glass with amalgamated tinfoil, in forming mirrors. The tinfoil is rubbed over with quicksilver, and more of the latter poured over it: the plate of glass, perfectly clean and dry, is then applied to it in such a way as to exclude all air bubbles, and to bring the glass and foil into perfect contact. The plate, after being inclined so as to allow the superfluous quicksilver to drain off, is loaded with weights, under which it remains till the adhesion is complete. To convex and concave mirrors the amalgamated foil is applied by means of accurately-fitting plaster moulds. The interior of globes is silvered by introducing a liquid amalgam (see AMALGAM, p. 313,) and turning about the globe till every part is covered with it. But a method of literally silvering glass has lately been patented by Mr. DRAYTON. He mixes 1 oz. of nitrate of silver, 3 oz. of water, 1 oz. of liquid ammonia, and 3 oz. of spirit of wine, and filters the solution after it has stood 3 or 4 hours. To every ounce of the solution he adds ¼ oz. of sugar (*grape* sugar, if possible,) dissolved in equal quantities of water and alcohol. The surface to be silvered is covered with this liquid, and a temperature of 160° F. maintained till the deposition of silver is complete. When quite dry, the coated surface is covered with mastic varnish. Other substances besides sugar occasion the deposition of silver from the ammoniacal solution; as oil of cassia, oil of cloves, and other essential oils, aldehyde, &c.; but M. VOHL prefers an alkaline solution of gun-cotton. Dissolve gun-cotton in a solution of caustic potash, pour it into a solution of nitrate of silver, and add ammonia sufficient to redissolve the precipitate. The liquor being slowly heated in a water-bath becomes brown, effervesces, and deposits silver of superior brilliancy.

GLAZES. Common earthenware is glazed with a composition containing lead, on which account it is unfit for many pharmaceutical purposes. The following glaze has been proposed, among others, as a substitute:—100 parts of washed sand, 80 of purified potash, 10 of nitre, and 20 of slaked lime; all well mixed, and heated in a black-lead crucible, in a reverberatory furnace, till the mass flows into a clear glass. It is then to be reduced to powder. The goods to be slightly burnt, placed under water, and sprinkled with the powder.

GLAZE FOR PORCELAIN. Feldspar 27 parts, borax 18, Lynn sand 4, nitre 3, soda 3, Cornwall China clay 3 parts. Melt together to form a frit, and reduce it to a powder, with 3 parts of calcined borax.—ROSE.

GLUE is made by boiling parings of ox-hides and other skins in water, evaporating the solution to a due consistence, allowing it to gelatinize in wooden boxes, cutting it into layers with a wire, and drying them on nets stretched on wooden frames. *Bones* also yield a pale glue, described under GELATINE. Bank-note glue, or mouth glue, is made by dissolving 1 ℔ of fine glue, or gelatine, in water, evaporating it till most of the water is expelled, adding ½ ℔ of brown sugar, and pouring it into moulds. Some add a little lemon juice. It is also made with 2 parts of dextrine, 2 of water, and 1 of spirit.

GLUE LIQUID. 1. Dissolve bruised orange shell-lac in ¾ of its weight of rectified spirit, or of rectified wood naphtha, by a gentle heat. It is very useful as a general cement and substitute for glue. 2. Another kind may be made by dissolving 1 oz. of borax in 12 oz. of soft water, adding 2 oz. of bruised shell-lac, and boiling till dissolved, stirring it constantly. 3. Dissolve 1000 parts of glue in 1000 parts by weight of water in a glazed pot, over a gentle fire. When it is melted, add nitric acid (sp. gr. 1·32) 200 parts, pouring it in very gradually. An effervescence is caused by the escape of hyponitrous acid. When all the acid is added, allow the mixture to cool. (This glue is found to remain unaltered on exposure to the air. It is applied cold, and is recommended as very convenient in chemical operations.)—M. DUMOULIN.

GLUE, MARINE. Cut caoutchouc into small pieces, and dissolve it, by heat and agitation, in coal naphtha. Add to this solution powdered shell-lac, and heat the whole with constant stirring, until combination takes place, then pour it while hot on metal plates, to form sheets. When used it must be heated to 248° F., and applied with a brush.

GLUTEN, VEGETABLE. Form wheat flour into a stiff paste with cold water; then knead it under a stream of water till all the starch is washed away. What remains is impure gluten.

GOLDEN COMPOUND. Anhydrous tungstate of soda, or the salt obtained by fusing 2 equivalents of tungstic acid with 1 of carbonate of soda, is to be melted in a porcelain crucible, over a spirit lamp, at a temperature not more than sufficient: then add small pieces of pure tin to the melted mass. Cubes of a golden colour instantly form. The process should not be continued too long, or they acquire a purple hue. (See AURUM MUSIVUM.)

GUM, BRITISH. (See DEXTRINE.) It is also prepared by heating starch alone, or previously mixed with an acid. PINEL directs half a gallon of nitric and half a pint of muriatic acid to be mixed with 100 gallons of water, and as much potato fecula added as will form a paste. In 2 hours remove the paste in buckets, prepared for the purpose, to drain off all the water. Then place the paste in small lumps in a drying room till dry; pulverize it, and expose the powder the first day to the temperature of 100°, the next day raise it to 150°, on the third day to 190°. It is then powdered, sifted, and heated from 300° to 350°. To give it the appearance of gum, after it has gone through the stove, and it is powdered and sifted, mix it to a paste with water to which 1 per cent. of nitric acid has been added, spread it on copper plates in layers ¾ of an inch thick, and heat it in an oven from 240° to 300°, then remove it to the open air to cool.

GUM ARABIC, PURIFICATION OF. PICCIOTTO'S process. The gum is dissolved in water, and sulphurous acid gas passed into it. The sulphurous acid is sufficiently removed for common purposes by gently boiling the mucilage in a retort with a receiver attached. But to obtain the gum in a purer state, carbonate of barytes is added, the mixture is filtered, afterwards agitated with gelatinous alumina, again filtered, and evaporated.

GUN BARRELS, TO STAIN. (See BROWNING LIQUIDS, page 325.)

GUN COTTON. Mix 1½ fluid oz. of each of the strongest nitric and sulphuric acids; put the mixture in a Wedgewood mortar, and when cool, add 100 gr. of cotton wool. Stir it with a glass rod, and when it is fully soaked, squeeze out the acid with the pestle or a porcelain spoon, throw the cotton into a large quantity of water, squeeze it again, and wash it under a stream of water till quite free from acid. In the specification, the patentee directs 1 measure of nitric acid, sp. gr. 1·45 or 1·50, to be mixed with 3 measures of sulphuric acid, sp. gr. 1·85; the cotton to be soaked in the acid, then squeezed from it, and left in a covered vessel for an hour; and after washing, to be dipped in a solution of 1 oz. carbonate of potash in a gallon of water, then pressed, and partially dried; again dipped in a weak solution of nitre, then dried in a room heated to 150°. This destructive compound has already fallen into disuse as to the purposes for which it was introduced; but seems likely to be usefully applied to other objects. See COLLODION.

GUN POWDER. A compound of nitre, charcoal, and sulphur. The nitre should be purified by recrystallization, the sulphur by distillation, and the charcoal selected of the best quality; that of the dog wood, alder, poplar, chestnut, or willow, is preferred. The following is the composition of some of the most approved kinds:—

	Nitre.	Charcoal.	Sulphur.
Royal Mills, Waltham Abbey	75	15	10
Marsh's Sporting	76	15	9
——— Mining	65	15	20
French (Government). . .	75	12·5	12·5
——— Sporting	78	12	10
Chinese	75	14·4	9·9

GUN POWDER, WHITE. Well-dried ferro-prussiate of potash 1 part, white sugar 1 part, chlorate of potash 2 parts. Let the ingredients be separately reduced to a fine powder, and the powders mixed by the hand, or by means of a leathern barrel turning on its axis. Or they may be moistened with water, and granulated by passing the paste through a wire sieve.

GYPSUM, TO HARDEN. KEATING'S patent process is to moisten calcined gypsum with a solution of 1 ℔ of borax, 1 ℔ of tartar, in 11 ℔ of water; it is then heated to redness for 6 hours, and pulverized. ERDEMANN recommends plaster figures, &c., to be soaked in a solution of FUCHS'S soluble glass.

HAHNEMANN'S WINE TEST. See TESTS.

HARNESS JET. Take 4 oz. best glue, 1½ pint good vinegar, 2 oz. best gum Arabic, ½ pint good black ink, 2 dr. best isinglass. Dissolve the gum in the ink, and melt the isinglass in another vessel in as much hot water as will cover it. Having first steeped the glue in the vinegar until soft, dissolve it completely by the aid of heat, stirring to prevent burning. The heat should not exceed 180°. Add the ink and gum, and allow the mixture again to rise to the same temperature. Lastly, mix in the solution of isinglass, and remove from the fire. When used, a small portion must be heated until fluid, and then applied with a sponge, and allowed to dry on.

HARNESS, WATERPROOF PASTE FOR. Put into a pipkin black rosin 2 oz., place on a gentle fire, and when melted add bees'-wax 3 oz. When this is melted, remove from the fire, and stir in ½ oz. fine lamp black, and ½ dr. Prussian blue finely powdered. When completely mixed, add spirits of turpentine to form a thin paste, and let it cool. To be applied like blacking.

HEADING FOR BEER. Equal parts of alum and sulphate of iron.—GRAY.

INCENSE. Olibanum 2 parts, benzoin 1 part.

INDIA RUBBER COURT PLASTER. A stout frame of wood must be made, about 3 yards long and about $1\frac{1}{4}$ yard wide. Within this frame must be placed two sides of another frame, running longitudinally and across, so fixed in the outer frame that the two pieces may slide independently of each other backwards and forwards about 6 inches. Tapes of canvass must be tacked round the inside of the inner frame and the corresponding sides of the outer frame, so as to form a square for the material to be sewn in, which when done, the two loop frames must be drawn tightly to the outer by means of a twine passed round each, in order to stretch perfectly free from irregularities the silk or satin previous to laying on the composition.

To make the Plaster. Dissolve India rubber in naphtha or naphtha and turpentine, lay it on with a flat brush on the opposite side to that which is intended for the plaster. When the silk is perfectly dry, and the smell in a great measure dissipated, it will be ready for the adhesive material; to make which, take equal parts of Salisbury or fine Russian glue and the best isinglass, dissolve in a sufficient quantity of water over a water-bath, and lay on with a flat hogtool while warm. It is requisite to use great caution to spread the plaster evenly and in one direction, and a sufficient number of coatings must be given to form a smooth surface, through which the texture of the fabric is not perceptible. Each coating should be perfectly dry before the succeeding one is given, after which the frame is to be placed in a situation free from dust, and where a draught of air would facilitate the drying. The quantity of water used and the weight of the two materials must be a little varied according to the season and the gelatine strength they possess. Lastly, the plaster being ready to receive the polishing coat, which gives also the balsamic effect to it, a preparation is made in nearly the same manner as the Tinct. Benz. Co. of the P. L., with the addition of more gums. This preparation must be laid on once only, and with a brush kept for the purpose. For making plasters on coloured silk it is only necessary to select the silk a shade deeper than the colour required, as the plaster causes it to appear a little lighter.

INDIGO. The principal preparations of indigo are described under CHEMIC BLUE, and DYES. Indigo may be purified by several methods, of which the following is the most simple:—Mix indigo with half its weight of Paris plaster and sufficient water to form a thin paste. Spread this evenly on an iron plate, about 2 inches wide, to the depth of one-eighth of an inch, and let it dry in the air. Then apply the flame of a large spirit lamp to the under side of the plate, beginning at one end and advancing it to the other as the sublimation proceeds. The violet vapour condenses on the surface in brilliant prisms or plates. Good indigo yields from 15 to 17 per cent.—Mr. T. TAYLOR.

Purified indigo is also obtained from the alkaline solution of reduced indigo, described under DYES; or by dissolving indigo in a mixture of 1 part of caustic soda, 1 of grape sugar, and 20 of water. To the clear solutions thus obtained add muriatic acid to throw down the indigo, wash this perfectly with pure water, and finally with alcohol. If care be taken to exclude the air before and after adding the acid, and to wash it with recently boiled water, to drain it rapidly and dry it *in vacuo*, the indigo is obtained nearly white, but becomes blue on exposure to the air.

INKS. The following are specimens of the most useful kinds:—

Black Writing Inks. 1. BRANDE'S. Bruised Aleppo galls 6 oz., soft water 6 pints; boil together, add 4 oz. of sulphate of iron, and 4 oz. of gum Arabic. Put the whole in a bottle, and keep it in a warm place, shaking it occasionally. In 2 months pour it off into glass bottles; and add to each pint a grain of corrosive sublimate, or 3 or 4 drops of creasote.

2. Dr. WOLLASTON'S. Galls 1 oz., gum ½ oz., cloves ½ dr., sulphate of iron ½ oz., water 8 oz. Digest, with frequent shaking, till it has sufficient colour. A good durable ink, and will bear diluting.

3. *Prerogative Court Ink.* Galls 16 oz., gum 6 oz., alum 2 oz., sulphate of iron 7 oz., kino 3 oz., logwood in powder 4 oz., water 8 ℔.—GRAY.

4. Dr. URE'S *Ink.* For 12 gallons of ink take 12 ℔ of bruised galls, 5 ℔ of gum Senegal, 5 ℔ of green sulphate of iron, and 12 gallons of rain water. Boil the galls in a copper with 9 gallons of water for 3 hours, adding fresh water to replace what is lost by evaporation. Let the decoction settle, and draw off the clear liquor: add to it a strained solution of the gum; dissolve also the sulphate of iron separately, and mix the whole. Instead of boiling the galls, they may be macerated in a portion of hot water for 12 hours, then put into a percolator, and the rest of the water passed through it.

5. *Anti-corrosive Ink.* Aleppo galls 10 ℔, logwood 5 ℔, pomegranate-peel 2½ ℔, cloves 2½ oz., soft water 8 gallons. Let the whole boil gently for an hour or two, then cover the copper and leave it for 12 or 24 hours, stirring it now and then. Strain off the decoction and add 2 gallons more water to the ingredients; simmer gently for an hour, and strain. Mix the liquors, and let them settle; draw off the clear liquor from the dregs; dissolve in a portion of it 2½ ℔ of gum Arabic, and ½ ℔ of sugar candy; and in another portion 2½ ℔ of green sulphate of iron. Strain both solutions and mix the whole together; then add 1 oz. of calcined borax, and ¼ oz. of creasote dissolved in ¼ pint of spirit of wine. [Dr. HARE recommends an ink free from acid, to be made with galls and "finery cinder;" but we are not sure what is intended by this name.]

6. RIBAUCOURT'S *Ink.* Galls 1 ℔, logwood ½ ℔, gum 6 oz., sulphate of iron ½ ℔, sulphate of copper 2 oz., sugar 2 oz., water 12 ℔ (or 5 quarts.) This has the disadvantage of corroding the steel pens and the penknives with which it comes in contact.

7. Galls 3 oz., sulphate of iron 1 oz., logwood ½ oz., gum ½ oz., ale a quart. Let it stand in a loosely corked bottle, in a warm place, for a week or more, shaking it daily.

8. Boil 4 oz. of logwood for an hour in 6 quarts of

water; adding boiling water as it evaporates: then add 16 oz. of blue galls coarsely bruised, 4 oz. of dried sulphate of iron (i. e. heated till it becomes whitish and pulverulent,) 3 oz. of brown sugar, 6 oz. of gum Arabic, and ¼ oz. of acetate of copper ground with a little of the decoction. Keep the whole in a bottle uncorked for a fortnight, shaking it twice a day.

9. READE'S *Patent.* This differs from common black ink, in containing a portion of soluble Prussian blue.

10. *Chrome Ink.* Extract of logwood ½ oz., gum ¼ oz., water a pint. Dissolve also in 12 oz. of water ½ oz. of yellow chromate of potash (or ¼ oz. each of bichromate and bicarbonate of potash;) and mix the two solutions. The ink is ready for immediate use.

11. Dr. LEWIS'S *Writing Ink.* Powdered sulphate of iron 1 oz., powdered logwood 1 oz., powdered galls 3 oz., gum Arabic 1 oz., white wine or vinegar 1 quart.

12. BERZELIUS recommends a solution of vanadiate of ammonia in infusion of galls. Dr. URE states that this forms the most perfect ink that can be desired; but the scarcity and high price of the vanadiate prevent its use.

13. RUNGE'S *Black Writing Fluid.* Boil logwood 22 lb, in enough water to yield 14 gallons of decoction. To 1000 parts of this decoction, when cold, add 1 part of chromate of potash. The mixture is to be well stirred. The proportions are to be carefully observed, and the yellow chromate, not the bi-chromate, employed. (This ink is said to possess some great advantages; to adhere strongly to paper, so that it can neither be washed off by water, nor even altered by weak acids; to form no deposit; and not to be in the least acted upon by steel pens.) Steel pens should be washed in an alkaline solution before being used with this ink.

(*Packers' Marking Ink* is merely the dregs of black ink, for marking parcels with a brush.

Copying Ink. Mr. BRANDE directs 1 oz. of brown sugar to be added to No. 1, for copying. Another kind is made by dissolving ½ oz. of gum, and 20 gr. of Spanish liquorice, in 13 dr. of water, and adding to it a drachm of lamp-black, previously mixed with a teaspoonful of sherry. If the lamp-black is greasy, it should be heated to redness in a covered crucible. Another published form is—Black ink 3 oz., sugar candy 1 oz.

Ink Powder. This consists of the dry ingredients for ink, powdered and mixed. 1. Powdered galls 4 oz., sulphate of iron (heated till it becomes white and pulverulent) 1 oz., powdered gum 1 oz., white sugar ½ oz.; mix. To make a quart of ink, with water or beer.

2. Powdered galls 2 ℔, green vitriol 1 ℔, powdered gum 8 oz. In 2 oz. packets, each for 1 pint of ink.—GRAY.

Red Writing Inks. 1. Best ground Brazil wood 4 oz., diluted acetic acid a pint, alum ½ oz. Boil them slowly in a covered tinned copper, or enamelled saucepan, for an hour; strain, and add ½ oz. gum. Some direct the Brazil wood to infuse for 2 or 3 days before boiling.

2. WEBER'S *Red Ink*. Boil 4 oz. of Pernambuco wood with 16 oz. of dilute acetic acid and an equal quantity of water, until 24 oz. remain. Add an ounce of alum, and evaporate again to 16 oz.; add gum Arabic 1 oz., strain; and to the cold liquid add lastly 1 dr. of protochloride of tin. (Said to be of a finer colour, and more permanent, than cochineal ink.)

3. Boil 2 oz. of good Brazil wood, ½ oz. of alum, and ½ oz. of cream of tartar, in 16 oz. of rain water, till reduced to half; strain, and dissolve in it ½ oz. of gum Arabic, and add a tincture made with 1½ dr. of cochineal in 1½ oz. of spirit of wine.—HENSELER.

4. Brazil 4 oz., alum 2 oz., water a quart. Boil for an hour, and strain; then add 1 oz. of gum.

5. Triturate 1 dr. of cochineal and 1 dr. of subcarbonate of potash, with a little boiling water; then add 1 dr. of burnt alum and 2 dr. of cream of tartar, and water to bring it to the desired colour. [Not so permanent as the Brazil ink.]

6. *Carmine Ink*. Heat a scruple of carmine with 3 oz. of water of ammonia for some minutes, a little below boiling, and add 15 or 20 gr. of gum. (The inkstand must be kept well closed.)

7. STEPHENS' *Red Ink*. Patent. Take some common

soda, potash, or carbonate of ammonia, and add to it, at intervals, twice its weight of crude argol in powder. When effervescence has ceased, pour off the solution, or filter it from insoluble matter. Add to it next, by measure, half the quantity of oxalate of alumina, prepared by adding to precipitated alumina in a damp state as much oxalic acid as will dissolve it. Into this mixture, when cold, put as much powdered cochineal as will give it a fine red colour, and after letting it stand for 48 hours, strain it for use.

Blue Inks. 1. READE'S Patent. Prepare a solution of iodide of iron, from iodine, iron, and water; add to the solution half as much iodine as first used. Pour this solution into a semi-saturated solution of ferro-prussiate of potash, containing nearly as much of the salt as the whole weight of iodine. Collect the precipitate, wash it, and finally dissolve it in water, to form the blue ink. The solution from which the precipitate is separated, evaporated to dryness, and the residue fused, re-dissolved, and crystallized, yields pure iodide of potassium. [This process being patented, ink must not be prepared by it for sale.]

2. Add a pint of a cold solution of persulphate of iron (prepared as directed, page 387) to a solution of 6 oz. of ferro-cyanide of potassium in 2 pints of water. Collect the precipitate, wash it with distilled water until it begins to dissolve, then triturate it in a mortar with sufficient distilled water to form a blue ink.

3. Chemic, or Saxon blue (sulphate of indigo,) diluted with water to the desired shade, with a little gum.

4. Pure Prussian blue, triturated with a sixth part of its weight of oxalic acid, with a little water, to a smooth paste, and more water added to bring it to the proper colour. A larger proportion of the acid is ordered in some recipes.

5. Dr. NORMANDY'S *Blue Ink.* Chinese blue (ferro-cyanide of iron) is ground in water with binoxalate of potash and gum Arabic, in the following proportions:— 7 oz. of water to 3 dr. of Chinese blue, 1 dr. of binoxalate of potash, and 1 dr. of gum Arabic.

6. STEPHENS' *Patent Blue Ink.* Common Prussian blue is first macerated in strong sulphuric acid, then repeatedly washed in water, and afterwards dried. This process is to render it more soluble in oxalic acid, which is now to be gradually added in the proportion of about 1 part to 6 of the Prussian blue (as before maceration,) together with sufficient water to yield a dense blue solution.

7. Digest 2 oz. of the cuttings of tin plate with 4 oz. of nitrous acid, and add the solution to a gallon of water in which 2 oz. of prussiate of potash have been dissolved. [This requires frequent shaking, to keep the precipitate (which is Prussian blue) suspended.]

Violet Inks. 1. Boil 8 oz. of logwood in 3 pints of rain or distilled water to 1½ pint. Strain, and add 1½ oz. of clean gum, and 2½ oz. of alum in fine powder. Agitate frequently till dissolved.

2. Cudbear 1 oz., pearlash 1½ oz., mucilage 2 oz., soft water to make a pint. Pour the water hot on the cudbear and pearlash, allow the mixture to stand for 12 hours, then strain, and add the mucilage. 1 oz. of rectified spirit may also be added.

Purple Inks. 1. Add a little muriate of tin to a strong decoction of logwood. A little gum may be added.

2. Dr. NORMANDY'S *Purple Ink.* To 12 ℔ of Campeachy wood add as many gallons of boiling water, pour the solution through a funnel, with a strainer made of coarse flannel, on 1 ℔ of hydrate or acetate of deutoxide of copper finely powdered, (having at the bottom of the funnel a piece of sponge;) then add immediately 14 ℔ of alum, and for every 340 gallons of liquid add 80 ℔ of gum Arabic or gum Senegal. Let these remain for 3 or 4 days, and a beautiful purple colour will be produced.

Brown Ink. 1. Boil ½ oz. of catechu with 8 oz. of water until dissolved, and strain. Dissolve 60 gr. of bichromate of potash in 1½ oz. of water, and add it gradually to the solution of catechu until the desired shade is obtained. It requires no gum.

2. By adding to the violet ink, finely powdered bichromate of potash, in the proportion of from 15 to 30 grains to an ounce, various shades of brown and snuff colour are obtained.

Yellow Ink. 1. Gamboge triturated with water, and a little alum added.

2. Boil 8 oz. of French berries with 1 oz. of alum in a quart of water; strain, and add 1 oz. of gum.

Green Ink. 1. Dissolve 3 dr. of bichromate of potash in 1 oz. of water; add to the hot solution ½ oz. of alcohol, and decompose the mixture by a little strong sulphuric acid till it assumes a brown colour. Evaporate the liquid to half, let it cool, dilute with a sufficient quantity of water, and filter; add to the filtered liquid 4 dr. of alcohol, decompose it with a few drops of sulphuric acid, and let it rest. After some time it assumes a fine green colour. A little gum may be added. [There is danger of the paper, and steel pens, suffering from an excess of sulphuric acid.]—WINCKLER.

2. Distilled verdigris 2 oz., cream of tartar 1 oz., water 8 oz.; boil to half and filter.—KLAPROTH.

3. Add to the yellow ink No. 2 sufficient sulphate of indigo.

4. Dissolve sap green in water with a little alum.

5. Rub 3½ dr. of Prussian blue, and 3 dr. of gamboge, with 2 oz. of mucilage, and add ½ pint of water.

Gold and Silver Ink. Fine bronze powder, or gold or silver leaf, ground with a little sulphate of potash, and washed from the salt, is mixed with water and a sufficient quantity of gum.

Indestructible Writing Fluids. The common writing inks being liable to be obliterated by many chemical agents, several compounds more capable of resisting these agents have been proposed; of which the following appear deserving of notice.

1. *Carbon Ink.* Dissolve real Indian ink in common black ink; or add a small quantity of lamp-black, previously heated to redness, and ground perfectly smooth with a small portion of the ink.

2. STEPHENS' (*patent*) *Carbon Ink.* Common soda of commerce is mixed with resinous matters (as shell-lac or rosin,) in about equal parts by weight. Water being added according to the strength required, the solution is boiled until the resin has become dissolved. Mix in

a mortar with the requisite quantity of fine lamp-black, and add any suitable coloured solution.

3. *Shell-lac Ink, or* COATHUPE'S *Writing Fluid.* To 18 oz. of water add 1 oz. of powdered borax, and 2 oz. of bruised shell-lac, and boil them in a covered vessel, stirring them occasionally, till dissolved. Filter, when cold, through coarse filtering paper; add 1 oz. of mucilage; boil for a few minutes, adding sufficient finely powdered indigo and lamp-black to colour it. Leave the mixture for 2 or 3 hours for the coarser particles to subside; pour it off from the dregs, and bottle it for use.

4. *Gluten Ink.* Dissolve wheat gluten, free from starch, in weak acetic acid of the strength of common vinegar; mix 10 gr. of lamp-black and 2 gr. of indigo with 4 oz. of the solution, and a drop or two of oil of cloves.

5. HAUSMANN'S. Dissolve 1 part of genuine asphaltum with 4 parts of oil of turpentine, and sufficient lamp-black. If sufficient lamp-black be used to give it a suitable consistence, it may be used with types.

6. BRACONNOT'S *Indelible Ink.* Take 20 parts of Dantzig potash, 10 of tanned leather-parings, and 5 of sulphur; boil them in an iron pot with sufficient water to dryness: then raise the heat, stirring the matter constantly, till the whole becomes soft, taking care that it does not ignite. Add sufficient water, and filter through cloth. It must be kept from the air. It flows freely from the pen, and resists many chemical agents; but it is not strictly indelible.

7. Dr. NORMANDY'S *Indelible Ink.* Frankfort lamp-black 24 ℔, to be ground with mucilage, made by adding 24 ℔ of gum to 60 gallons of water, and the mixture filtered through a very coarse flannel; 4 ℔ of oxalic acid are then added, with as much decoction of cochineal and sulphate of indigo as will yield the shade of colour desired.

8. *Indian Ink.* Real lamp-black, produced by combustion of linseed oil, ground with gum, and infusion of galls. It is prepared both in a liquid and solid form, the latter being dried in the sun.

Ink for writing on Zinc Labels. Horticultural ink:

1. Dissolve 100 gr. of chloride of platinum in a pint of water. A little mucilage and lamp-black may be added.

2. Sal ammoniac 1 dr., verdigris 1 dr., lamp-black ½ dr., water 10 dr. Mix.

Ink for writing on Steel or Tin Plate, or Sheet Zinc. 1. Mix 1 oz. of powdered sulphate of copper and ½ oz. of powdered sal ammoniac, with 2 oz. of diluted acetic acid; adding lamp-black or vermilion.

2. Dissolve 1 part of copper in 10 of nitric acid, and dilute with 10 parts of water.

White Marking for Black Bottles, in cellars. Grind flake-white, or sulphate of barytes, with a little oil of turpentine, and any light-coloured varnish, to a proper consistence.

Lithographic Ink. 1. LASTEYRIE'S: Dried soap 1 oz.; melt, and add shell-lac 5 oz., then common soda 1 oz., mastic 1 oz., and lastly, lamp-black 3 dr. Melt, stir together, and when completely melted, pour into moulds: to be used as Indian ink.

2. *Autographic.* White soap 100 parts, white wax 100, mutton suet 30, shell-lac 50, mastic 50, lamp-black 30 or 35. Melted as above.

3. *Lithographic Ink.* Heat 40 parts of yellow wax until its vapour kindles on coming in contact with a burning match; then remove it from the fire, and add gradually, in small parts, Marseilles soap 22 parts, gum-lac 28 parts, and mastic 10 parts. Extinguish the flame, and incorporate perfectly with this mixture lamp-black 9 parts. Then again heat until the vapour can be ignited, when remove it from the fire, and after the flame has been extinguished, pour it upon a stone. The mass is then cut into pieces.—M. WEISHAUPT.

4. *Crayons.* White wax 8 oz., white soap 2 oz., shell-lac 2 oz., lamp-black 3 tablespoonfuls. Melt the wax and soap with a brisk fire; stir in the lamp-black; allow the mixture to burn for half a minute, then extinguish the flame, and add the shell-lac by degrees, stirring continually. Put the mixture on the fire till it kindles, or nearly so. Extinguish the flame, let the mixture cool a little, and pour it into moulds.

Inks for Marking Linen. Some of these are used with types; others with a clean quill pen.

1. Sulphate of manganese 1 dr., water 1 dr., powdered sugar 2 dr., lamp-black ½ dr. Triturate them together and stamp it on the linen with types. When dry, wash the part with liquor potassæ; dry; and wash with plenty of water.

2. Dr. SMELLIE'S. Sulphate of iron 1 dr., linseed oil 1 oz., vermilion ½ oz.: grind perfectly smooth. Printer's ink is also used with type.

3. Heat to redness equal weights of black oxide of manganese and caustic potash, and mix it with an equal weight of pipe-clay, and sufficient water to give it a due consistence. To be applied with types or stencils. It becomes brown, and does not wash out. The following are used with a quill pen:—

4. Nitrate of silver 100 gr., distilled water 1 oz., gum Arabic 2 dr., sap green a scruple. Dissolve. The linen is first to be wetted with the following *pounce*, dried and rubbed smooth, then written on by a clean quill or bone pen dipped in the ink. *Pounce* or *Mordant.* Subcarbonate of soda 1 oz., water 8 oz. [A great variety of recipes might be given, slightly differing from the above in the proportion of the ingredients, and in the colouring matter. GRAY directs 2 dr. of nitrate of silver, 6 dr. of water, and 2 of mucilage, and a pounce of 1 oz. of subcarbonate of soda in 16 of water, with a little sap green. Another form is—nitrate of silver 1 oz., distilled water 5 oz., powdered gum 1¼ oz., sap green sufficient to colour it. The linen to be first wet with the following preparation:—subcarbonate of soda 1 oz., water 6 oz., gum 1 oz.; dissolve. Some add a little powdered bole to the preparation; the object in colouring it being merely that the part which has been wetted may be more readily distinguished. The quantity of nitrate of silver should not be much less than 100 grains in an ounce of ink; the proportion of the other ingredients is of less importance. Some direct the addition of a drop or two of nitric acid.]

5. *Italian.* Moisten the linen with a solution of recently prepared muriate of tin, and write with a neutral solution of salt of gold.

Marking Ink, without Preparation. These merely require to have a hot iron passed over the part written on, or to be held pretty near the fire till the writing assumes a dark colour.

1. Nitrate of silver 3 dr., water 1½ oz.; dissolve, and add as much strong liquid ammonia as will redissolve the precipitate formed by it; add 2 dr. of mucilage, a little sap green, and water, if required, to make up the measure to 2 oz. A little ivory black, Indian ink, or indigo, is sometimes used to colour it. Some recipes contain nitrate of copper in addition to nitrate of silver. Several recipes might be given, but they will all probably be superseded by Mr. REDWOOD'S. [In operating with ammonia and nitrate of silver, fulminating silver is sometimes unexpectedly formed, and may prove a source of danger. Perhaps in this respect, as well as others, Mr. REDWOOD'S preparation claims a preference.]

2. Mr. REDWOOD'S. Rub together 1 oz. nitrate of silver, and 1 oz. of bitartrate of potash; add 4 ounces of liquor ammoniæ, and when dissolved mix in 6 dr. of white sugar, 10 dr. of powdered gum Arabic, ½ oz. of archil, and water to make up 6 oz. by measure. [Instead of archil, ¼ oz. of sap green may be used to colour the ink; or 40 grains of fine vegetable black, previously triturated with a little water or mucilage.]

3. Rev. J. B. READE'S patent. This differs from the last in using tartaric acid instead of bitartrate of potash. The quantities may be 1 oz. of nitrate of silver, 3 drachms of tartaric acid, and the above quantities of the other ingredients. The use of tartaric acid he claims an exclusive right to.

4. Add to the last an ammoniacal solution of an oxide or salt of gold.—READE. [This addition prevents its being acted on by cyanide of potassium, and some other agents which the silver ink fails to resist.]

5. In addition to the above recipes, the following of M. HENRY may deserve attention in large establishments where economy is an object:—Take 1 oz. of iron filings, and 3 oz. of vinegar or diluted acetic acid. Mix the filings with half the vinegar, and agitate them continually until the mixture becomes thick, then add

the rest of the vinegar, and 1 oz. of water. Apply heat to assist the action, and when the iron is dissolved, add 3 oz. of sulphate of iron, and 1 oz. of gum previously dissolved in 4 oz. of water; and mix the whole with a gentle heat. To be used with a brush and stencil plates.

Printing Ink. This is usually made by boiling linseed oil in a large iron pot, setting fire to it, and letting it burn for half an hour or more. Various additions are made to it by some manufacturers, the use of which is not very evident. A viscid varnish is obtained, which is ground with lamp-black, vermilion, or other colouring matters, till perfectly smooth. 2½ oz. of lamp-black are sufficient for each pound of varnish. See VARNISHES.

Printer's Ink from Rosin Oil. Melt together 13 ounces of rosin, 1 ℔ of rosin oil, and 1½ oz. of soft soap; when cold, add lamp-black or other colouring matters.

Copper-plate Printing Ink. This is not rendered so viscid as the former, and is coloured with Frankfort black.

READE'S *Patent Printing Inks.* The *blue* consists of his soluble Prussian blue (see BLUE WRITING INK, above) ground with oil as above. The *black*, by evaporating his black ink, and mixing the product with oil as usual. The *red* in the same manner, from his patent red ink.

Sympathetic or Secret Inks. The solutions used should be so nearly colourless that the writing cannot be seen till the agent is applied to render it visible.

1. Digest 1 oz. of zaffre, or oxide of cobalt, at a gentle heat, with 4 oz. of nitro-muriatic acid till no more is dissolved, then add 1 oz. of common salt, and 16 oz. of water. If this be written with, and the paper held to the fire, the writing becomes green, unless the cobalt should be quite pure, in which case it will be blue. The addition of a little nitrate of iron will then impart the property of becoming green. It is used in chemical landscapes, for the foliage.

2. Put into a phial ½ oz. of distilled water, 1 dr. of bromide of potassium, and 1 dr. of pure sulphate of copper. The solution is nearly colourless, but becomes brown when heated.

3. Boil oxide of cobalt in acetic acid. If a little common salt be added, the writing becomes green when heated; but with nitre it becomes a pale rose-colour.

4. A solution of acetate of lead. Colourless, but becomes brown when exposed to sulphuretted hydrogen gas.

5. A weak solution of sulphate of copper. The writing becomes blue when exposed to the vapour of ammonia.

6. A solution of sulphate—or preferably, persulphate—of iron. It becomes black when washed with infusion of galls; *blue*, by prussiate of potash. [This constitutes colourless ink, which becomes visible when written with on paper containing galls, or tannin, or prussiate of potash.]

7. Mix equal quantities of sulphate of copper and sal ammoniac, and dissolve in water. It becomes yellow when heated.

8. A weak solution of nitrate of mercury. Becomes black by heat.

9. Rice water, or any solution of starch. It becomes blue when washed over with an alcoholic solution of iodine.

10. Lemon juice, milk, juice of onions, and some other liquids become black when the writing is held to the fire.

INK, to preserve from mouldiness. Add a small quantity of a solution of creasote in pyroligneous acid or rectified spirit.

IODATE OF POTASH. Fuse iodide of potassium in a capacious hessian crucible, remove it from the fire, and add to it, while still semi-fluid, successive portions of pulverized chlorate of potash, stirring after each addition, till no further action takes place. One part of iodide of potassium will require $1\frac{1}{2}$ of the chlorate. Wash the residuum in warm water, which leaves only iodate of potash.

IODIDE OF POTASSIUM. In addition to the process given in the Pocket Formulary, the following, by M. CRIQUELON, may deserve attention:—Slake 40 parts of lime with sufficient water, and add 24 parts of iron filings; mix, and add 94 parts of iodine by degrees, so as to avoid too violent action, stirring after each addition, and adding water, if necessary, to moderate the action. Triturate the mixture till starch paper ceases to become brown when touched with it, but only shows an ochreous spot. Throw it on a filter, and wash it till the water which passes gives no precipitate with acetate of lead. Treat the liquors with solution of carbonate of potash till it no longer occasions a precipitate. Filter, and evaporate the solution. 94 parts of iodine yield 119 parts of iodide of potassium. Another method is that of Mr. READE, described under INK (READE'S BLUE.)

IODINE. See Pocket Formulary. Other methods of obtaining it are the following:—

To the mother liquor of kelp (after the crystallizable salts have been separated) add sulphuric acid to render the liquor sour. Introduce the acid liquor into a leaden still, heat to 140 FAHR., add binoxide of manganese, and lute on with pipe-clay a leaden head, fitted to a series of spherical glass condensers, each having two mouths opposite each other, and inserted the one into the other. A stopper in the head of the still allows the contents to be occasionally inspected, and additions of acid or oxide made, if necessary. See Dr. PEREIRA'S "Elements" for a drawing of the apparatus. SOUBEIRAN proposes to add sulphate of copper to the ley, which precipitates half the iodine. He then decants the clear liquor, and adds more sulphate of copper with some iron filings. An iodide of copper is formed, which is separated from the iron filings and suspended in the liquor by agitation, collected on a filter, and heated with oxide of manganese and sulphuric acid.

IRON LIQUOR. See DYES, page 347.

IRON, PERSULPHATE OF. Dissolve 16 ounces of sulphate of iron in 4 pints of water, to which has been added 14 fluid drachms of oil of vitriol. Heat to boiling, and add (by small portions, boiling the solution after each addition) 4 ounces of nitric acid, or so much that the solution yields with ammonia a brown precipitate unmixed with black. Continue the boiling for some time, let the solution cool, filter, if necessary, and add water to make up the measure exactly 4 pints. If required in a dry state, evaporate to dryness by a gentle heat.

ISINGLASS. The air bags or sounds, of several kinds of fishes, washed, dried, and otherwise prepared. They are either dried without opening (purse, pipe, and lump isinglass,) or opened and not folded (leaf and honeycomb isinglass,) or folded (book isinglass,) or twisted into the shape of a lyre or horse-shoe (short and long staple.) The leaf isinglass is sometimes rolled out into thin plates (ribbon and rolled leaf isinglass.) The inner membrane, which is insoluble, is removed from the opened air bags, in the best kinds. The Russian isinglass, which is most esteemed, is made from the air bags of several species of ACIPENSER (*sturgeon;*) particularly A. Huso (the *Beluga;*) A. GULDENSTADTII (the *Osseter;*) A. RUTHENUS (the *Sterlet;*) A. STELLATUS (the *Sewruga;*) and also from the Silurus glanis (the *Som*) which yields the Samovey isinglass. Brazilian and East India isinglass are of inferior quality; it is not certainly known from what genera or species of fish they are obtained. New York isinglass is the air-bladder of the common hake, macerated in water and rolled out into ribbons. The sounds of the cod yield an inferior kind. Prepared sole skins are used as a cheap substitute for isinglass. See Dr. PEREIRA'S "Elements," for the description of each variety.

IVORY BLACK. Burn shavings and waste pieces of ivory from the ivory turners, in a covered crucible, till no more smoke issue. Cover it closely while cooling. It should be afterwards washed with diluted muriatic acid, then with water till no longer acid, dried, and again heated in a covered crucible. It is of a deeper colour than bone-black, and is used as a pigment, a tooth powder, and to decolorize syrups and other liquids.

IVORY, FLEXIBLE. The pieces of ivory or bone, already manufactured into the shape required, are to be steeped for some time in dilute muriatic acid, until they have lost their earthy parts so far as to become yellowish, flexible, and elastic. When dry they become again inflexible, but their flexibility may at any time be restored by steeping them in water. In this manner flexible tubes, probes, bougies, &c., may be constructed.

IVORY, TO STAIN. Ivory is stained with the usual dyeing

materials; it should be first steeped in the mordant and afterwards in the hot colour. Nitromuriate of tin is the mordant for red, with decoction of brazil or cochineal; for yellow, with fustic; for violet, with logwood. After being plunged in hot liquor it should be placed in cold water. A black stain is given by nitrate of silver.

Ivory may be *gilded* by immersing it in a fresh solution of protosulphate of iron, and afterwards in solution of chloride of gold. It may be *bleached* by solution of sulphurous acid.

JAPAN. See VARNISHES.

JELLIES. See DIETETIC ARTICLES.

KID-GLOVE CLEANER. Add 15 drops of strongest solution of ammonia to spirits of turpentine ½ pint. (Having fitted the gloves on wooden hands, apply this mixture with a brush. Follow up this application with some fine pumice powder. Rub with some flannel or sponge dipped in the mixture. Rub off the sand, and repeat the same process twice or thrice. Hang in the air to dry, and, when dry, place in a drawer with some scent.)

KYAN'S SOLUTION, for preventing the dry rot. Dissolve 1 ℔ of corrosive sublimate in 5 gallons of water.

LABARRAQUE'S CHLORO-SODAIC LIQUOR is nearly identical with the Liquor Sodæ Chlorinatæ of the London Pharmacopœia. It is made by passing the chlorine gas from 2 oz. black oxide of manganese, and 8 oz. of muriatic acid, into a solution of 15 oz. of crystallized subcarbonate of soda in 3 pints of water; or sufficient to bring it to the density of 12° Baumé, or 1·09 specific gravity.

LAC, PREPARATIONS OF. Stick-lac consists of twigs of several kinds of trees encrusted with a resinous matter produced by the puncture of an insect (the coccus lacca.) This triturated with water and dried, forms seed-lac. The seed-lac heated and pressed in cotton bags forms shell-lac. Lac dye is the colouring matter extracted from stick-lac by water, and evaporated to dryness with the addition of earthy matters, and formed into square cakes. Seed-lac and shell-lac are chiefly used in varnishes, dissolved in rectified spirit, or rectified wood naphtha. The alcoholic solution is rendered paler, so that it may be used for polishing light-coloured woods, by digesting it in the sun, or near a fire, for 2 or 3 weeks, with good animal charcoal, and then filtering it through paper in a funnel heated with hot water. Shell-lac may be bleached by dissolving it in a solution of potash or soda, and passing chlorine into the solution. The precipitated lac is collected and well washed. KASTNER directs 3 parts of carbonate of potash to be dissolved in 24 of water, and 3 of lime added, and the whole digested in a close vessel for 24 hours. The clear liquor is poured off, and boiled with 4 parts of shell-lac. When cold, dilute with 4 times its bulk of water, and filter; then add chloride of lime, and afterwards diluted muriatic acid.

LACQUERS. See VARNISHES.

LAKE LIQUOR. Boil 1 oz. each of cochineal and salt of tartar in 8 oz. of water; then add 1 oz. of cream of tartar, and the same of alum.

LAKES. These consist of vegetable colours in combination with alumina. Alum is usually added to an infusion or decoction of the colouring ingredient, and afterwards potash added, which throws down the colouring matter combined with alumina. Some of the lakes are noticed under PIGMENTS.

LEMON JUICE, FACTITIOUS. Dissolve 4 oz. of citric acid in 3 pints of water, with 8 drops of essence of lemon, rubbed with the acid, or dissolved in a little spirit. After standing a few days, filter it, and preserve it in well-closed bottles.

LENSES, EXTEMPORANEOUS. Procure a piece of thin platinum wire, and twine it once or twice round a pin's point, so as to form a minute ring with a handle to it. Break up a piece of flint glass into fragments a little larger than mustard seed; place one of these pieces on the ring of wire, and hold it in the point of the flame of a candle or gas-light. The glass will melt, and assume a complete lens-like or globular form. Let it cool gradually, and keep it for mounting. Others are to be made in the same manner; and if the operation be carefully conducted, but very few will be imperfect. The smaller the drop melted, the higher in general will be its magnifying power. It may be mounted by placing it between two pieces of brass, which have corresponding circular holes cut in them, of such a size as to hold the edge of the lens. They are then to be cemented together. —FRANCIS.

LINSEED OIL, CLARIFIED, FOR VARNISHES. Heat in a copper boiler 50 gallons of linseed oil to 280° F.; add 2½ ℔ of calcined white vitriol, and keep the oil at the above temperature for half an hour; then remove it from the fire, and in 24 hours decant the clear oil, which should stand for a few weeks before it is used for varnish.

LINSEED OIL, REFINED. (WILKES' Patent.) In 236 gallons of oil pour 6 ℔ of oil of vitriol, and stir them together for 3 hours; then add 6 ℔ of fullers' earth, well mixed with 14 ℔ of hot lime, and stir for 3 hours. Put the oil into a copper boiler, with an equal quantity of water, and boil for 3 hours; then extinguish the fire, and when the materials are cold, draw off the water, and let the oil stand to settle for a few weeks before using.

LIQUORICE, PURIFIED EXTRACT OF. Italian or Spanish juice may be purified by the following method:—Take a sugar mould, close the vent hole with a stopper, place inside some coarse tow, and over this some clean straw, laid crosswise in layers of an inch each, then the sticks of liquorice placed upright, and packed closely in the mould with chopped straw cut rather long. When this arrangement is completed to within an inch of the brim, pour water over the liquorice, allow it to remain for 24 hours, then draw it off, and add more. The liquor, on evaporation, yields an extract perfectly soluble in water.

LITMUS. A preparation of some kind of lichen, probably Lecanora tartarea, or Roccella tartarea, or both. The exact mode of preparing it is kept secret. It is imported in small cubical masses, many samples of which Dr. PEREIRA found to contain, besides the colouring matter and tissues of the lichen, indigo, chalk, &c. See TESTS.

LOZENGES. See Trochisci, P. F., and LOZENGES, under PATENT MEDICINES, in this volume.

LUBRICATING COMPOUNDS. See ANTI-ATTRITION. The French compound termed *Liard* is thus made:—Into 50 parts of finest rape oil put 1 part of caoutchouc cut small, and apply heat until it is nearly all dissolved.

MANKETTRICK'S Lubricating Compound consists of caoutchouc (dissolved in spirit of turpentine) 4 ℔, common soda 10 ℔, glue 1 ℔, oil 10 gallons, water 10 gallons. Dissolve the soda and glue in the water by heat, then add the oil, and lastly the caoutchouc, stirring them until perfectly incorporated.

LUCIFERS. See MATCHES, below.

LUMINOUS PHIALS. Nearly fill a bottle with olive or almond oil, and heat it in a water-bath. Drop into it small slices of phosphorus so long as it is dissolved. Let the solution cool, and pour off the oil from the undissolved phosphorus into clean dry phials, which should not be quite filled. When uncorked they emit light.

LUTES. See CEMENTS.

MANURES, ARTIFICIAL. These constitute a new and important branch of manufacture; but a few of the more simple and readily prepared kinds are all that can be noticed here.

Powder for Coating Seeds. Fine bone dust 20 parts, gypsum 1 part. The seeds are steeped in water from the dunghill, then strewed over with the powder, so that each shall receive a layer of it, and afterwards dried.

Sulphated Bones. See *Bones, Sulphated.* A usual proportion is 33 of sulphuric acid to 1 cwt. of bones.

Saline Mixture, as a top-dressing for potatoes, &c. Equal weights of nitrate of soda and dry sulphate of soda. 1½ cwt. to an acre.

Mr. HUXTABLE'S *Mixture.* Bone-dust 4 cwt., gypsum 4 cwt., salt 2 cwt., ashes 2 quarters, wood ashes 30 bushels.

Another Saline Mixture. Sulphate of ammonia 42 ℔, sulphate of lime 56 ℔, sulphate of potash 56 ℔, carbonate of magnesia 14 ℔, salt 56 ℔, to 1 acre.

Dr. ANDERSON'S *Manure for Clover.* Sulphate of ammonia 98 ℔, gypsum 172 ℔, sulphate of potash 174 ℔, sulphate of soda 333 ℔, sulphate of magnesia 246 ℔, sulphuric acid 98 ℔, saltpetre 202 ℔, common salt 107 ℔, muriate of potash 149 ℔.

Dr. JOHNSTONE'S *Substitute for Guano.* Bone-dust 7 bushels, sulphate of ammonia 100 ℔, wood ashes 20 ℔, salt 100 ℔, dry sulphate of soda 11 ℔.

To Promote the Blowing of Flowers. See page 352.

MARBLE, TO CLEAN. Mix soft soap, solution of potash, and slaked lime, to a paste; spread it over the marble, and leave it for a day or two. Then wash it off.

MARBLE, TO STAIN. Make the marble hot, and pour on it the coloured liquid, also made hot. The stains usually employed are, archil, solution of indigo, solution of verdigris, decoction of Brazil wood, logwood and sulphate of iron, tincture of dragon's blood, &c. But the most penetrating medium is wax, which may be coloured with alkanet, annatto, verdigris, &c.

MARINE GLUE. See GLUE.

MARINE SOAP. See SOAP.

MATCHES FOR INSTANTANEOUS LIGHT. 1. *Chlorate Matches (without sulphur.)* Chlorate of potash, separately powdered, 6 dr., vermilion 1 dr., lycopodium 1 dr., fine flour 2 dr.; mix carefully the chlorate with the flour and lycopodium, avoiding much friction, then add the vermilion, and mix the whole with a mucilage made with —1 dr. powdered gum Arabic, 10 gr. of tragacanth, 2 dr. of flour, and 4 oz. of hot water; mix; add sufficient water to bring it to a proper consistence, and dip in it the wood, previously dipped into a solution of 1 oz. of gum thus, and ½ oz. of camphor, in 6 oz. of oil of turpentine.

2. *With Sulphur.* Chlorate of potash 9 gr., sulphur 2 gr., sugar 3 gr., vermilion 1 gr., flour 2 gr., spirit of wine q. s. The chlorate of potash, &c. must be separately reduced to powder, and the whole mixed with as little friction as possible. The wood should be previously prepared as above, or with camphorated spirit. [These are ignited by dipping them in sulphuric acid, and instantly withdrawing them. The acid should be absorbed by asbestos.] They are now become obsolete, having given place to—

Lucifer Matches. These contain phosphorus in a finely divided state, to which it is reduced by agitating it in some warm solution of gum or glue, then adding the other ingredients, so as to form a paste, into which the wood or card is dipped. It is said that urine and artificial urea have the property of readily dividing phosphorus when warmed and agitated together. The following are some of the published recipes:—

1. Form 6 parts of glue into a smooth jelly, and rub it with 4 parts of phosphorus, at a temperature of 140° or 150° F.; add 10 parts of nitre, 5 of red ochre, and 2 of fine smalts. The matches are first dipped in melted wax to the depth of $\frac{1}{10}$th of an inch, first rubbing their ends on a hot iron plate.

2. *Noiseless Congreves.* Triturate 9 parts of phosphorus with a solution of 16 parts of gum, and add 14 parts of nitre, and 16 of vermilion.—Dr. BOETTGER.

3. Glue 6 parts, phosphorus 4, nitre 10, red lead 5, smalts 2; the glue is soaked in water for 24 hours, then liquefied in a warm mortar, and the phosphorus added, taking care that the temperature is not above 167° F.

4. Glue 21, phosphorus 17, nitre 38, red lead 24; proceed as before.

Promethean Matches. These consist of a composition similar to that of the chlorate matches, enclosed at the end of a paper spill, with a minute glass bulb filled with oil of vitriol in the centre of the composition. When struck, the vessel of acid is broken, and kindles the match.

MILK, PRESERVED (Bethel's Patent.) The milk or cream is first scalded, and, when cold, strongly charged with carbonic acid gas, by means of a soda-water machine. [Attempts have also been made to preserve milk by evaporating it to dryness; but it is necessary to remove the cream in order to effect it.]

MINERAL, CHAMELEON. See CHAMELEON MINERAL.

MOIRÉE METALLIQUE. A method of ornamenting the surface of tin plate by acids. The plates are washed with an alkaline solution, then in water, heated, and sponged or sprinkled with the acid solution. The appearance varies with the degree of heat and the nature and strength of the acids employed. The plates, after the application of the acids, are plunged into water slightly acidulated, dried, and covered with white or coloured varnishes. The following are some of the acid mixtures used:—Nitro-muriatic acid, in different degrees of dilution; sulphuric acid, with 5 parts of water; 1 part of sulphuric, 2 of muriatic acid, and 8 of water; a strong solution of citric acid; 1 part nitric acid, 2 sulphuric, and 18 of water. Solution of potash is also used.

MORDANTS. See DYES, p. 346.

MULTUM. A name given to a compound of liquorice and quassia, sold by druggists to brewers.

NITRATE OF BARYTES. This may be made from the carbonate by dissolving it in dilute nitric acid, evaporating, and crystallizing; but more cheaply from the sulphate of barytes, by converting it into a soluble sulphuret by heating it with charcoal, and decomposing the filtered solution with nitric acid. M. WEISS recommends mixing the pulverized sulphate of barytes (cawk or heavy spar) with one-eighth of charcoal and one-fourth of flour, heating it in a covered crucible, pulverizing the product and forming it into balls, with one-eighth of charcoal and a little water, and again heating them placed between layers of charcoal. Hot water extracts the sulphuret, which crystallizes from the filtered solution. By decomposing this by nitric acid (avoiding the gas which escapes) the nitrate is obtained. The other salts of barytes are obtained in a similar manner.

NITRATE OF SILVER. See ARGENTI NITRAS, P. F. It may be prepared from impure silver by the following process:—Dissolve it in nitric acid, add common salt till no more silver remains in solution. Wash the precipitate thoroughly; then add water and a very little hydrochloric acid, and introduce some pieces of zinc; let them remain together 24 hours, stirring frequently. Remove the zinc, and wash the reduced silver thoroughly. Again dissolve it in nitric acid, diluted with 2 or 3 parts of water; filter, and evaporate, that it may crystallize.

NITRATE OF STRONTIAN. This may be obtained from the native carbonate of strontian, or more cheaply from the native sulphate, by the processes employed for Nitrate of Barytes.

NITRIC AND NITRO-MURIATIC ACIDS. See ACIDS.

NITRITE OF POTASH. It is obtained mixed with a little nitre and potash by heating nitre to redness. To purify the residuum, dissolve it in boiling water, set aside for 24 hours, pour off the liquid from the deposited nitre, neutralize the free alkali with acetic acid, and add twice its volume of alcohol. In a few hours more nitre crystallizes, and the liquid separates into two layers; the upper is alcoholic solution of acetate of potash, the lower is solution of nitrate of potash, which may be evaporated to dryness, or kept in solution. *Used as a test for iodine, with starch paste and hydrochloric acid.* CORENWINDER passes nitrous acid gas, formed by acting on 1 part of starch with 10 of nitric acid, through a solution of caustic potash, sp. gr. 1·38, until it becomes acid; then add a little caustic potash, so as to render it distinctly alkaline.

NITRO-PRUSSIDE OF SODIUM. To 213 parts of powdered ferro-prussiate of potash, in a porcelain basin, add 450 parts of nitric acid of 1·42 density (or 337½ parts at 1·50,) adding all the acid at once. When dissolved, transfer to a bolt-head, and digest in a water-bath until the solution precipitate salts of protoxide of iron of a slate colour. Neutralize, when cold, with a cold solution of carbonate of soda; then boil, and separate the precipitate by filtration. Evaporate the liquid again, filter, and allow the nitrates of potash and soda to crystallize out. Evaporate the liquid again, and remove the prismatic crystals of nitro-prusside as they form. They may be dissolved in water and recrystallized by cooling.

NOVARGENT. This is said to consist of a solution of fresh precipitated chloride of silver in hyposulphite of soda (or, according to the Pharmaceutical Journal, of oxide of silver in cyanide of potassium,) mixed with prepared chalk.

OILS, PURIFICATION AND BLEACHING OF. Fish and other fat oils are improved in smell and colour, by passing hot air or steam through them. DUNN'S method is to heat the oil by steam to 170° or 200°, and force a current of air through it, under a chimney, till it is bleached and purified. Mr. CAMERON'S method of bleaching palm oil is to keep it at 230° with continual agitation by passing into it high-pressure steam, through leaden pipes of two inches diameter. Four tons of oil require 10 hours' steaming. Palm oil is also bleached by chloride of lime. Take from 7 to 14 ℔ of chloride of lime, triturate it in a mortar, adding gradually 12 times the quantity of water, so as to form a smooth cream. Liquefy 112 ℔ of palm oil, remove it from the fire, add the solution of chloride of lime, and stir well with a wooden stirrer. Allow it to cool, and when become solid, break it into small fragments, and expose it to the air for 2 or 3 weeks. Then put into a cast-iron boiler, lined with lead, and add sulphuric acid in equal weight to the chloride of lime, and diluted with 20 parts of water. Boil with a moderate heat till the oil drops clear from the stirrer; then let it cool.

To remove the fœtor from fish oils treat them in the same way (except the exposing to the air,) using only 1 ℔ chloride of lime to 112 ℔ of oil. It does not remove the natural smell of the oil.

Fresh burnt animal charcoal has some effect in improving the colour and smell of most kinds of oil; but its effects are limited.

Calcined magnesia has been used to deprive oils of their rancidity.

Mr. Watt's patented method of bleaching oil is by chromic acid. For palm oil it is thus used:—The oil is heated in a steam vessel, allowed to settle and cool down to 130° F., then removed into wooden vessels, taking care that no water or sediment accompany it. For a ton of palm oil make a saturated solution of 25 ℔ of bichromate of potash; add 8 ℔ sulphuric acid, and 50 ℔ muriatic acid (or an equivalent quantity of salt and sulphuric acid.) Put the muriatic into the oil, and let it be constantly stirred till it becomes of a light-green colour. If not sufficiently decoloured, add more of the mixture. Let the oil settle for half an hour, then pump it into a wooden vat, boil it for a few minutes with fresh water, by means of a steam-pipe, and let it settle. For linseed, rape, and mustard oil, a dilute solution of chromic acid is used, with a little muriatic acid: for olive, almond, and castor oil, no muriatic acid is required. Fish oils and fats are first boiled in a steam apparatus with a weak soda ley (½ ℔ soda for every ton of fat) for half an hour; then ½ ℔ sulphuric acid, diluted with 3 ℔ of water, is added; the whole boiled for 15 minutes, and allowed to settle for an hour or more, when the water and sediment are drawn off, and the oil further bleached by a solution of 4 ℔ of bichromate of potash and 2 ℔ of sulphuric acid properly diluted.

Mr. DAVIDSON treats whale oil first with a solution of tan, next with water and chloride of lime, and lastly, with diluted sulphuric acid and warm water. Rape and other seed oils are also refined by means of sulphuric acid and twice as much water. Mr. GRAY directs 2 ℔ of oil of vitriol to 112 ℔ of oil. The oil should be carefully washed from the acid, and filtered.

Mr. BANCROFT'S process for refining common olive oil, lard, oil, &c., for lubricating purposes, is to agitate them with from 3½ to 8 per cent. of caustic soda ley, of 1·2 specific gravity. If on trial of a small quantity the ley be found to settle clear at the bottom, enough has been added. The oil is allowed to rest for 24 hours, for the soapy matter to subside; the supernatant oil is then filtered.

Another plan of purifying oils (especially lamp oils,) is to agitate them with a strong solution of common salt.

The above methods of treating oil are of doubtful propriety in reference to such as are to be used as medicines. Oils which have been so carefully prepared from sound and fresh materials as to require no purification should be selected for this purpose. This is especially important in reference to cod-liver oil. See LINSEED OIL.

OIL FOR MACHINERY. Sperm oil, palm oil, and olive oil, are used. Care should be taken that they are not adulterated. For compound lubricants see *Anti-attrition*, and LUBRICATING COMPOUNDS.

OLEINE. This may be prepared by boiling fine olive oil with absolute alcohol, and evaporating the solution.

OXYGENATED WATER, OR DEUTOXIDE OF HYDROGEN. THENARD'S oxygenated water is thus made:—Expose fragments of perfectly pure barytes to a current of oxygen gas, in a green glass tube heated to dull redness, to form a deutoxide of barium. To 7 oz. of water add as much pure muriatic acid as will dissolve 4 dr. of barytes; add to this, by degrees, 3 dr. of pulverized deutoxide of barium, and when this is dissolved, add sulphuric acid, drop by drop, till the barytes falls down in the state of sulphate. Then add more deutoxide, and precipitate by sulphuric acid as before. Then filter the solution; and repeat the solution and precipitation several times, till about 3 oz. of deutoxide of barium is used, filtering the liquid after every second repetition. Sulphate of silver is then added to remove the hydrochloric acid, and afterwards pure barytes, to throw down the sulphuric acid, and a few drops of diluted sulphuric acid to remove any excess of barytes.

This energetic compound must not be confounded with the oxygen water formed by impregnating water with oxygen gas; nor with the oxygenous aerated water of Searle, which is water strongly charged with protoxide of nitrogen.

OXYGEN GAS. See GASES.

PAPER, COPYING. Mix lard with black lead or lamp-black, into a stiff paste, and rub it over writing paper with flannel, and wipe off the superfluous quantity with a soft rag. These sheets alternated with writing paper, and written on with a solid pen, produce 2 or 3 copies of a letter at once.

Lithographic Paper. Give the paper 3 coats of thin size, 1 of starch, and 1 of solution of gamboge. Each to be applied with a sponge, and allowed to dry before the next is applied.

Hydrographic Paper. This name has been given to paper which may be written on with water. It may be made by rubbing paper over with a mixture of finely powdered galls and sulphate of iron heated till it becomes white. The powder may be pressed into the paper by passing it between rollers, or passing a heavy iron over it. A mixture of dried sulphate of iron and ferro-prussiate of potash may be used for blue writing.

Or the paper may be imbued with a strong solution of one ingredient, thoroughly dried; and the other applied in powder. Paper which has been wet with a solution of ferro-prussiate of potash also serves for writing on with a colourless solution of persulphate of iron.

Iridescent Paper. Nut-galls 8 parts, sulphate of iron 5, sal ammoniac 1, sulphate of indigo 1, gum Arabic ⅛th. To be boiled in water, and the paper washed with it exposed to ammonia.

Photographic Paper. See PHOTOGRAPHIC PREPARATIONS, below.

Tracing Paper. Paper well wetted with Canada balsam and camphine, and dried. Another kind is made with nut oil and oil of turpentine; the paper is moistened with it, and then rubbed with flour. A temporary tracing paper is made by moistening paper with pure alcohol: it must be used while wet.

Waxed Paper. Lay the paper on a clean hot iron plate, and rub it over with a piece of white wax enclosed in a muslin.

FIRE PROOFING FOR PAPER. Dip it in a strong solution of alum, and then dry it. Should the paper be extra thick, the same process may be repeated.

PAPER PASTE. Boil white paper in water for 5 hours; then pour off the water, and pound the pulp in a mortar; pass it through a sieve, and mix with some gum water or isinglass glue. It is used in modelling by artists and architects.

PAPIER-MACHÉ. A plastic material, formed of cuttings of white or brown paper, boiled in water, and beaten to a paste in a mortar, and then mixed with a solution of gum Arabic in size, to give tenacity. It is variously manufactured by being pressed into oiled moulds, afterwards dried, covered with a mixture of size and lamp-black, and varnished.

PAPYRINE. Dip white unsized paper for ½ a minute in strong sulphuric acid, and afterwards in water containing a little ammonia. When dried it has the toughness and appearance of parchment.

PARAFFINE. Liquid and solid paraffine are obtained from

the tarry product of the distillation of peat, by first distilling off the lighter tar oil, then the residue separately. The crystallized paraffine is separated by a hair sieve, melted, cast into moulds, pressed in a stearine hot-press, at a temperature not exceeding 100°; then re-distilled, and the same process repeated till it is obtained perfectly pure. The liquid paraffine is re-distilled, and burned in lamps. The solid is made into candles.

PASTES. See BLACKING PASTE, FURNITURE PASTE, &c., above. For flour paste, see CEMENTS. For almond paste, honey paste, and tooth pastes, see COSMETICS.

Paste for Cleaning Brass, &c. 1. Rotten stone in very fine powder 2 oz., soft soap 1 oz., oil of amber 1 dr.

2. Neat's-foot oil 16 oz., water of ammonia 1 oz., powdered rotten stone sufficient to form a paste.

3. Rotten stone 4½ ℔, oxalic acid (dissolved in the water) 2 oz., soft soap 8 oz., sweet oil 8 oz., oil of amber 1 oz., boiling water 1 ℔. Some substitute oil of turpentine for oil of amber.

Paste for Razors. 1. Emery very finely levigated in the same manner as prepared chalk, mixed with lard, or tallow, or a mixture of these with neat's-foot oil.

2. Equal parts of jewellers' rouge, black lead, and prepared suet.

3. PRADIER'S. Best putty powder 1 oz., jewellers' rouge 1 oz., scales of iron ½ oz., levigated Turkey stone 3 oz., beef suet 1½ oz.

4. Mix equal parts of dried sulphate of iron and salt, and apply a gradually increased heat, in a closed vessel. Pulverize, elutriate, and mix with lard or tallow.

PASTILLES, AROMATIC. See PERFUMERY.

PAYNE'S PROCESS FOR RENDERING WOOD FIRE-PROOF. The wood is introduced into a close vessel, which is exhausted of air; the liquid is then admitted, and forced in by the pump till the pressure is from 110 to 140 ℔ to the square inch. The liquids employed are the liquid sulphuret of calcium, or of barium; a solution of sulphate of iron is afterwards forced into the wood.

PERCUSSION CAPS, Priming for. 100 gr. of fulminating mercury are triturated, with a wooden muller on marble, with 30 gr. of water and 60 gr. of gunpowder. This is sufficient for 400 caps. Dr. URE recommends a solution of gum mastic in turpentine as a medium of attaching the fulminate to the cap.

PHOSPHORESCENT OIL. Dissolve 1 gr. of phosphorus in 1 oz. of olive oil in a test tube by the heat of hot water, or add a larger quantity to some oil of lavender, in which it will dissolve spontaneously. Keep in a close phial.

PHOSPHORUS. See Pocket Formulary.

PHOSPHORUS MATCHES. See LUCIFERS. The old phosphorus bottles with sulphur matches were made by melting phosphorus with a fourth part of wax in the bottles placed in warm water, and turning them about so as to coat the sides.—GRAY.

PHOSPHORUS PASTE FOR VERMIN. Introduce 1 dr. of phosphorus into a Florence flask, and pour over it 1 oz. of rectified spirit. Immerse the flask in hot water, until the phosphorus has melted, then put a well-fitting cork into the mouth of the flask, and shake briskly until cold. The phosphorus is now reduced to a finely divided state. This, after pouring off the spirit, is to be mixed in a mortar with 1½ oz. of lard. Five oz. of flour and 1½ oz. of brown sugar, previously mixed together, are now added, and the whole made into a paste with a little water. Cheese may be substituted for sugar when the paste is intended for rats or mice. (There is said to be no danger whatever of spontaneous ignition, either during or after the preparation of this paste.)—PHARM. JOURNAL.

PHOTOGRAPHIC COMPOUNDS. For the manipulations of the art, see the several treatises on the subject.

PHOTOGRAPHIC SOLUTIONS. 1. *Solution of Common Salt.* This is made of various strengths, with 1 part of salt to 6, 8, 10, 20, and 25 parts of water.

2. *Solution of Nitrate of Silver.* This consists of pure crystallized nitrate of silver dissolved in distilled water. The strength varies from 20 to 120 gr. of the nitrate to each ounce of water.

3. *Gallo-nitrate of Silver.* Dissolve 100 gr. of crystallized nitrate of silver in 2 oz. of distilled water, and add 2 fluid dr. and 40 minims of acetic acid. Mix these

at the time of using with an equal measure of cold saturated recently prepared solution of gallic acid. It is used in preparing Calotype paper.

4. *Bromide Solution.* This consists of 40 gr. of bromide of potassium to 1 oz. of distilled water.

5. *Iodide Solution.* Dissolve 100 gr. of iodide of potassium in 4 oz. of distilled water.

6. *Hyposulphite Solution.* Dissolve 1 oz. of pure hyposulphite of soda in a pint of distilled water.

7. *Barytic Solution.* Muriate of barytes (chloride of barium) 35 gr., distilled water 2 oz.

8. *Sal Ammoniac Solution.* Dissolve 40 gr. of muriate of ammonia in 4 oz. of water.

9. *Chromate Solution* (*simple.*) A saturated solution of bichromate of potash. A little sulphate of indigo is sometimes added to vary the colour.

10. *Compound Chromate Solution.* Dissolve 10 gr. of bichromate of potash and 20 gr. of sulphate of copper in an ounce of water.

11. *Hydriodate of Iron and Barytes Solution.* Hydriodate of barytes 40 gr., water 1 oz., pure sulphate of iron 5 gr.; mix, filter, add a drop or two of diluted sulphuric acid, and when settled, decant the clear liquor for use.

12. Mr. TALBOT'S *Aceto-nitrate of Silver.* Nitrate of silver 60 grains, acetic acid 80 gr., distilled water 1 ounce.

For solution of Chlorate of Potash, and of Ammonio-Citrate of Iron, no definite formulæ have been met with.

PHOTOGRAPHIC ETCHING ON STEEL. Process of Mr. FOX TALBOT. Some bichromate of potash is dissolved in a strong solution of gelatine, and this is poured on the surface of the steel plate, and dried. A yellow coating is thus formed. Upon this is placed the object to be copied, as fern leaves, grasses, or pieces of lace; they are pressed closely by a piece of glass, and exposed to sunshine. By this the salt is decomposed, and the chromic acid, by acting on the gelatine, produces in the exposed parts a brown opaque surface, which is comparatively insoluble in water. The plate being placed in water, the gelatine is dissolved off the steel opposite the super-imposed object. A solution of bichloride of platinum being now poured on the plate, the lines are rapidly etched in. The plate being then washed until all the gelatine is removed, it is submitted to the operation of the copper-plate printer. Very beautiful prints of grasses, textile fabrics, &c., have been obtained in this way.

PHOTOGRAPHIC PAPERS. [The paper should be the finest satin post paper, of uniform texture, free from the maker's mark, specks, and all imperfections. The papers must be prepared by candle-light, and kept in the dark till used.]

1. *Simple Nitrated Paper.* This is merely paper brushed over with a strong solution of nitrate of silver. In brushing over the paper, it must not be crossed. Its sensitiveness is increased by using spirits of wine instead of water. This paper only requires washing in water to fix the drawing.

2. *Muriated Paper.* The paper is first soaked in solution of common salt, pressed with a linen cloth or blotting-paper, and dried. It is then brushed over on one side (which should be marked near the edge) with the solution of nitrate of silver, and dried at the fire. The stronger the solution, the more sensitive the paper. If the barytic solution, No. 7, be used instead of common salt, richer shades of colour are obtained. The sal ammoniac solution, No. 8, gives a very sensitive paper. A due proportion must be observed in the silver and salt solutions.

Mr. HUNT gives the following as proper proportions:—Sensitive paper for the camera. 50 gr. of common salt to 1 oz. of water; and 120 gr. of nitrate of silver to 1 oz. of water. Or, 60 gr. of the nitrate, with the solution No. 8. Or, 100 gr. with the solution No. 7.—Less sensitive for copying engravings, botanical and entomological specimens, &c. The salt solution to contain 25 gr. of salt to 1 oz. of water. The silver solution, 90 gr. in 1 oz.—Common, for copying lace-work, feathers, patterns, &c. The salt solution 20 gr., the silver solution, 40 gr. to an ounce. To fix the drawings on these papers, they must be first washed in lukewarm water, then dipped twice in the solution of hyposulphite of soda, No. 6; then in pure water, and dried.

3. *Iodized Paper.* Brush over the paper on one side (which should be marked) with strong solution of nitrate of silver (100 gr. to 1 oz.;) then dip it in the solution No. 5; wash it in distilled water, drain, and dry it.

4. *Bromide Paper.* Soak the paper in the solution No. 4; then brush it over with strong solution of nitrate of silver, and dry in the dark.

5. *Calotype Paper.* Brush iodized paper (3) with the gallo-nitrate of silver (solution No. 3,) and mark the side; in half a minute dip it into water, and press it between blotting paper. It is then ready for the camera, where it remains from half a minute to five minutes. When removed from the camera, dip it into water, press it between blotting paper, and wash it with a solution of 100 gr. of bromide of potassium in 8 or 10 oz. of water.

6. *Chromatype Paper.* Soak the paper in the solution No. 9, and dry it at a brisk fire. To fix the drawing, careful immersion in warm water is all that is required. It is not sufficiently sensitive for the camera.

7. *Compound Chromatype Paper.* Wash the paper with the solution No. 10, and dry it. After the paper has been exposed to the sun with the article to be copied superposed upon it, it is washed over in the dark with a solution of nitrate of silver of moderate strength. A vivid picture makes its appearance, which is sufficiently fixed by washing in pure water. For copying engravings, &c. Another method is to brush writing paper over with a solution of 1 dr. of sulphate of copper in 1 oz. of water; and when dry, with a strong but not saturated solution of bichromate of potash.

8. *Cyanotype Paper.* Brush the paper over with a solution of ammonio-citrate of iron. Expose the paper in the usual way, then wash it over with a solution of ferrocyanide of potassium.

9. *Crysotype Paper.* Wash the paper with solution of ammonio-citrate of iron, dry it, and afterwards brush it over with a solution of ferrocyanide of potassium. Dry

it in a dark room. The image is brought out by brushing it over with a neutral solution of gold or of silver.

10. *Catalisotype.* Steep paper in water with a drop or two of hydrochloric acid, absorb the superfluous moisture with blotting paper; brush over with a mixture of ½ dr. syrup of iodide of iron, 2½ dr. of water, and a drop or two of tincture of iodine. Dry with blotting paper, and brush over with a solution of 12 gr. of nitrate of silver to 1 oz. of distilled water. It is then ready for the camera. The picture is fixed by washing in water and afterwards in a solution of bromide of potassium (20 grains to 1 ounce.)

11. *Paper for Positive Photographs.* Most of the preceding give negative pictures, the lights and shadows being reversed; in the following they are correct. Wash highly-glazed paper with the solution No. 8, dry it, and brush it over with the following solution:—Dissolve 120 grains of crystallized nitrate of silver in 1½ oz. of distilled water; and add 1½ oz. of alcohol; after it has stood a few hours, filter it. Expose the paper thus washed to the sunshine till it is darkened; if mottled, wash it a second time, and expose it again. To use this paper, wash it over with the solution No. 11, expose it in the damp state, with the engraving or other object on it to the light, and fix the drawing by washing with water only. [To copy objects, lay them on a plate of clear glass fixed in a frame, place the prepared paper over them, and fix a back with a cushion attached to it so as to press the paper closely on the glass. The glass is then exposed to the light, and the drawing afterwards fixed, as described above. For feathers, lace-work, and other objects which freely admit light through them, the nitrated paper and less sensitive muriated papers may be used. For copying engravings, leaves and other botanical objects, or entomological specimens, the more sensitive muriated papers, or the bromide paper, or other sensitive kinds, may be used. Engravings should be wetted and placed with their face to the prepared side of the paper, and kept in close contact with it. Leaves should have their under surface next the glass. For the camera the most sensitive

samples of the muriated papers, made with not less than 100 grains of the nitrate of silver to the ounce, are selected. The calotype is still more certain. The papers intended for the camera require to be very carefully prepared. Glass is used instead of paper, after being coated with white of egg, or collodion, with which the compounds of silver are mixed, or over which they are brushed.

PHOTO-LITHOGRAPHY. Process of M. NIEPCE. Dissolve some of the bitumen called Jew's pitch in essential oil of lavender, and spread over the surface of the stone a uniform layer of this solution. Having obtained a camera picture by any of the calotype processes, adjust it over the stone by means of a glass, and expose it thus to the sunshine for about ¾ of an hour. The parts of the resin exposed to the rays are rendered more soluble in spirit than the rest. The stone is next immersed in spirit for a brief period, and then placed under flowing water, and well washed. The parts acted on by the sun should alone be dissolved, and the remainder left. The lithographic stone is now prepared for printing in the ordinary way, and the resin is removed from the other parts.

PIGMENTS. A few of these have been noticed before; see INDIGO, LAKES, PRUSSIAN BLUE, PURPLE OF CASSIUS. They generally constitute a distinct branch of manufacture, but a brief account of the composition of some of them may be useful. Those of which the colouring matter is derived from the animal and vegetable kingdoms will first be noticed; then the mineral colours.

Carmine. Several processes have been published for this beautiful pigment, but probably some minute precautions, not generally known, may be necessary to the production of the finest quality. The climate and state of the atmosphere are said to influence the result.

1. *Madame* CENETTE'S *process.* Into 6 pails of boiling clear, soft water, in a copper vessel, throw 2 ℔ of powdered cochineal of good quality; boil for 2 hours, add 3 oz. of purified nitre, and after a few minutes, 4 oz. of salt of sorrel. Remove the vessel from the fire, let the contents settle for 4 hours, draw off the clear

liquor with a syphon into flat plates, and leave it at rest for 3 weeks. Carefully detach the pellicle of mould from the surface, withdraw the liquid with a syphon and pipette, and dry the deposit in a stove.

2. Boil 4 quarts of soft water in a pewter kettle, add to it 4 oz. of finely powdered cochineal; boil for 5 minutes, adding 2 dr. of powdered cream of tartar; then add 8 scruples of Roman alum, and keep the whole on the fire for a minute longer. Let the decoction settle, decant it into cylindrical glasses, and cover them. When the carmine has subsided, pour off the clear liquor, and dry the sediment. By adding solution of tin to the liquid, more carmine is obtained.

3. Into a 14-gallon boiler of tinned copper put 10 gallons of distilled water, or filtered rain water; when it boils, sprinkle in, by small quantities, 1 ℔ of powdered cochineal, and keep it boiling for half an hour. Then add 3½ oz. of crystallized carbonate of soda; in a minute or two, draw the fire, and add 1½ oz. of Roman alum in fine powder; stir with a glass rod till the alum is dissolved, leave it to settle for 25 minutes, draw off the liquor with a glass syphon, and strain the rest through a coarse linen cloth. Clean the boiler, return into it the clear coloured liquor, and stir into it the whites of 2 eggs, previously well beaten with a quart of warm (not hot) water. Then light the fire, and heat the liquor till it begins to boil; separate the coagulum by filtration, wash it on the filter with distilled water, spread it thinly on earthen plates, and dry it in a stove.

Inferior carmine may be improved by dissolving it in water of ammonia, and precipitating it by acetic acid and alcohol.

Cochineal Lake. Add 2 ℔ of pearlash to the red liquor from which the carmine has been prepared in the last process, and return it to the boiler with the dregs of the cochineal; boil for half an hour, draw the fire, and when the sediment has subsided, draw off the clear liquor into an earthen vessel. Pour on the sediment a solution of 1 ℔ of pearlash in 2 gallons of water, and boil for half an hour. Filter, and return both liquors into the copper. When as hot as the hand can bear, add to the liquor, by little and little, 3 ℔ of powdered Roman alum, and let it simmer for 5 minutes. Allow it to settle, draw off the clear liquor, collect the sediment on a filter, wash it with clean rain water, and leave it covered with a cloth for a few days, till half dry; form it into small lumps, and dry them in a stove.

Carthamine, or Safflower Lake. Wash safflower till the water comes off colourless; mix it with water holding 15 per cent. of carbonate of soda in solution, so as to form a thick paste; leave it for several hours, then press out the red liquid, and nearly neutralize it with acetic acid. Then put cotton into it, and add successive small portions of acetic acid, so as to prevent the liquid becoming alkaline. In 24 hours take out the cotton, wash it, and digest it for half an hour in water holding 5 per cent. of crystallized carbonate of soda in solution. Immediately on removing the cotton, supersaturate the liquid with citric acid, and collect the precipitate, which must be repeatedly washed in cold water. For pink saucers the liquid is allowed to deposit in the saucers. Mixed with the scrapings of French chalk it constitutes rouge.

Lakes are also obtained from Brazil-wood and madder, by adding alum to a concentrated decoction of the former, or to a cold infusion of the latter (made by triturating the madder, enclosed in a bag, with the water,) and afterwards sufficient subcarbonate of potash or soda to throw down the alumina in combination with the colouring matter. The precipitate is to be washed and dried. A little solution of tin added with the alum improves the colour. Lakes may be obtained from most vegetable colouring matters by means of alum and an alkaline carbonate. *Yellow Lake* is made from French or Persian berries, by boiling them in water, with a little soda or potash, and adding alum to the strained liquor as long as a precipitate is thrown down. Or by boiling weld, or quercitron bark, in water, and adding alum and chalk in a pasty state.

Rose Pink. Boil 6 ℔ of Brazil-wood and 2 ℔ of peach-wood in water, with ¼ ℔ of alum; and pour the strained decoction on 20 ℔ of sifted whiting.

Bistre. It is obtained from the soot of beech-wood.

Sap Green. The expressed juice of buckthorn berries (and sometimes of other species of rhamnus, and also of privet berries) is allowed to settle, and the clear liquid evaporated to dryness. A little gum-Arabic is sometimes added to the juice.

MINERAL PIGMENTS. *Azure Blue, or Smalts.* The common is made by fusing zaffre (roasted cobalt ore calcined with siliceous sand) with potash. A finer quality is obtained by precipitating a solution of sulphate of cobalt by a solution of silicate of potash. Another cobalt blue is obtained by adding a solution of phosphate of soda to a solution of nitrate of cobalt, and mixing the precipitate, washed, but not dried, with eight times its weight of fresh hydrated alumina. When dry, heat it to a cherry red.

Ægyptian Azure. Carbonate of soda 16 oz., calcined flints 24 oz., copper filings 4 oz. Pulverize, mix, and fuse in a crucible for two hours. When cold reduce to powder.

Blue Verditer. It is generally stated to be made by adding chalk to a solution of nitrate of copper produced in the process of refining silver: but Mr. PHILLIPS did not succeed in making it by this means, and found no lime in the best samples.

New Blue. Mix equal parts of common arseniate of copper (see Mineral Green, below,) and neutral arseniate of potash, fuse by heat in a large crucible, then add to the fused salt ⅕ of its weight of nitre. Effervescence takes place, and the salt becomes blue. Cool, pulverize, and wash.

Chrome Yellow. To a solution of bichromate of potash add a solution of nitrate of lead as long as a precipitate forms. Wash the precipitate, and dry it with a gentle heat. An inferior kind is said to be made by 4 ℔ of pure white lead, 1 ℔ of bichromate of potash, and 20 ℔ of water, and boiling till the water becomes colourless.

Chrome Red. Melt saltpetre in a crucible heated to dull redness, and add chrome yellow, by small portions, till no more red fumes arise. Allow the mixture to settle; then pour off the melted salt from the heavy sediment, and wash the latter with water, which should be quickly poured off, and dry the pigment. The liquefied salt poured off contains chromate of potash, and is reserved for making chrome yellow.

Orange Chrome is chrome yellow acted on by an alkali, which deprives it of part of the chromic acid.

King's Yellow. This is a yellow sulphuret of arsenic, now almost superseded by chrome yellow, but occasionally used for killing flies.

Naples Yellow. Mix 12 parts of metallic antimony, 8 parts of red lead, and 4 of oxide of zinc, and calcine in a reverberatory furnace. The mixed oxides are rubbed together, fused, and the fused mass elutriated into a fine powder.—Dr. URE. M. GUIMEL recommends 1 part of well washed antimoniate of potash to be ground into a paste with 2 parts of red lead, and the powder exposed to a red heat for 4 or 5 hours, keeping the heat moderate.

Brighton Green. An inferior colour, made with 28 ℔ of whiting, or white lead, 7 ℔ sulphate of copper, 3 ℔ sugar of lead, and ¼ oz. of bichromate of potash.

Brunswick Green. Pour a saturated solution of muriate of ammonia over copper filings in a close vessel placed in a warm situation; add more of the solution from time to time till three parts of the muriate have been used to two of copper. After standing for a few weeks the pigment is separated from the unoxidized copper by washing through a sieve. It is then to be well washed, and dried slowly in the shade. It is often reduced with white lead; some samples contain arsenic.

Arsenical Copper Greens. Of these there are several varieties.

Mineral Green, Scheele's Green, or Arsenite of Copper. 1. Dissolve 11 oz. of white arsenic and 2 ℔ of carbonate of potash, by heat, in a gallon of water. Dissolve also 2 ℔ of sulphate of copper in 3 gallons of water. Filter each solution separately, and add the former gradually to the latter as long as it occasions a precipitate. Wash the precipitate, drain it and dry it.

2. Dissolve 50 lb of sulphate of copper and 10 lb of lime in 20 gallons of good vinegar, and add quickly a boiling hot solution of 50 lb of white arsenic. Stir repeatedly, then allow it to settle; decant the clear liquor (which is reserved to dissolve the arsenic next time,) and wash the precipitate, and dry it.

3. *Emerald Green.* Mix 10 parts of pure verdigris with sufficient boiling water to form a soft pulp, and strain this through a sieve. Dissolve 9 or 10 parts of white arsenic in 100 parts of boiling water, and, whilst boiling, let the verdigris pulp be gradually added, constantly stirring the mixture till the precipitate becomes a heavy, granular powder.

Green without Arsenic. Dissolve 48 lb of sulphate of copper and 2 lb of bichromate of potash in water, and add to the clear solution 2 lb of pearlash and 1 lb of chalk.

Rinman's Green Pigment. Dissolve together in sufficient water 1 part of sulphate of cobalt, and 3 of sulphate of zinc; precipitate with carbonate of soda, wash the precipitate, and calcine it.

Chrome Green. A mixture of chrome yellow and Prussian blue. [See also Chrome Oxide, p. 336.]

Barth's Green. A mixture of Prussian blue and yellow lake.

Ultramarine, Factitious. Take 70 parts of silica, or pure siliceous sand, in fine powder; 240 parts of recrystallized alum, calcined; 144 parts of sulphur; 48 parts of finely powdered charcoal; 240 parts of dry carbonate of soda. These are mixed together with the greatest care till the mixture appears of uniform colour under a powerful magnifier, and the mixture exposed to a moderate red heat in a closely covered crucible for an hour and a half. Wash the product with boiling water. Mix the powder with its own weight of sulphur and 1½ its weight of dried soda, and burn as before; heat it again with sulphur and soda, and wash it till the filtered fluid no longer colours acetate of lead. If a sample of the dried powder becomes blue when burnt with sulphur, it is ready for the last operation. Spread over a cast iron plate a layer of sulphur a line in thickness, and over it an equal layer of the dried powder after having passed it through a gauze sieve. Heat the plate so as to burn away the sulphur at the lowest possible temperature. Reduce the pigment to powder and repeat the burning with sulphur and pulverization till the colour is perfect.

White Lead is carbonate of lead, prepared by various processes. *Zinc White* is oxide of zinc, prepared by combustion. *Antimony White* is oxide of antimony.

PLATES, DAGUERREOTYPE, are prepared by cleaning and polishing the silver surface, exposing it to the vapour of dry iodine or tincture of iodine, or iodide of bromine, or bromide of lime. After having the image thrown on them, they are exposed to the vapour of mercury. But the manipulations and precautions necessary to the success of the operation are too numerous to detail here.

PLATE-BOILING POWDER. Equal parts of cream of tartar, alum, and common salt. A small quantity added to the water in which plate is boiled gives it a silvery whiteness.

PLATE POWDERS. 1. *Jewellers' Rouge.* Dissolve green vitriol in hot water, and add a solution of pearlash, as long as it throws down a precipitate. Wash the precipitate repeatedly with warm water, drain it on calico, and finally calcine it till it assumes a bright colour. It is sometimes made by calcining the sulphate of iron with a strong heat till oxide of iron only remains. Let it be triturated with water, and prepared in the same way as prepared chalk. See POLISHING POWDER, below.

2. *French Plate Powder.* Mix one part of jewellers' rouge with 12 of carbonate of magnesia.

3. Finely prepared chalk, or burnt hartshorn. One way in which these are used is to boil them with water, with pieces of rag; the finer particles are entangled in the fibres of the rags, which are dried and kept for use.

4. Quicksilver with chalk 1 oz., prepared hartshorn 8 oz., prepared chalk 4 oz. Powders containing quicksilver, besides the necessary wearing of the surface, are

supposed to render the plate more brittle. If used, it should not be in larger proportion than the above.

5. Finest putty powder 1 oz., levigated chalk 5 oz.; a little rouge may be added to colour it.

See NOVARGENT, SILVERING POWDER, &c., for restoring the silver to plated goods.

PLATINA, BLACK (OXIPHOROUS.) Dissolve protochloride of platinum in a boiling solution of potash, add alcohol in small portions till all effervescence ceases. Boil the black precipitate successively with alcohol, muriatic acid, and potash, and finally 4 or 5 times with water.

PLATINATED ASBESTOS. Dip asbestos in a solution of chloride of platinum, and heat it to redness. It causes the inflammation of hydrogen in the same manner as sponge platina.—Dr. HARE.

PLATINIZED SILVER. Silver plates for SMEE'S voltaic battery are covered with pulverulent platinum by adding a little bichloride of platinum to acid water, and decomposing the solution by the use of a platinum terminal in connexion with the copper of a battery, the silver plate to be platinized being in connexion with the zinc. Platinum itself is sometimes platinized in the same way. Sometimes the plates are platinized without the battery. The following solution is used by Dr. WRIGHT for the plates of his battery: Saturated solution of chloride of platinum ½ drachm, sulphuric acid 1½ drachm, water 2 drachms. Dip the plates in it for a few seconds, and wash them quickly.

PLATINUM, CHLORIDES OF. Dissolve platinum in nitro-muriatic acid, and evaporate with a gentle heat to dryness. The red bichloride remains. Heated to 450° the protochloride remains.

PLATINUM SPONGE. Dissolve separately in rectified spirit chloride of platinum and sal ammoniac. Mix the solutions, and heat the precipitate to redness. For balls for hydrogen lamps, form the precipitate into balls while moist, and afterwards burn them.

POISON. See BEETLE WAFER, BUG POISONS, and RAT POISON.

POLISH. See FRENCH POLISH.

POLISH FOR BOOTS, &c. See BLACKING.

POLISHING POWDER FOR SPECULA. LORD ROSS. Precipitate a dilute solution of sulphate of iron by ammonia in excess; wash the precipitate, press it in a screw press till nearly dry; then expose it to heat until it appears of a dull red colour in the dark.

POT POURRI. See PERFUMERY.

POTASH, CARBONATE OF. *Salt of Tartar.* Mix 10 parts of pearlash with 6 of water; let them stand in a cool place for 24 hours, stirring them frequently: filter, concentrate the solution by a gentle heat, stirring constantly; remove from the fire as soon as the liquor begins to appear opaque, and continue the stirring until cold. To procure it purer redissolve it in an equal weight of distilled water, filter, and evaporate to dryness. It is free from sulphate of potash, but contains 1·1 per cent. of chloride of potassium.

POTASH, CHLORATE. See CHLORATE OF POTASH.

POUNCE. Powdered gum juniper is used under this name for preparing parchment for writing on. For liquid pounce, see INK, MARKING.

POUDRE CLARIFIANT. Beat together the whites and yolks of eggs, dry them with a very gentle heat, and reduce to powder. For clarifying wines and syrups.

POWDERS. See TOOTH POWDERS, AND HAIR POWDERS, under COSMETICS; SCENT POWDERS, under PERFUMERY, &c.

PRESERVATIVE LIQUIDS. See ANATOMICAL SUBJECTS, and ANIMAL SUBSTANCES, TO PRESERVE.

PRUSSIATE OF POTASH (YELLOW.) What is known in commerce by this name is the ferro-prussiate of potash, or ferrocyanide of potassium. It is prepared by fusing in an egg-shaped iron pot a mixture of 2 parts of pearl-ash, and 5 parts of dry animal matters, such as horns, hoofs, tallow-chandler's greaves, &c., till fetid vapours cease to be produced. Iron filings are sometimes added, but usually the iron necessary to the formation of this salt is derived from the iron pots and stirrers. The fused mass (*prussiate cake*) is allowed to cool, dissolved in warm water, and the clear filtered or decanted solution evaporated, that crystals may form. These are dissolved in hot water, and the solution allowed to cool very slowly, that large crystals may form.

RED PRUSSIATE OF POTASH. *Ferrid-cyanide of Potassium.* Into a dilute solution of the above prussiate of potash a current of chlorine gas is passed, till the solution ceases to give a blue precipitate with persalts of iron. It is then evaporated, crystallized, and recrystallized till quite pure. [M. POSSELT advises to add a few drops of solution of potash to the boiling liquor, to decompose the green matter that is formed; to filter the hot solution, to separate some peroxide of iron which is thrown down, and to let the liquor cool very slowly.] Or, boil yellow prussiate of potash with 12 or 15 parts of water, and while boiling add good chloride of lime until a filtered sample no longer yields a blue precipitate with persalts of iron. Filter quickly, and add carbonate of potash till the liquid has a faintly alkaline reaction, then evaporate for crystallization.—CHEMIST, vol. viii.

PRUSSIAN BLUE. *Percyanide, ferrocyanide, or ferro-prussiate of iron.* Commercial Prussian blue is made by adding to a solution of prussiate of potash, or of prussiate cake, a solution of 2 parts of alum and 1 of sulphate of iron, washing the precipitate repeatedly with water, to which a little muriatic acid has been added, and exposing it to the air till it assumes a deep blue colour. A purer kind is made by adding a solution of persulphate or perchloride of iron to a solution of pure ferroprussiate of potash. TURNBULL'S Prussian blue (ferridcyanide of iron) is made by adding a solution of red prussiate of potash to one of proto-sulphate of iron; or by adding proto-sulphate of iron to a mixture of yellow prussiate of potash, chloride of soda, and hydrochloric acid.

SOLUBLE PRUSSIAN BLUE. Add a solution of proto-sulphate of iron to a solution of prussiate of potash, and expose the precipitate to the air till it becomes blue, and wash it till the soluble salts are washed away. By continuing the washing, the blue itself dissolves, forming a deep blue solution, which may be evaporated without decomposition. Or add a solution of persulphate of iron to a solution of ferro-prussiate of potash, keeping the latter in excess; wash the precipitate until it begins to dissolve, and dry it. See INK, READE'S *patent Blue*, for another method.

PURPLE OF CASSIUS. See Aurum Stanno-paratum, Pocket Formulary. Many other processes have been proposed, of which the following is one:—Dissolve 3 gr. of gold in aqua regia, avoiding excess, and dilute with 3 oz. of water. Mix 30 gr. of pink salt (the bichloride of tin with sal ammoniac) with 3¼ gr. of tin filings and 2 dr. of water till the tin is almost entirely dissolved; add 7 dr. of water, and add this solution to the gold solution, slightly warmed. Wash the precipitate, and dry it.

PYROLIGNEOUS ACID, PYROXYLIC SPIRIT, PYROACETIC SPIRIT, &c. By the destructive distillation of dried wood, chiefly that of the beech and birch, in iron cylinders, an acid liquor and tar are produced. These are received in proper reservoirs, and are afterwards separated. The tar is subjected to distillation, and yields *oil of tar* (containing creasote, eupione, &c.,) and leaves a residuum of pitch, or English asphalt. The acid liquor, separated from the tarry deposit, is also distilled; the first portion which comes over contains the pyroxylic spirit, which is rectified by one or more distillations. It may be further purified by distilling it with dried muriate of lime, and finally with quicklime. This constitutes one of the articles sold under the name of naphtha, and is regarded by chemists as a hydrated oxide of methule. After the pyroxylic spirit has come over, the crude pyroligneous acid distils, which still holds some tar and empyreumatic oil in solution. It is purified by saturating it either directly with common soda, or first with lime, or rather chalk, and when the neutral solution has become clear, evaporating it to 1·114 sp. gr., and adding sufficient saturated solution of sulphate of soda to decompose the impure acetate of lime. The clear solution obtained by either process is then evaporated, that the acetate of soda may crystallize. This is afterwards roasted at a temperature of about 500° Fahrenheit, to destroy the tar, and again dissolved and crystallized. The purified acetate is then distilled with sulphuric acid, to obtain a purer pyroligneous or acetic acid. See Acidum Aceticum, P. F. For some manufacturing purposes, an impure acid is obtained by merely saturating the crude pyroligneous acid with lime, evaporating to dryness, and distilling with sulphuric acid.

If acetate of lime or acetate of lead be distilled without addition, and the liquid which comes over be rectified over lime, *pyroacetic spirit* is obtained: this is also termed *acetone*.

PYROPHORUS. This name is given to several compounds, prepared by calcination, which take fire when exposed to the air, especially when breathed upon. The following are perhaps some of the best:—

1. Heat tartrate of lead in a tube of hard glass, and securely close the tube before the charred residuum becomes cold. A little poured out and breathed upon takes fire. The tartrate of lead is made by dissolving separately 2 dr. of tartaric acid and 5 dr. of crystallized acetate of lead in sufficient water, mixing the solutions, and collecting, washing, and drying the precipitate.

2. Calcine tartar-emetic in a similar manner, or in a close crucible.

3. Mix 11 parts of lamp-black with 2 of powdered sulphate of potash, and heat the mixture strongly in a closely-covered crucible. The product is so combustible that it can scarcely be transferred to a bottle without danger.

4. Mix 3 parts of powdered alum with 1 of flour, and calcine the mixture in a common phial, coated with clay or placed in sand, till it ceases to emit a blue flame. Before it is cold, close it securely with a sound cork or glass stopper.

5. Mix neutral chromate of lead with 1-6th its weight of sulphur; triturate them with water sufficient to form a paste, and make it into pellets; dry these perfectly, then heat them in a tube till the sulphur is all driven off, and secure as the last.

RAT AND MICE POISONS. [Such as contain *arsenic* are placed first, and afterwards several compounds which have been introduced as substitutes for that mineral, which has proved so destructive of human life. According to a recent act of Parliament, this dangerous compound can only be purchased in wholesale quantities. Among other precautions taken to prevent accident, it is provided that it be mixed with colouring matters, such as soot and indigo, in order to prevent its being taken by mistake, or ensure detection if designedly administered.]

Arsenical Paste (authorized by the Government of France.) Melt 2 ℔ of suet in an earthen vessel over a slow fire, and add 2 ℔ of wheat flour, 3 oz. of levigated white arsenic, 2½ dr. of lamp-black, 15 drops of oil of aniseed. It may be used alone, or mixed with bread crumbs, &c. [For destroying rats and mice.]

2. For barn floors. Mix a pint of good flour with as much yellow arsenic as will lie on a shilling; put this in a small heap on the floor, and over this put another pint of good flour unmixed. Draw a track up to the heap with a feather dipped in oil of aniseed and oil of caraways, and sprinkle this over with a little flour.*

3. Mix a quart of the best oatmeal, 2 oz. of powdered loaf sugar, 6 drops each of the oils of rhodium, caraway, and aniseed, and ¼ gr. of musk. Mix them very perfectly without touching the mixture with the hands. Place in a retired place 6 or 8 pieces of clean board, and on each two tablespoonfuls of the powder, for a few successive nights, without disturbing the rats. About the sixth night, if they are found to eat freely, mix a teaspoonful of white arsenic with the powder. What remains in the morning should be burnt, avoiding the fumes.—THE CHEMIST, vol. vi.

4. White arsenic 2 oz., carbonate of barytes 2 oz., white sugar 3¾ oz., rose pink ¼ oz., oil of aniseed and oil of rhodium, of each 5 drops.

5. Malt flour 1 ℔, oil of rhodium 3 drops, sugar 2 oz., 8 cloves, a tablespoonful of caraway seeds, all beaten in a mortar. Lay it in small parcels where they frequent, for 3 or 4 nights, till they eat freely, then add some arsenic dissolved in spirit of salts.—MAYER.

6. *Ointment for Rats in Ricks.* Mix together 1 ℔ of fresh butter, free from salt, 1½ oz. of calomel, 8 oz.

* The following is an old rat-catcher's receipt for oils to attract rats:—Two dr. of oil of aniseed, 2 drops of nitrous acid, and 2 gr. of musk. Oil of rhodium is also supposed to be very attractive to these vermin. Assafœtida with these oils is also used.

of crumbs of white bread, 2 oz. of sugar, 5 drops each of oils of nutmeg and rhodium, and 2 drops of oil of aniseed. To use it, make a hole with the arm under the ridge; into this hole insert a stick, and on the middle of it, where it does not touch the rick, put a lump of the ointment. *For Traps.* Put the same, with 2 or 3 drops of oil of thyme.

7. *Hampshire Millers' Rat Powder.* Mix 1 oz. of nux vomica in powder with a pound of fresh oatmeal, and add a few drops of oil of rhodium, or what answers better, oil of aniseed with musk.

8. *Philanthrope Muophobon.* A French preparation so called consists of 1 part of emetic tartar to 4 of farinaceous and other ingredients.

9. Put into a flask 2 dr. of phosphorus and 5 or 6 oz. of water, put the flask in warm water (about 150° Fahrenheit) till the phosphorus is liquefied; pour the contents into a mortar, and immediately add 5 or 6 oz. of rye-meal; when cool, add the same quantity of melted fresh butter, and 4 oz. of sugar.

10. Another form of the phosphorus compound is—Melt 1 ℔ of lard in a bottle plunged in water, and heated to 150° Fahrenheit. Introduce into it ½ oz. of phosphorus, and add a pint of proof spirit. Cork the bottle securely after its contents have been heated to 140° or 150°, and taking it out of the water-bath, agitate it briskly till the phosphorus is uniformly diffused; repeat the agitation occasionally as it cools, and when cold, pour off the spirit which has separated (which may be reserved for the same purpose,) and incorporate with the fatty compound wheat, flour and sugar. Oil of rhodium or aniseed may be added. Place little lumps of this in the rat-holes, and set some water near for them to drink. For a third receipt, see *Phosphorus Paste for Vermin*, p. 402.

11. Valentia almonds 1 oz., treacle 2 oz., carbonate of barytes 1 oz., oil of aniseed 5 drops, flour enough to form a paste.

12. Powdered squill ½ oz., strong cheese 2 oz. Mix, and form into balls. *For Mice.*

RENNET. The stomach of a calf, washed, salted, and dried.

RENNET LIQUID. ESSENCE OF RENNET. Fresh Rennet 12 oz., salt 2 oz., proof spirit 2 oz., white wine a quart; digest for 24 hours, and strain. A quart of milk requires 2 or 3 teaspoonfuls. WISLIN directs, 10 parts of a calf's stomach, salt 3 parts. The membrane of the stomach is to be cut with scissors, and kneaded with the salt, and the rennet found in the interior of that organ; the whole left in a cool place in an earthen pot till the cheesy odour is replaced by the proper odour of rennet, which will be in 1 or 2 months. Then add 16 parts of water and 1 of spirit. Filter, and colour with burnt sugar.

RUST, TO PREVENT AND REMOVE. Steel goods are rubbed over with a mixture of lime and oil, to preserve them from rusting. Mercurial ointment has been recommended for the same purpose. M. PAYEN recommends plunging the articles into a solution of common soda. Spots of rust are removed by rubbing them with fine emery and sweet oil. As a chemical means of removing them, the ammoniacal chloride of zinc may be found useful. See ZINC.

SAXON BLUE. See CHEMIC BLUE. The solution of indigo in sulphuric acid, diluted with twice its weight of water, is so termed.

SCOURING DROPS, FOR REMOVING GREASE. 1. Alcohol (pure) 6 oz., camphor 2 oz., rectified essence of lemon 8 oz.

2. Camphine 3 oz., essence of lemon 1 oz.; mix. Some direct them to be distilled together.

3. *French.* Camphine 8 oz., pure alcohol 1 oz., sulphuric ether 1 oz., essence of lemon 1 drachm.

4. Spirit of wine a pint, white soap 3 oz., ox-gall 3 oz., essence of lemon ¼ oz.

SEALING-WAX. 1. *Blue.* Shell-lac 2 parts, dammar rosin 2 parts, Burgundy pitch 1 part, Venice turpentine 1 part, artificial ultramarine 3 parts.

2. *Light Blue.* As the last, with 1 part of dry sulphate of lead.

3. *Dark Blue.* Venice turpentine 3 oz., finest shell-lac 7 oz., clear amber or black resin 1 oz., Prussian blue 1 oz., carbonate of magnesia 1½ dr. The last two to be made into a stiff paste with oil of turpentine, and added to the melted shell-lac and Venice turpentine.

Black. 1. Venice turpentine 4½ oz., shell-lac 9 oz., colophony ½ oz., lamp-black mixed to a paste with oil of turpentine q. s.

2. Inferior. Venice turpentine 4 oz., shell-lac 8 oz., 3 oz. of colophony, and sufficient lamp-black mixed with oil of turpentine to colour it.

3. Shell-lac 8 oz., Venice turpentine 4 oz., lamp-black 6 oz.

4. Common, for bottles. Rosin 6 oz., shell-lac 2 oz., Venice turpentine 2 oz., lamp-black q. s.

Brown. 1. *Light Brown.* Venice turpentine 4 oz., shell-lac 7½ oz., brown earth (English umber?) ½ oz., cinnabar ½ oz., prepared chalk ½ oz., carbonate of magnesia moistened with oil of turpentine 1½ drachm.

2. *Light Brown*—Second quality. Venice turpentine 4 oz., shell-lac 7 oz., rosin 3 oz., English umber 3 oz., cinnabar ¼ oz., prepared chalk 1 oz., magnesia as the last.

3. *Dark Brown.* Venice turpentine 4 oz., fine shell-lac 7½ oz., English umber 1½ oz., magnesia as before.

4. *Dark Brown.*—Second quality. Venice turpentine 4 oz., shell-lac 7 oz., colophony 3 oz., English umber 1½ oz., magnesia as before.

Green. Venice turpentine 2 oz., shell-lac 4 oz., colophony 1¼ oz., King's yellow ½ oz., Prussian blue ¼ oz., magnesia as for brown.

Gold. 1. Venice turpentine 4 oz., fine shell-lac 8 oz., leaf-gold 14 sheets, bronze powder ½ oz., magnesia (made into a paste with oil of turpentine) 1½ drachm.

2. Use gold talc instead of gold leaf and bronze.—GRAY.

Marbled. Melt each coloured wax separately, and just as they begin to grow solid, mix together.—GRAY.

Red. 1. *Fine Carmine Wax.* Venice turpentine 2 oz., finest shell-lac 4 oz., colophony 1 oz., Chinese vermilion 1½ oz., magnesia (moistened with oil of turpentine) 1½ dr.

Finest Red. Venice turpentine 4 oz., shell-lac 7 oz., cinnabar 4 oz., carbonate of magnesia (with oil of turpentine) 1½ dr.

3. As the last, with only 3½ oz. of cinnabar.

4. Venice turpentine 4 oz., shell-lac 6½ oz., colophony

½ oz., cinnabar 2½ oz., magnesia (with oil of turpentine) 1½ dr.

5. Venice turpentine 4 oz., shell-lac 6 oz., colophony ¾ oz., cinnabar 1¾ oz., magnesia as before.

6. As last, but use colophony and cinnabar each 1½ oz.

7. Venice turpentine 4 oz., shell-lac 5½ oz., colophony 1½ oz., cinnabar 1¼ oz., magnesia as before.

8. *English.* Venice turpentine 2 oz., shell-lac 4 oz., vermilion 1 oz.

9. *Spanish.* Venice turpentine 8 oz., shell-lac 2 oz., colophony 4 oz., vermilion 1 oz. Remove from the fire, and add ½ oz. rectified spirit.

Yellow. Venice turpentine 2 oz., shell-lac 4 oz., colophony 1¼ oz., King's yellow ¾ oz., magnesia as before.

Perfumed Wax. Add to any of the above a small quantity of fine benzoin.

Common Bottle Wax. 1. Dark rosin 18 oz., shell-lac 1 oz., bees'-wax 1 oz. Melt together, and colour with red lead, Venetian red, or lamp-black.

2. Rosin 19 oz., bees'-wax 1 oz.; colour as before.

SHELL-LAC, to bleach. See LAC, page 389.

SILK CLEANER. Mix well together a ¼ ℔ of soft soap, a teaspoonful of brandy, ½ pint of proof spirit, and ½ pint of water. It is to be spread with a sponge on each side of the silk without creasing it; the silk is then rinsed out two or three times, and ironed on the wrong side.

SILVERING POWDER, &c., for silvering copper, covering the worn parts of plated goods, &c. 1. Nitrate of silver 30 gr., common salt 30 gr., cream of tartar 3½ dr. Mix. Moistened with water and rubbed on dial plates or other copper articles, it coats them with silver.

2. Silver precipitated from its nitric solution by copper 20 gr., alum 30 gr., cream of tartar 2 dr., salt 2 drachms.

3. Precipitated silver ½ oz., common salt 2 oz., muriate of ammonia 2 oz., corrosive sublimate 1 dr.; make it into a paste with water. Copper utensils are previously boiled with tartar and alum, and rubbed with this paste, then made red-hot, and afterwards polished.

4. Dissolve muriate of silver in a solution of hyposulphite of soda, and mix this with prepared hartshorn or other suitable powder.

SILVERING PASTE. Nitrate of silver 1 part, cyanide of potassium (Liebig's) 3 parts, water sufficient to form a thick paste. Apply it with a rag. A bath for the same purpose is made by dissolving 100 parts of sulphite of soda, and 15 of nitrate of silver, in water, and dipping the article to be silvered into it.

For SILVERING GLASS, see GLASS.

SILVER, TO PURIFY AND REDUCE. Silver, as used in the arts and coinage, is alloyed with a portion of copper. To purify it, dissolve the metal in nitric acid slightly diluted, and add common salt, which throws down the whole of the silver in the form of chloride. To reduce it into a metallic state several methods are used:—1. The chloride must be repeatedly washed with distilled water, and placed in a zinc cup; a little diluted sulphuric acid being added, the chloride is soon reduced. The silver when thoroughly washed is quite pure. In the absence of a zinc cup, a porcelain cup containing a zinc plate may be used. The process is expedited by warming the cup.

2. Digest the washed chloride with pure copper and ammonia. The quantity of ammonia need not be sufficient to dissolve the chloride. Leave the mixture for a day, then wash the silver thoroughly.—HORNUNG.

3. Boil the washed and moist chloride in solution of pure potash, adding a little sugar: when washed, it is quite pure.

SILVER, SOLVENT FOR. See page 427.

SIZE. *Oil size* is made by grinding yellow ochre or burnt red ochre with boiled linseed oil, and thinning it with oil of turpentine. *Water size* (for burnished gilding) is parchment size ground with yellow ochre.

SMALTS. See PIGMENTS.

SMOKING FLUID. One drop of creosote in a pint of water imparts a smoky flavour to fish or meat dipped into it for a few minutes.

SOAP. For PERFUMED AND TOILET SOAPS, see page 241. For the manufacture of soaps generally see Dr. URE'S Dictionary of the Arts, and other similar works. Hard soaps are made by boiling oils or fats with a ley of caustic soda. Soft soaps consist of oil and potash; and as they do not separate from the ley like the hard soaps, they generally contain an excess of caustic alkali. Silica soap has silicate of soda incorporated with it. Soap is adulterated by earthy matters, as pipe-clay, &c.; these and other impurities remain when soap is dissolved in alcohol.

SOAP, MARINE. *Patent.* This is made by substituting cocoa-nut oil for the fats and oils used in the manufacture of common soap. It has the advantage of forming a lather with salt water.

SODA. For its medical and pharmaceutical compounds, see Pocket Formulary.

SODA, HYPOSULPHITE OF. Dissolve 1 ℔ of crystallized carbonate of soda in a quart of boiling water. Slake ½ ℔ of lime in another quart of water. Mix the solutions, let them stand in a covered vessel until cold, pour off the clear liquid, and boil it with more sulphur than it will dissolve. Pour off the clear solution into a deep vessel, and pass sulphurous acid gas through it until it becomes nearly colourless. While still a little yellow, filter, and evaporate it quickly in an earthen vessel to a syrupy consistence. Shake this with half its bulk of rectified spirit, and allow the lower layer to crystallize under the alcoholic solution which floats on it. It must be kept from the air and light.

SOLVENTS FOR INDIAN RUBBER. *Æther* for this purpose should be agitated with water, and decanted. *Benzole* will dissolve caoutchouc with warmth and long digestion. *Rectified coal naphtha* forms an imperfect solution employed in MACKINTOSH'S water-proof fabrics. *Oil of turpentine,* rendered pyrogenous by absorbing it with bricks or porous ware, and distilling it without water, and treating the product in the same way, is also used for this purpose. It is stated that the solution on evaporation does not leave the caoutchouc in a sticky state. Another method is to agitate oil of turpentine repeatedly with a mixture of equal weights of sulphuric acid and water; and afterwards expose it to the sun for some time. *Bisulphuret of carbon* is a good solvent, dissolving the gum without heat. This constitutes PARKES' Patent Solvent. *Chloroform* is an excellent but rather expensive solvent. *Caoutchoucine* has also been employed as a solvent. It is prepared by distilling Indian rubber without addition, increasing the heat to 600° Fahr. The product is rectified by distilling it with one-third of water. It is then a colourless fluid of ·680 specific gravity. Its smell is improved by agitating it with 5 oz. of nitro-muriatic acid to each gallon. Indian rubber is rendered more readily soluble by first digesting it with a solution of carbonate of soda, or water of ammonia.

SOLVENTS FOR GUTTA PERCHA. Benzole readily dissolves it. So do chloroform and bisulphuret of carbon.

SOLVENT FOR OLD PUTTY AND PAINT. Soft soap mixed with solution of potash or caustic soda; or pearlash and slaked lime mixed with sufficient water to form a paste. Either of these laid on with an old brush or rag, and left for some hours, will render it easily removable.

SOLUBLE GLASS. See GLASS.

SOLUTIONS USED IN ELECTROTYPE MANIPULATIONS, &c.

For the Decomposing Cell. 1. Saturated solution of sulphate of copper 2 parts, sulphuric acid 2 parts, water 6 or 8 parts. 2. Mr. WALKER directs 2 measures of a saturated solution of sulphate of copper, and 1 measure of acidulated water (1 part of sulphuric acid to 9 of water.) 3. ROBELL'S solution consists of 2 parts of a saturated solution of sulphate of copper, and 1 part of a saturated solution of Glauber's salt, to which as much sulphate of copper has been added as it will take up.

2. *Gold Solution.* Dissolve 2 oz. of cyanide of potassium (by LIEBIG'S method) in a pint of warm distilled water, add ¼ oz. of oxide of gold, and agitate together.

3. *Silver Solution.* Dissolve 2 oz. of LIEBIG'S cyanide of potassium in a pint of distilled water; add ¼ oz. of moist oxide of silver (precipitated by lime-water from a solution of the crystallized nitrate,) and agitate together till the oxide is dissolved.

4. *Solution in which Steel Articles are dipped before Electroplating them.* Nitrate of silver 1 part, nitrate of mercury 1 part, nitric acid (sp. gr. 1·384) 4 parts, water 120 parts.

5. *Solution, or Pickle, for immersing Copper Articles*

in before Electroplating. Sulphuric acid 64 parts, water 64, nitric acid 32, muriatic acid 1. Mix. The article, free from grease, is dipped in the pickle for a second or two.

SOLUTION FOR MULLINS' VOLTAIC BATTERY. *In contact with the Zinc:* 1 part of sal ammoniac to 5 of water. *In contact with the copper;* a saturated solution of sulphate of copper. M. BACHHOFFNER uses a saturated solution of common salt and a saturated solution of sulphate of copper.

SOLUTION FOR SOLDERING. Dissolve zinc in muriatic acid to saturation, add pulverized sal ammoniac, and boil for a short time. Applied with a sponge or feather it facilitates the flow of the solder.

SOLUTIONS FOR THE WATER-BATH. Various salts dissolved in water materially raise the boiling point, and thus afford the means of obtaining a steady temperature at different degrees above 212°. The following are some of the most useful:—

A saturated	solution of	nitrate of soda	boils at	246
"	"	Rochelle salts ·	"	240
"	"	nitre . . .	"	238
"	"	muriate of soda	"	224
"	"	sulphate of magnesia	"	222

SOLVENT FOR SILVER. *Nitro-sulphuric Acid.* Dissolve 1 part of nitre in 10 parts of oil of vitriol. Used for dissolving the silver from plated goods, &c. It dissolves silver at a temperature below 200°, and scarcely acts upon copper, lead, and iron, unless diluted. The silver is precipitated from the solution, after moderately diluting it, by common salt, and the chloride reduced as directed page 424.

SPIRIT OF NITRIC ETHER. See P. F. It need only be added here, that its acidity is removed and prevented by rectifying it from neutral tartrate of potash.

SPONGE, BLANCHED. Soak the sponges for several days in cold water, renewing the water and squeezing the sponges occasionally. Then wash them in warm water, and place them in cold water to which a little muriatic acid has been added. Next day take them out and wash them thoroughly in soft water; then immerse them in aqueous sulphurous acid (sp. gr. 1·034) for a week. They are afterwards washed in plenty of water, squeezed, and allowed to dry in the air. For burnt, prepared, and waxed sponge, see SPONGIA, P. F.

STAINS, FOR WOOD, IVORY, &c. See IVORY, TO STAIN; WOOD, STAINS FOR; BOOKBINDERS' STAINS, &c.

STAINS, TO REMOVE. Stains of *iodine* are removed by rectified spirit. *Ink* stains by oxalic acid or superoxalate of potash. *Iron Moulds* by the same; but if obstinate, it has been recommended to moisten them with *ink*, then remove them in the usual way.

Grease Spots. See SCOURING DROPS.

Red Spots on black cloth from acids, are removed by spirits of hartshorn, or other solutions of ammonia.

Stains of Marking Ink or Nitrate of Silver, to remove. 1. Wet the stain with fresh solution of chloride of lime, and after 10 or 15 minutes, if the marks have become white, dip the part in a solution of ammonia or of hyposulphite of soda. In a few minutes wash with clean water.

2. Stretch the stained linen over a basin of hot water, wet the mark with tincture of iodine.

3. They may also be removed by cyanide of potassium; but this should be done by the druggist, and not intrusted to any one else.

STARCH. Starch is procured from various roots and seeds. Its varieties are numerous; but a few of the most important only can be noticed here.

Arrow-root (West Indian.) The fæcula of the tubers of the Maranta arundinacea. The fresh tubers are washed and beaten to a pulp, which is well stirred in a large tub of cold clean water, and the fibrous part wrung out by the hands, and thrown away. The water in which the fæcula is suspended is passed through a hair sieve or coarse cloth, allowed to settle, and the water poured off. After being repeatedly washed, the wet starch is drained, and afterwards dried in the sun. [The other varieties of arrow-root (see page 282) are prepared by analogous processes from the roots which yield them.]

Potato Starch. The tubers are washed and peeled, usually by machinery, rasped by a revolving grater, and the pulp washed on hair sieves till freed from the starchy matter. Successive portions of the pulp are thus treated till the vessel over which the sieves are placed is sufficiently full. The starch held in suspension in water subsides to the bottom; the water is then drawn off, and the starch stirred up with fresh water, and again allowed to subside. This is repeated several times till the starch is sufficiently pure. The fibres and the washing waters are used as manures. The washed fibres have also been recommended as an ingredient in bread for diabetic patients.

Wheat Starch. Wheat flour is steeped in water for a week or two and allowed to ferment. The acid liquor is drawn off, and the residue washed on a sieve: what passes through is allowed to settle, the sour liquor drawn off, and the starch thoroughly washed from the slimy matter. It is then drained in perforated boxes, cut up into square lumps, placed on bricks to absorb the moisture, and dried in a stove. See Dr. PEREIRA'S Elements.

Various means are adopted to free the starch from gluten and other impurities. In the patent rice starch, and probably other kinds of starch, alkaline solutions are used. Ammonia has been recommended, as it does not, like potash and soda, dissolve any portion of pure starch.

The various kind of fæcula are distinguishable by the form of their particles or grains. By a microscopical examination of these the mixture or substitution of potato starch with the more expensive kinds is readily detected. Figures of the different kinds of starch grains are given in the Pharmaceutical Journal, vol. iv., in Dr. PEREIRA'S Elements, &c. M. GOBLEY has proposed to distinguish them by the coloration produced when the several kinds are exposed to the vapour of iodine; but the effect seems to depend greatly on the relative dryness of the samples.

STEARINE, STEARIC ACID. Fat is saponified, and the soap decomposed by an acid, with a large quantity of water, the mixture being kept warm and well stirred. The water being drawn off, the fatty matter is well washed, allowed to cool, and submitted to strong pressure.

STORM GLASS. Take 2½ dr. of camphor, 38 gr. of nitre, and 38 gr. of sal ammoniac; dissolve them in 9 dr. of water, and 6 dr. of rectified spirit, with a gentle heat. It is placed in a glass tube covered with a brass cap, with a small hole to admit air. Or it may be put in an eau de Cologne or other long bottle, tied over with bladder. Its various changes are supposed to indicate changes of weather, but the indications are not to be relied on.

STUFFING BIRDS AND ANIMALS, PREPARATIONS FOR. 1. Camphor 1 oz., corrosive sublimate 1 oz., alum ½ oz., sulphur 1 oz.; all finely powdered and mixed.

2. Tanner's bark dried and powdered 2 oz., burnt alum 1 oz., snuff 1 oz.; mix, and add arsenic ¼ oz., camphor ¼ oz., sulphur 1 dr.

3. BÉCŒUR'S *Arsenical Soap.* Camphor 5 dr., arsenic 4 oz.; white soap 4 oz., carbonate of potash 12 oz., air-slaked lime 4 oz.; make a stiff paste with a little water.

STYROL. Mix 20 parts of storax with 7 of carbonate of soda, and put them into a retort with water, and apply heat. A limpid fluid distils, which becomes when heated to a certain point a transparent solid.

SUGAR RESIN. Mix 16 parts of strong sulphuric acid with 8 of the strongest nitric acid; when cooled to 70° Fahr. stir in 1 part of finely powdered sugar. In a few seconds, when the sugar has become pasty, take it out of the acid and plunge it into cold water. Add more sugar to the acid, and proceed as before. Wash the resinous matter carefully, and dissolve it in alcohol or ether. Evaporate the solution with a gentle heat. It is very combustible. Its solution may be used to render gunpowder, lucifer matches, &c., waterproof.

SULPHATE OF COPPER. To a concentrated solution of bisulphate of potash, add a cold solution of sulphate of copper, filter, and heat gently.

SULPHO-CYANIDE OF AMMONIUM. Saturate 2 parts of common water of ammonia (sp. gr. ·950) with sulphuretted hydrogen; and add 6 parts of the same ammonia. To this mixture add 2 parts of sulphur, and the product of the distillation of 6 parts of prussiate of potash, 3 of sulphuric acid, and 18 of water. Digest till the sulphur is no longer acted on, and the liquid becomes yellow. Boil the liquid till it becomes colourless, filter, evaporate, and crystallize.

SULPHURET OF CARBON. See BISULPHURET OF CARBON.

SYRUP OF MILK. Evaporate with constant stirring, 6 ℔ of skimmed milk to 3 ℔; add 4½ ℔ of sugar; dissolve with a gentle heat, and strain. It may be flavoured with the addition of 1 oz. of cherry-laurel water. [For other Syrups see P. F.] Milk may be preserved by first heating it, and when cold, charging it with carbonic acid gas.

TANNIN. See ACID, TANNIC, page 310.

TERPINE. Leave oil of turpentine for a long time in contact with a mixture of nitric acid and alcohol. Crystals of terpine form. By boiling an aqueous solution of terpine with a small quantity of sulphuric or other acid, *terpinole* is formed, and may be separated by distillation. It has the odour of hyacinths.

TEST LIQUORS, TEST PAPERS, &c. Distilled water only should be used in these preparations. In preparing the papers, the liquid should be placed in an earthenware plate or dish, and the paper carefully immersed in it so as to be uniformly wetted, then dried out of the reach of acid, ammoniacal, or other vapours, likely to affect it: and afterwards kept in bottles, jars, or cases. Dr. FARADAY recommends unsized paper, but Mr. PARNELL and other good authorities direct good letter paper to be used.

Brazil Paper. Dip paper in a strong decoction of Brazil wood, and dry it. [It is rendered purple or violet by alkalies; generally yellow by acids.]

Cabbage Paper. Make a strong infusion of red cabbage leaves, strain it, and evaporate it by a gentle heat till considerably reduced. Then dip the paper in it, and dry it in the air. [This paper is of a grayish colour; alkalies change it to green, acids to red. It is a very delicate test: if rendered slightly green by an alkali, carbonic acid will restore the colour.]

Dahlia Paper. From the petals of violet dahlias, as cabbage paper.

Elder-berry Paper. This is merely paper stained with the juice of the berries. Its blue colour is changed to red by acids, and to green by alkalies.

Indigo Paper. Immerse paper in sulphate of Indigo, wash it with water rendered slightly alkaline, then with pure water, and dry it in the air.

Iodide of Potassium and Starch Paper. Mix starch paste with solution of iodide of potassium, and moisten bibulous paper with it. [It becomes blue when exposed to ozone. Chlorine has the same effect.]

Lead Paper. Paper dipped in a solution of acetate of lead. [When moistened it detects sulphuretted hydrogen, which renders it black.]

Blue Litmus Paper. Bruise 1 oz. of litmus in a mortar, and add boiling water; triturate together, put them in a flask and add boiling water to make up to half a pint; when cool, strain it, and dip paper in it. More colour may be extracted from the litumus by hot water, but the liquid will require to be concentrated by evaporation. [Acids change the colour to red, but it does not become green with alkalies.]

Red Litmus Paper. As the last, adding to the strained infusion a few drops of nitric acid, or of pure acetic acid. Dr. FARADAY recommends holding blue litmus paper over a large jar, into which a few drops of muriatic acid have been introduced, till sufficiently reddened.

Rose Paper. Make a strong infusion of the petals of the red rose, and dip unsized paper in it. Dipped in an alkaline solution, so weak as not to affect turmeric paper, it assumes a bright green colour.

Manganese Paper. Dip paper in a solution of sulphate of manganese. [It becomes black in an ozonized atmosphere.]

Rhubarb Paper. Dip paper in a strong infusion of rhubarb, and dry it. [Alkalies render it brown. It is not, like turmeric paper, affected by boracic acid.]

Starch Paper. This is merely paper imbued with starch paste. Cotton cord is sometimes used instead of paper. [As a test for iodine, which turns it blue.]

Turmeric Paper. Boil 1 oz. of coarsely powdered turmeric root in half a pint of water for half an hour, and strain: dip paper in the liquid, and dry it. [It is rendered brown by alkalies, and also by boracic acid and borates.]

TEST SOLUTIONS, &c. [The vegetable preparations are here placed first.]

Tincture and Infusion of Red Cabbage. Digest red cabbage with rectified spirit in a warm place for a few days; strain, and distil off most of the spirit, and evaporate what remains to the consistence of syrup. It will keep for years. When required for use, dilute it with a little water; or the concentrated infusion directed above for the paper may have a little spirit added to it. [If the cabbage leaves be well dried, they may be kept in a close vessel for use, and a strong infusion made when wanted.]

Acid Infusion of Red Cabbage. Dr. FARADAY directs one or more red cabbages to be cut up in strips, and boiling water poured on them, and a little dilute sulphuric acid (equal to ½ oz. of oil of vitriol to a large cabbage) to be added, and the whole kept for an hour or two in a copper or earthen vessel. It is then strained, the cabbage infused in a little more water and acid, and the mixed infusion evaporated to one-third its first bulk, allowed to settle, and put into bottles. When required for use, the acid is neutralized by caustic potash or soda. Another plan is to dry the leaves at 120°; and when required for use to make a strong infusion, adding a drop of sulphuric acid, to neutralize the strained infusion with marble, filter, and add a little spirit, if required to be kept.

Infusion of Tincture of Litmus. This is made as directed above for litmus paper. Or an ounce of powdered litmus may be triturated with 6 oz. of boiling water, digested near the fire for an hour, and mixed, when cool, with 2 oz. of spirit. Or digest 1 oz. of powdered litmus in a pint of proof spirit for 7 days. If required red, a few drops of acetic acid are added to either of these. The next day, decant the clear liquor. Dr.

PEREIRA directs 1 part of litmus to 25 of water. When made very strong, it must be diluted when used.

Tincture of Galls, Infusion of Galls, &c. Fresh powdered blue galls 1 oz., proof spirit 8 oz.; digest in a close vessel for a week, and filter. A watery infusion of galls may be made in the same proportion with boiling water for immediate use. PETTENKOFER directs 1 oz of powdered galls to be infused in 3 or 4 ounces of boiling water for several hours, and 2 oz. of salt added. After filtration, it retains its transparency and power of precipitating gelatine for years. [These are used to detect iron, with the salts of which it produces a black colour; for gelatine, which it precipitates in brownish-white flocks; and several of the organic alkaloids.]

MARSH'S *Dahlia Test.* Make a strong infusion of the petals of dark dahlias; strain, and add to every pint ½ oz. of strong sulphuric acid; stir with a glass rod, and when cold, add to each pint 2 gr. of corrosive sublimate. Filter through coarse cloth and bottle. When required for use, neutralize it carefully with ammonia, and use the liquid by dipping paper in it.

Syrup of Violets. On 4 oz. of fresh petals of violets pour half a pint of water at 104° Fahrenheit, stir them together, and in a minute or two strain off the water with gentle pressure, and pour 8 oz. of boiling distilled water on the flowers. In 12 hours, strain through linen, let the infusion settle, and decant, then dissolve in it twice its weight of refined sugar, by a gentle heat. [A delicate test for acids and alkalies.]

Dr. CLARK'S *Test for Hardness of Water.* Dissolve 1 oz. of Hawe's best white soap in a gallon of proof spirit. If not of such strength that it requires 32 measures to be added to 100 measures of solution of chloride of calcium of 16 degrees of hardness (see below) before it lathers, it must be adjusted to that strength. [The chloride of calcium solution is thus made:—Dissolve 16 grains of pure carbonate of lime in a small quantity of pure hydrochloric acid, avoiding loss from effervescence; evaporate the solution to dryness, and dissolve the residue in water, and again evaporate till a neutral solution is obtained; then dissolve in a gallon of water. This forms the standard solution of 16 degrees of hardness. One measure of this solution with 15 of distilled water constitutes a solution of one degree of hardness; and so on up to 16 degrees. The degree of hardness expresses the number of grains of carbonate of lime per gallon contained in the water. For the mode of using this test, see Dr. CLARK'S pamphlet, or PARNELL'S Chemical Analysis.]

Solution of Carbonate of Ammonia. Mr. PARNELL directs this test to be prepared by dissolving 1 part of sublimed carbonate of ammonia in 3 of water, and adding 1 part of water of ammonia.

Solution of Oxalate of Ammonia. Dissolve 1 oz. of crystallized oxalate of ammonia in a pint of water.

Solution of Sulphuretted Hydrogen. Pass sulphuretted hydrogen gas (see GASES, page 363) through cold distilled water, which has been recently boiled, till it will absorb no more. Keep it in small bottles securely closed.

Solution of Hydrosulphuret of Ammonia. Pass sulphuretted hydrogen gas (see page 363) through water of ammonia till the liquid occasions no precipitate in a solution of sulphate of magnesia.

Solution of Ammonio-nitrate of Silver. To a solution of nitrate of silver (1 part crystallized nitrate to 20 of distilled water) add gradually weak water of ammonia till a mere trace of the oxide first precipitated is left undissolved. Let it settle, decant it into a clean, stoppered bottle, and keep it from the light. The Edinburgh Pharmacopœia directs 44 grains of nitrate of silver to be dissolved in a fluid-ounce of water, and sufficient ammonia added, as above. [It gives a pale yellow precipitate with arsenious acid, and a chocolate red with arsenic acid; the same with their salts.]

Solution of Nitrate of Silver. The Edinburgh Pharmacopœia directs this test to be prepared by dissolving 40 grains of the nitrate in a fluid-ounce of distilled water. The London Pharmacopœia directs 60 grs. to a fluid-ounce. Mr. PARNELL recommends 1 part to 15 or 20 of water. [It is used chiefly for the detection of chlorine or muriatic acid. The precipitate, chloride of silver, is insoluble in nitric acid. Also for hydrocyanic acid, with which it gives a white precipitate, which is decomposed by heat, the silver being reduced.]

Solution of Ammonio-sulphate of Copper. Dissolve 1 drachm of sulphate of copper in 2 oz. of water, and add ammonia till the precipitate first thrown down is nearly all dissolved. Let it settle, and pour off the clear solution. [Chiefly used as a test for arsenical compounds, with which it gives a green precipitate.]

Solution of Chloride of Barium. Dissolve 60 grains of the chloride in a fluid ounce of distilled water.

Solution of Nitrate of Barytes. (Ed. Ph.) Dissolve 40 grains of nitrate of barytes in 800 grains of distilled water.

Solution of Indigo. Digest 1 part of fine indigo in 10 parts of oil of vitriol, and dilute with water.

HAHNEMANN'S *Wine Test, for detecting lead in wine.* Sulphuret of lime 3 oz., tartaric acid 3 oz., water 2 ℔, mix, decant, and add 1 oz. of tartaric acid. Or, simple sulphuretted hydrogen water 4 oz., tartaric acid 1 dr.

TROMMER'S *Test* for sugar in urine. Put some of the suspected urine into a large test-tube, and add a few drops of solution of sulphate of copper, then sufficient solution of potash to render it strongly alkaline. If sugar be present, the precipitated oxide redissolves into a blue liquid, and on boiling *red* oxide of copper is precipitated. [White merino that has been wet with a solution of bichloride of tin, is said to form a ready test for sugar in urine, &c. A portion wet with the suspected liquor, and exposed to 260 to 300° of heat, becomes blackened if sugar is present.] The following is proposed as a quantitative test for sugar: Dissolve 400 grains of pure crystallized sulphate of copper in 1600 grains of distilled water; add this gradually to a solution of 1600 grains of neutral tartrate of potash in a little water mixed with 6 or 7 thousand grains of solution of caustic soda, of 1·12 sp. gr. Add water to make up the whole 11,544 grain measures (26 fl. oz., 2 fl. dr., 54 minims.) 1000 grain measures are equivalent to 5 grains of grape sugar.

PETTENKOFER'S *Test* for bile, in urine, &c. Put a

small quantity of the suspected liquid into a test-tube, and add to it, drop by drop, strong sulphuric acid till it becomes warm, taking care not to raise the temperature above 122° Fahr. Then add from 2 to 5 drops of syrup, made with 5 parts of sugar to 4 of water, and shake the mixture. If the liquid contain bile, a violet coloration is observed. Acetic acid, and those substances which are converted into sugar by sulphuric acid, may be substituted for sugar.

TOBACCO WATER. See WASHES for vermin on plants.

TOUCH PAPER. Dip a piece of white blotting-paper, or printing-paper, in a solution of 1 oz. of nitre in 8 oz. of water. Dry it perfectly.

TREES, METALLIC. *Lead Tree.* Dissolve 1 oz. of sugar of lead in a quart of distilled or filtered rain-water, adding a few drops of acetic acid. Filter, and put the clear solution into a decanter or bottle. Suspend in it a piece of zinc, and set it aside.

Silver Tree. Dissolve 20 gr. of crystallized nitrate of silver in an ounce of distilled water; put it into a phial, and add about ½ a drachm of pure quicksilver.

Tin Tree. Dissolve 3 dr. of muriate of tin in a pint and a half of water, with 10 or 15 drops of nitric acid; and suspend in it a rod of zinc.

TURPENTINE, VENICE (factitious.) It is usually made by dissolving black resin in oil of turpentine. Dr. PEREIRA states the proportion to be 5 fluid oz. of the oil to 16 oz. of resin; but some makers put as much as 8, 10, or even 12 oz. of oil of turpentine to each pound of resin. [We have introduced this factitious preparation, because no genuine Venice (or larch) turpentine is now to be obtained.]

TURPENTINE, OIL OF. Common turpentine, chiefly American, is distilled with water; the oil comes over with the water, and is found floating on it. It is rectified by distilling it again with water. See CAMPHINE and SOLVENTS FOR INDIA RUBBER, for further modifications of this oil.

URN POWDER. Oxide of iron, crocus, or jeweller's rouge.

VARNISHES. These constitute a distinct branch of manufacture, and many of them can be advantageously or safely made only on the large scale on premises adapted for the purpose. A few of the most easily prepared and useful varnishes have been selected for insertion. For fuller information see Dr. URE's Dictionary of Arts, DUMAS' Chemie appliqué aux Arts, &c. Some practical information on the subject will be found in Mr. REDWOOD's edition of GRAY's Supplement, and in the 49th vol. of the Transactions of the Society of Arts.

Spirit Varnishes. The spirit employed should not be less than 60° overproof. In preparing and using them, they should be kept at a distance from a candle or other flame. Respecting the gums (resins) employed, it may be useful to mention that shell-lac is rendered more soluble by being powdered and exposed for a long time to the air; sandarach gives hardness to varnishes; mastic gives a gloss to a solution of other gums; benzoin still more, but its colour is objectionable; anime readily dissolves, but renders the varnish long in drying; copal and amber are scarcely soluble in spirit, but are rendered partially so by other gums, and also by being previously fused by heat. Shell-lac gives a durable varnish, objectionable only on account of its colour, which may be rendered paler by charcoal. See LAC.

1. *White Spirit Varnish.* Rectified spirit 2 gallons, gum sandarach 5 lb. Put them into a tin bottle, cork securely, and agitate frequently, placing the tin occasionally in hot water till the gum is dissolved, then add a quart of pale turpentine varnish.

2. *Brown.* Rectified spirit 2 gallons, sandarach 3 lb, shell-lac 2 lb, pale turpentine varnish a quart. Proceed as the last.

3. Sandarach 2 oz., shell-lac ½ oz., rectified spirit 16 fluid oz.

4. *White.* Gum sandarach 1½ oz., mastic ½ oz., elemi ¼ oz., foreign oil of lavender ¼ oz., rectified spirit 8 oz.

Copal Spirit, or Drying Varnish. Copal, fused and pulverized, 3 oz., sandarach 6 oz., mastic 3 oz., Venice turpentine 2½ oz., highly rectified spirit a quart, powdered glass 3 oz. Mix the powdered glass and resins, and sift them; introduce them into a matrass with the spirit, and heat to boiling, constantly agitating till the gums are dissolved; then add the turpentine. Heat the varnish for half an hour, and when removed from the fire, agitate till cold.

Brilliant Amber Spirit Varnish. Fused Amber 4 oz., sandarach 4 oz., mastic 4 oz., highly rectified spirit a quart. Expose to the heat of a sand-bath, with occasional agitation, till dissolved. [The amber is fused in a close copper vessel, having a funnel-shaped projection, which passes through the bottom of the furnace by which the vessel is heated.]

Chinese Varnish. Mastic 2 oz., sandarach 2 oz., rectified spirit a pint. Close the matrass with bladder, with a pin-hole for the escape of vapour; heat to boiling in a sand or water bath, and when dissolved strain through linen.

Crystal Varnish. Picked mastic 4 oz., rectified spirit a pint, animal charcoal 1 oz. Digest and filter.

French Polish and *Lacquers* are varieties of spirit varnishes. The former have already been noticed (page 354.) A few formulæ for the latter are here added:—

Pale or Gold Lacquers. To a pint of rectified spirit add as much gamboge as will give it a bright yellow colour, then add 12 oz. of seed-lac in fine powder, and set it in a sand-bath till dissolved. Or a tincture of annatto (1 part to 8 of spirit) may be added to give the desired colour.

Dark Lacquer. Clear seed-lac 1 ℔, dragon's blood 1 oz.; pulverize together, and add them to a pint and half of rectified spirit. Set in a warm place till dissolved.

Lacquer for Brass Work. Turmeric 1 oz., saffron ¼ oz., Spanish annatto ¼ oz., rectified spirit a pint. Digest at a gentle heat for several days; strain through coarse linen, put the tincture in a bottle, and add 3 oz. of good seed-lac coarsely powdered. Place in a moderate heat, and shake frequently till dissolved; if wanted of a redder shade, increase the quantity of annatto, or add a little dragon's blood. [Some makers prepare a strong tincture of the various colouring ingredients, and add them to the lacquer to produce the required shade.]

Oil of turpentine, and other essential oils, are used as solvents, forming essence varnishes, as the following:—

Mastic Varnish. Clean mastic 5 oz., rectified oil of turpentine (camphine) a quart. Digest in a warm place, shaking frequently till the solution is complete, then strain.

Picture Varnish. Chio turpentine 2½ oz., mastic 12 oz., camphor ½ dr., pounded glass 4 oz., rectified oil of turpentine 3 pints. For oil paintings.

Canada Varnish. Clear balsam of Canada 4 oz., camphine 8 oz.; warm gently, and shake together till dissolved. For maps, drawings, &c.; they are first sized over with a solution of isinglass, taking care that every part is covered; when dry, the varnish is brushed over it.

TINGRY'S *Essence Varnish.* Mastic in powder 12 oz., pure turpentine 1½ oz., camphor ½ oz., powdered glass 5 oz., rectified oil of turpentine a quart.

Common Turpentine Varnish. This is merely clear pale resin dissolved in oil of turpentine; usually 5 ℔ of resin to 7 ℔ of turpentine.

Oil Varnishes. These consist of copal and other gums dissolved by heat in boiled linseed oil; generally with the addition of oil of turpentine.

Cabinet Varnish. Fuse 7 ℔ of African copal, and pour on it 4 pints of hot clarified linseed oil (see OILS;) in 3 or 4 minutes, if it feels stringy, take it out of the building where there is no fire near, and when it has cooled to 150° mix in 3 gallons of oil of turpentine of the same temperature, or sufficient to bring it to a due consistence. [Various qualities of copal varnish are made for different purposes; inferior gums are often substituted for or mixed with copal.]

Amber Varnish. Amber 16 oz.; melt in an iron pot, and add ½ pint of drying linseed oil, boiling hot, and add 3 oz. of resin and 3 oz. of asphalte, each in fine powder. Stir till they are thoroughly incorporated; remove from the fire, and add a pint of warm oil of turpentine.

Common Oil Varnish. Resin 3 ℔, drying oil ½ a gallon; melt together, and add, when removed from the fire, 2 quarts of warm oil of turpentine.

Varnish for Printers' Ink. To every 10 ℔ of clarified linseed oil (page 391) add 5 ℔ of clear black resin, and ½ ℔ oil of turpentine. It is then ready for mixing with lamp-black or other colouring matter. A twelfth part of Canada balsam is sometimes added for the finer sorts.

A few miscellaneous varnishes are added.

Varnish for Engraving on Copper. Yellow wax 1 oz., mastic 1 oz., asphaltum ½ oz.; melt, pour into water, and form into balls for use. A softer varnish for engravers is made with 1 part of tallow and 2 of yellow wax; or with 2 oz. of wax, 1 dr. of common turpentine, and 1 dr. olive oil. See ETCHING VARNISHES, p. 350.

Varnish for Engraving on Glass. 1. Wax 1 oz., mastic ½ oz., asphaltum ¼ oz., turpentine ½ dr.

2. Mastic 15 parts, turpentine 7, oil of spike 4 parts.

LE BLOND'S *Varnish.* Keep 4 ℔ of balsam of copaivi warm in a sand or water bath, and add 16 oz. of copal, previously fused and coarsely powdered, by single ounces daily, and stir it frequently; when dissolved add a little Chio turpentine.

BESSEMER'S *Varnish,* for metallic paint. This is made with 8 ℔ of copal, 2½ gallons of drying oil, and 25 gallons of oil of turpentine. These are made into a varnish nearly as directed for Cabinet Varnish; and afterwards mixed with a gallon of slaked lime, and left for 3 days to settle. The clear portion is then drawn off, and 5 parts of varnish mixed with 4 parts of bronze powder.

MACKINTOSH'S *Caoutchouc Varnish.* Dissolve 1 ℔ of India rubber cut in shreds in a quarter of a pint of rectified coal naphtha. [Caoutchouc varnishes may be made with either of the solvents noticed above, page 425. The following are also used:—

India Rubber Varnish, for boots. Dissolve ¼ oz. of caoutchouc in 2 oz. of mineral naphtha. Dissolve also ½ oz. of asphaltum in 1 oz. of oil of turpentine. Mix the solutions.

Balloon Varnish. Melt India rubber in small pieces

with its weight of boiled linseed oil, and thin it with oil of turpentine.]

Varnish for Frames for Hot Beds. Mix 4 oz. of pulverized white cheese, 2 oz. of slaked lime, and 4 oz. of boiled linseed oil. Mix, and add 4 oz. each of whites and yolks of egg, and liquefy the mixture by heat. This curious mixture is said to produce a pliable and transparent varnish.

Coloured Varnishes. Oil varnishes are coloured by grinding with them the most transparent colours, as distilled verdigris for green, &c. Spirit varnishes are also coloured with dragon's blood, gamboge, &c.

Sealing-Wax Varnish. Black or coloured sealing-wax broken small, and sufficient rectified spirit to cover it, digested till dissolved. An article called black lac is sold as an economical substitute for black sealing-wax.

Black Japan, for Leather, &c. Boil together a gallon of boiled linseed oil, 8 oz. of umber, and 3 oz. of asphaltum. When sufficiently cool, thin it with oil of turpentine.

Japan for Tin-ware. 1. Common copal varnish. 2. Dissolve copal 2 oz., and camphor 1 dr., in oil of turpentine 8 oz.

Brunswick Black. Melt 4 ℔ of asphaltum, add 2 ℔ of hot boiled linseed oil, and when sufficiently cool add a gallon of oil of turpentine.

Varnish for Gun Barrels after browning them. Shell-lac 1 oz., dragon's blood ¼ oz., rectified spirit a quart. Dissolve and filter.

Transfer Varnish. Alcohol 5 oz., pure Venice turpentine 4 oz., mastic 1 oz.

Hair Varnish. Dissolve 1 part of clippings of pigs' bristles, or of horsehair, in 10 parts of drying linseed oil, by heat. Fibrous materials (cotton, flax, silk, &c.) imbued with the varnish and dried, are used as a substitute for hair-cloth.

Glass Varnish. This is a solution of soluble glass, and should be thus made:—Fuse together 15 parts of powdered quartz (or of fine sand,) 10 parts of potash, and 1 of charcoal. Pulverize the mass and expose it for some days to the air; treat the whole with cold water, which removes the foreign salts, &c. Boil the residue in 5 parts of water until it dissolves. It is permanent in the air, and not dissolved by cold water. *Used to protect wood, &c., from fire.*

VINEGAR. Vinegar may be made from wine or ale, by keeping it for some weeks or months in a warm place, with access of air. In this country it is usually made from malt, or a mixture of malted and unmalted barley, which is mashed as for beer and fermented with yeast. The fermented liquor is then placed in a warm room for many weeks in unclosed casks, and finished by transferring it into larger vessels with false bottoms, on which are placed the refuse raisins, &c., from which wine has been prepared. A much quicker method of acetification is sometimes employed: the fermented liquor is made to pass in drops into tubs filled with beech chips, so as to expose an extended surface to the action of the air. In Germany it is also made by the direct acetification of spirit by means of platina black. The method of preparing wood vinegar has already been noticed. (See PYROLIGNEOUS ACID.) The following is one of the processes followed in making vinegar from sugar:—Boil 10 gallons of water for 10 minutes with a quart of bran; run it into a tub through flannel, and put into it 12 ℔ of coarse brown sugar, and when cooled to 70° add a quart of yeast at three different times. Let it work for four days, then take off the yeast, and run the liquor into a clean tub. Fill the tub nearly with the liquor, leaving room for 2 ℔ of bruised crab apples and 1 ℔ of raisins. If it ferments, add a little reserved liquor, or water boiled with sugar, till the fermentation ceases. Then place the cask upon a plank fronting the sun in summer, and near the fire in winter. Put into it 1 oz. of isinglass well beaten up with a quart of old vinegar, cover the bunghole with a piece of hop-bag (fastened to the edge of the hole by pitch,) and lay a tile over it. Leave it in this state till it becomes fit for use. On a small scale, Dr. TURNER states that vinegar may be made from 120 parts of water, 12 of brandy, 3 of brown sugar,

1 of tartar, and ½ of sour dough, left some weeks in a warm place.

WAFERS, GELATINE. Dissolve fine glue or isinglass in such a quantity of water as that the solution, when cold, may be consistent. Pour it hot on a plate of mirror glass (previously warmed with steam and slightly greased,) which is fitted in a metallic frame, having edges just as high as the wafers should be thick. Lay on the surface a second glass plate, also hot and greased, so as to touch every point of the gelatine while resting on the edges of the frame. By its pressure the thin cake is rendered uniform. When the glass plates have cooled, the gelatine will be solid, and may be removed. It is cut into disks of different sizes by means of proper punches.

WASHES FOR VERMIN IN PLANTS. 1. *Tobacco water.* Infuse 1 ℔ of tobacco in a gallon of boiling water, in a covered vessel till cold.

2. *For Lice on Vines.* Boil ½ ℔ of tobacco in 2 quarts of water; strain, and add ½ ℔ of soft soap, and ¼ ℔ of sulphur. Mix.

3. *For Aphides.* Boil 2 oz. of lime and 1 oz. of sulphur in water, and strain.

4. *For Red Spiders.* A teaspoonful of salt in a gallon of water. In a few days wash the plant with pure water. See BLIGHTS, remedies for.

WASHING POWDERS. These consist of soda-ash combined with gelatinous substances, as solution of glue, linseed jelly, &c., dried and powdered.

WASHING LIQUIDS are chiefly solutions of caustic soda.

WATER-PROOFING COMPOUNDS. *For Boots, &c.* 1. (ROOME'S patent.) Suet 8 oz., linseed oil 8 oz., yellow bees'-wax 6 oz., neatsfoot oil 1½ oz., lamp-black 1 oz., litharge ½ oz. Melt together, and stir till cold.

2. Linseed oil 8 oz., boiled ditto 10 oz., suet 8 oz., yellow wax 8 oz. Melt.

3. DR. HARVARD'S. Wax 8 oz., resin 4 oz., mutton suet 4 oz.; boil together, and apply warm to new boots.

4. COL. HAWKER'S. Drying oil 1 pint, wax 2 oz., Burgundy pitch 1 oz., oil of turpentine 2 oz. Melt over

a slow fire, and add a few drops of oil of lavender, or thyme. Brush the boots repeatedly with the composition before the fire, till they appear fully saturated.

5. *For Leather, &c.* Cut 3 drachms of India-rubber into small pieces, soak them for 24 hours in a solution of common soda; dissolve this and 3 oz. of asphaltum in 12 ounces of camphine, then add ½ oz. of boiled linseed oil.

For Cloth. It is alternately dipped in a solution of acetate of lead with a little gum, and solution of alum.

For Hats. Boil 8 ℔ shell-lac, 3 ℔ frankincense, and 1 ℔ borax in sufficient water.

For Canvass, &c. Gutta percha 3 parts is dissolved in resin spirit 9 parts, at a heat of 120° to 140° Fah., stirring occasionally.—Mr. CASTLEY.

WAX. Yellow bees'-wax is bleached by pouring the melted wax in a divided state on a revolving cylinder partly immersed in water so as to form it into fine ribbons, which are exposed to air and moisture till bleached, and subsequently refined by melting with water containing sulphuric acid.—Dr. PEREIRA. It has been proposed to bleach wax by adding to each pound of melted wax 2 oz. of powdered nitrate of soda, and afterwards stirring in, by little at a time, 1 oz. of sulphuric acid diluted with 10 parts of water, keeping the mixture warm, and constantly stirred with a glass rod in a capacious earthen vessel, till all the acid is added. It is then allowed to become somewhat cool, and the vessel filled with boiling water, well agitated and set aside. The cake of wax is removed into boiling water, till this no longer produces a precipitate with chloride of barium.—M. INGENHOL. [We have not found this render wax perfectly white.]

WAX FOR MODELLING. Lead plaster 8 oz., bees'-wax 8 oz., Burgundy pitch 8 oz.; melt together, stir in sufficient chalk to form a paste, and form it into small sticks for use. [For SEALING-WAX, see page 421.]

WELDING COMPOSITION. Mix borax with $\frac{1}{10}$ of sal ammoniac, fuse the mixture, and pour it on an iron plate. When cold, pulverize it and mix it with an equal weight of quicklime, sprinkle it on iron heated to redness, and replace it in the fire. It may be welded below the usual heat.

WHEAT, STEEP FOR. A pound of genuine sulphate of copper in sufficient water, for each sack of seed. Arsenic is also used; sulphate of zinc has been recommended; so has quicklime, which is thus used:—Soak the seed in a warm mixture of 36 to 48 ounces of quicklime to 6 or 7 gallons of water. This is for 4½ bushels of wheat: the solution should be sufficient to cover the seed 3 or 4 finger-breadths deep, and it should lie in it 24 hours. But sulphate of copper seems to give the most satisfactory results. It would be desirable, however, to find an innocuous substitute, as traces of copper have been found in wheat grown from the steeped seed. This appears to have been discovered in the use of a solution of sulphate of soda with lime, which has proved more successful in France than either arsenic or sulphate of copper. See *Blights, remedies for.*

WOOD, TO STAIN. 1. *Mahogany colour* (*dark.*) Boil ½ lb of madder, and 2 oz. of logwood, in a gallon of water; and brush the wood well over with the hot liquid. When dry, go over the whole with a solution of 2 drachms of pearlash in a quart of water.

2. (*Light.*) Brush over the surface with diluted nitrous acid, and when dry apply the following with a soft brush:—Dragon's blood 4 oz., common soda 1 oz., spirit of wine 3 pints; let them stand in a warm place, shaking frequently, then strain. Repeat the application until the proper colour is obtained.

3. (*To stain Maple a Mahogany colour.*) Dragon's blood ½ oz., alkanet ¼ oz., aloes 1 dr., spirit of wine 16 ounces. Apply it with a sponge or brush.

4. *Rosewood.* Boil 8 oz. of logwood in 3 pints of water until reduced to half; apply it boiling hot two or three times, letting it dry between each. Afterwards put in the streaks with a camel-hair pencil dipped in a solution of copperas and verdigris in decoction of logwood.

5. *Ebony.* Wash the wood repeatedly with a solution of sulphate of iron; let it dry, then apply a hot decoction of logwood and nutgalls for two or three times. When

dry wipe it with a wet sponge, and when again dry, polish with linseed oil.

6. *To Stain Wood Red.* Use a strong decoction of Brazil wood and alum. [Woods may be stained with the various dyes before described. See DYES.]

YEAST, ARTIFICIAL. Honey 5 oz., cream of tartar 1 oz., malt 16 oz., water at 122° F. 3 pints; stir together, and when the temperature falls to 65°, cover it up, and keep it at that temperature till yeast is formed.

ZINC, AMMONIO-CHLORIDE OF. By dissolving equal equivalents of chloride of zinc and sal ammoniac a crystallizable salt is formed, which dissolves oxides of copper and of iron, and is useful in tinning or zincing those metals.

ZINC, AMALGAMATED, (*for voltaic plates.*) Put a little mercury on the zinc plate, and pour on it dilute sulphuric acid; then rub the mercury over the surface by means of a piece of linen. Another method, which is said to give a more permanent coating, is that of Mr. WALENN. Having cleaned the plates by emery, and by immersion in diluted sulphuric acid, and then in clean water, dip them into a mixture of equal parts of a saturated solution of corrosive sublimate and a similar solution of acetate of lead; then rub them with a cloth.

ZINC, PLATINIZED, *for Dr. Wright's Battery.* Saturated solution of chloride of platinum ½ dr., sulphuric acid 1½ dr., water 2 dr. Mix; dip the zinc plates into the solution for a few seconds, and wash them quickly.

ZINC, OXIDE OF. It may be obtained from the purified sulphate by precipitating it from a *hot* solution by carbonated or bicarbonated alkalies. It cannot be obtained pure by caustic ammonia.—M. J. LEFORT. Mr. MIDGLEY prepares it on a large scale by the combustion of zinc in a muffle, heated by a furnace of peculiar construction; the zinc is introduced into the muffle from time to time, as the combustion proceeds; he is thus able to prepare one or two hundred weights at a time, by a continuous process.

ZINC, PURIFICATION OF. Granulate zinc by melting it, and pouring it while very hot into a deep vessel filled with water. Place the granulated metal in a hessian crucible, in alternate layers, with one-fourth its weight of nitre, with an excess of nitre at the top. Cover the crucible, and secure the lid; then apply heat. When deflagration takes place, remove from the fire, separate the dross, and run the zinc into an ingot mould. It is quite free from arsenic.

APPENDIX.

WEIGHTS AND MEASURES.

The weights and measures now employed in compounding medicines in Great Britain are derived from the *Troy Pound* and the *Imperial Gallon*, and are thus divided:—

Apothecaries' Weight.

℔ Pound.		℥ Ounces.		ʒ Drachms.		℈ Scruples.		Gr. Grains.		Minims. of water.
1	=	12	=	96	=	288	=	5760	=	6319·54
		1	=	8	=	24	=	480	=	526·62
				1	=	3	=	60	=	65·82
						1	=	20	=	21·94
								1	=	1·09

The Troy Pennyweight, 24 grains, is not used in compounding medicines.

Apothecaries' Measure.

C. Congius. Gallon.		O. Octarii. Pints.		f℥ Fluid Ounces.		fʒ Fluid Drachms.		♏ Minims.		Grains of water.
1	=	8	=	160	=	1280	=	76800	=	70000
		1	=	20	=	160	=	9600	=	8750
				1	=	8	=	480	=	437·5
						1	=	60	=	54·7
								1	=	0·9

Imperial Measure,—(*Common Divisions.*)

Quarter.		Bushels.		Pecks.		Gallons.		Quarts.		Pints.		Gills.
1	=	8	=	32	=	64	=	256	=	512	=	2048
		1	=	4	=	8	=	32	=	64	=	256
				1	=	2	=	8	=	16	=	64
						1	=	4	=	8	=	32
								1	=	2	=	8
										1	=	4

Avoirdupois Weight.

℔. Pound.		oz. Ounces.		dr. Drachms.		gr. Grains.		French Grammes.
1	=	16	=	256	=	7000	=	453·544
		1	=	16	=	437·50	=	28·346
				1	=	27·34	=	1·771

Other weights used are, the ton, 20 hundred weight; the hundred weight, 112 ℔; and the quarter, 28 ℔.

Table for converting Troy into Avoirdupois Weights.

(From Dr. Duncan's "Edinburgh Dispensatory.")

Troy ounces.		Avoirdupois ounces.	Avoirdupois grains.	Troy ounces.		Avoirdupois ounces.	Avoirdupois grains.
1	=	1	42½	7	=	7	297½
2	=	2	85	8	=	8	340
3	=	3	127½	9	=	9	382½
4	=	4	170	10	=	10	425
5	=	5	212½	11	=	11	30
6	=	6	255	12	=	13	72½

175 Troy ounces are equal to 192 Avoirdupois.

Troy ℔.	=	Avoirdupois ℔.	oz.	gr.	Troy ℔.	=	Avoirdupois ℔.	oz.	gr.
1	=	0	13	72½	18	=	14	12	430
2	=	1	10	145	19	=	15	10	65
3	=	2	7	217½	20	=	16	7	137½
4	=	3	4	290	30	=	24	10	425
5	=	4	1	362½	40	=	32	14	275
6	=	4	14	435	50	=	41	2	125
7	=	5	12	70	60	=	49	5	412½
8	=	6	9	142½	70	=	57	9	262½
9	=	7	6	215	80	=	65	13	112½
10	=	8	3	287½	90	=	74	0	400
11	=	8	0	360	100	=	82	4	250
12	=	9	13	432½	175	=	144	0	0
13	=	10	11	67½	200	=	164	9	62½
14	=	11	8	140	300	=	246	13	312½
15	=	12	5	212½	400	=	293	2	125
16	=	13	2	285	500	=	411	6	375
17	=	13	15	359½	1000	=	822	13	312½

The following are the divisions of the *old wine gallon* adopted in the London Pharmacopœia before 1836, and the Dublin Pharmacopœia before 1850. Its use in this kingdom is no longer legal.

Former Apothecaries' Measure.

C.		O.		f℥		fʒ		f℈		Minims.
1	=	8	=	128	=	1024	=	3072	=	61440
		1	=	16	=	128	=	384	=	7680
				1	=	8	=	24	=	480
						1	=	3	=	60
								1	=	20

Comparison between the Old and New Measure.

	Grains of distilled water. OLD.	NEW.	Cubic inches. OLD.	NEW.
Gallon .	58317·8	70000	231	277·274
Pint .	7289·7	8750	28·875	34·659
f℥j . .	455·6	437·5	1·804	1·733
fʒj . .	56·9	54.7	·225	·216

The old gallon was very nearly $\frac{5}{6}$ths of the new: the new is $\frac{6}{5}$ths of the old. The exact factor for converting the old measure into new is ·83311; and for converting new into old, 1.20032.

Relative value of the former and present Apothecaries' Measure.

(From the American Dispensatory.)

OLD.		NEW. O.	f℥	fʒ	♏.
Cong.	=	6	13	2	23
O.	=		16	5	18
f℥	=		1	0	20
fʒ	=			1	2½

NEW.		OLD. C.	O.	f℥	fʒ	♏.
Cong.	=	1	1	9	5	8
O.	=		1	3	1	38
f℥	=				7	41
fʒ	=					58

To find the weight of any given measure of a liquid, multiply the weight of the water it will contain by the specific gravity, water being 1·000. The weight of a gallon of any liquid, in avoird. ℔s and decimal parts, is at once seen from its density, merely removing the decimal point one place to the right. Thus a gallon of ether at ·750 weighs 7·50 (7½) ℔. A gallon of nitric acid at 1·500 weighs 15 ℔.

TABLE

SHOWING THE RELATIONS OF THE WEIGHTS AND MEASURES OF VARIOUS LIQUIDS.

	Specific Gravity.	A Fluid Ounce weighs	Imperial Pint weighs	Troy Ounce measures		Avoirdupois Ounce measures		A Gallon weighs in Avoirdupois	
		Grains.	Grains.	f℥	♏︎	f℥	♏︎	℔.	oz.
Water (distilled)	1·000	437½	8750	8	46	8	0	10	0
Alcohol. L. 1836. . .	·815	356½	7131	10	46	9	49	8	2½
Alcohol. E.	·796	348	6964	11	2	10	3	7	15⅜
Rectified Spirit. L. & E. .	·838	366½	7332½	10	28	9	33	8	6
Proof Spirit. L. & D. . .	·920	402½	8050	9	31	8	42	9	3 3/16
Proof Spirit. E. 1841 .	·912	399	7980	9	37	8	46	9	1⅞
Chloroform	1·480	647½	12950	5	56	5	24	14	12¾
Ether	·750	328⅛	6562½	11	42	10	40	7	8
Spirit of Nitric Æther. L.	·834	365	7297½	10	31	9	35	8	5 7/16
Olive Oil.	·9153	400½	8009	9	35	8	44	9	2 7/16
Syrup. (*Normal.* GUIBOURT)	1·320	577½	11550	6	39	6	4	13	3¼
Sulphuric Acid. L. . . .	1·845	807	16144	4	45	4	20	18	7 3/16
Nitric Acid. L.	1·420	621¼	12425	6	11	5	38	14	3 3/16
Nitric Acid, Pure. E. & D.	1·500	656¼	13125	5	51	5	20	15	0
Muriatic Acid	1·160	507½	10150	7	35	6	54	11	9 9/16

Weights and Measures of other Countries.

In the United States of America the weights are the same as in this country; but they have not adopted our imperial measure, and retain the old wine gallon and its divisions in the Pharmacopœia.

The unit of the British India ponderary system is the tola, equal to 180 Troy grains. 32 tolas are equal to ℔j Troy. The maund is equal to 100 Troy ounces.

In France the metrical or decimal system is now the only legal one. The following table shows the correspondence of the French metrical weights with English grains:—

		Troy Grains.			Troy Grains.
Milligramme	=	·0154	Decagramme	=	154·34
Centigramme	=	·1543	Hectogramme	=	1543·40
Decigramme	=	1·5434	Kilogramme	=	15434·00
Gramme	=	15·4340	Myriagramme	=	154340·00

The measures of capacity in France are multiples and divisions of the LITRE, which is the measure occupied by a kilogramme (15434 Troy grains) of distilled water at its greatest density. It exceeds the old Paris *pinte* by $\frac{1}{14}$th, and is equal to 35 fluid ounces and 103 minims, or 1·7608 imperial pints, or 61·028 English cubic inches. 4½ litres make an imperial gallon, within about fʒ xij.

The following table will show the relations between the litre and the imperial gallon of 277·2738 c. inches:—

Litres.			Cubic Inches.	Gall.	Pts.	Fl.℥	Fl.ʒ	Min.
$\frac{1}{1000}$	=	Millilitre	·061028					16·9
$\frac{1}{100}$	=	Centilitre	·61028				2	49
$\frac{1}{10}$	=	Decilitre	6·1028			3	4	10·36
1	=	Litre	61·028		1	15	1	43.69
10	=	Decalitre	610·28	2	1	12	1	16·9
100	=	Hectolitre	6102·8	22	0	1	4	49
1000	=	Kilolitre	61028·	220	0	16	6	40
10000	=	Myrialitre	610280·	2201	(or 275⅛ bushels.)			

French Measures of Length.

The standard unit is the *metre*, equal to 39·371 English inches, or 1 yard, 3 inches, and $\frac{37}{100}$ths. The *kilometre* (1000 metres) is 4 furlongs, 213 yards, 1 foot, 11 inches.

The following are some of the weights and measures formerly used in France.

The old French pound, *livre pois de marc*, was equal to 489·5 grammes, or 7561 Troy grains; but the metrical pound, *livre metrique*, substituted for it in 1812, contained exactly 500 grammes, or 7717 English grains. Both are now abolished. The following are their divisions:—

Livre.	Ounce.	Gros.	Scrupl.	Grs.			*Poids de Marc.*	*Metrique.*
1	16	128	384	9261	=	grammes	489·5	500
	1	8	24	576	=	"	30·6	31·25
		1	3	72	=	"	3·824	3.90
			1	24	=	"	1·274	1·30
				1	=	"	·053	·054

In the Paris Codex and medical works the grain is represented by 0·05 grammes (5 centigrammes,) 2 grains by 0·1 (1 decigramme;) the half drachm by 2 grammes; the drachm by 4 grammes; and the ounce by 32 grammes.

The old French measures used in pharmacy were—

		Litres.	Other Commercial Measures		Litres.
La Pinte	=	0·931	8 Pintes (un velte)	=	7·450
La Chopine	=	0.466	13·97 (ancien boisseau)	=	13·010
Le demi-Setier	=	0.233	288 = 1 muid	=	268.220
Le Poisson	=	0.116	576 = 1 tonneau d'Orléans, ou 2 muids	=	536·440
Le demi-Poisson	=	0.058			

(*From* GUIBOURT'S "*Pharmacopée Raisonnée.*")

The Litre, with its divisions and multiples, is the measure now used. It contains 1000 grammes of water; the number of grammes of other liquids corresponds with their specific gravity; water being 1000.

The former measures of length in France were the

Toise = 1·949 metres, or 6·3945 English feet.
Foot (pied) = 0·32484 metres = 12·785 Eng. inches.
Inch (pouce) = 0·02707 metres, or 1·0654 Eng. inches.
Line (ligne) or $\frac{1}{12}$ of an inch = ·002256 metres.

The metre is equal to 3 ft. 11 lines old French measure, or 3 ft. 3·7 in. English.

OTHER FOREIGN WEIGHTS AND MEASURES.

1.—*Medicinal pounds of* 12 *ounces, in English grains.*

(From Jourdan's "Pharmacopée Universelle.")

The following are divided as our Apothecaries' weight.

The pound of Austria weighs 6482·42 grains; Bavaria, 5556·24; Holland, 5787·75; Lubec, 5697·09; Nuremberg (German pound,) 5522·96; Poland, 5533·25; Prussia, 5113·99; Sweden, 5498·01; Venice (*sottile*,) 4649·17.

The division of the following differs in the scruple being divided into 24 grains.

Bologna, 5026·32; Lucca, 5162·67; Modena, 5254·61; Parma, 5062·35; Portugal, 5312·23; Rome, 5233·25; Spain, 5325·84; Tuscany, 5240·49; Piedmont [Turin,] 5123·49.

The Naples pound contains 5490·63 Troy grains; the ounce is divided into 10 drachms; the scruple into 20 grains.

2.—*Various Foreign Weights.*

The old Paris pound was divided into 16 ounces; the scruple into 24 grains. Its weight has been given above. The pound by which drugs are weighed in Turkey is the *Tchegy*, equal to 4957 English grains, and is divided into 100 drachms, each drachm, into 16 killos, and each killo into 4 grains.

The *obolo* is half a Spanish scruple; 3 *silicua* make 1 *obolo*, and 4 grains a *silicua*.

A *loth*, in Germany, Poland, &c., is half an ounce.

The commercial pound in several countries differs from the pharmaceutical. The civil pound of Bavaria and mark of Vienna are each about 19¾ avoirdupois ounces. That of Holland is the French kilogramme, or 12 grains more than 2 ℔ 3¼ oz. avoirdupois. The mark is half a kilogramme. The Coburg commercial pound is nearly 18 oz. avoirdupois.

3.—*Foreign Measures.*

The Austrian *mass* or *kanne* is equal to 1·415015 litres, or 2½ imperial pints, within 40 minims.

The *kanna* of Sweden = nearly 2·62 litres, or about 4 pints, 12 ounces, imperial.

Russian pound of water = 25·019 English cubic inches.

The *pott* (half kanne) of Denmark = 0·9653 litres.

The *arroba* of Spain = 16·073 litres.

The *almude* of Portugal = 16·451 litres.

The Prussian quart = 1·145 litres; or 1 qt., 3 fl. dr. imp.

The *barile* of Naples = 43·6216 litres; of Rome, 58·5416 litres; of Tuscany, 45·584 litres.

The *wedro* of Russia (10 *stof* or 30 Russian pounds) = 12·29 litres, or 21 pints, 12 oz., 12½ dr. imperial.

The *mass* of Wurtemburg = 1·537 litres, or about 3 pints, 14¾ oz. imperial.

Comparison of Thermometric Scales.

To convert the degrees of centigrade into those of Fahrenheit, multiply by 9, divide by 5, and add 32.

To convert degrees of centigrade into those of Reaumur, multiply by 4 and divide by 5.

To convert degrees of Fahrenheit into those of centigrade, deduct 32, multiply by 5, and divide by 9.

To convert degrees of Fahrenheit into those of Reaumur, deduct 32, divide by 9, and multiply by 4.

To convert degrees of Reaumur into those of centigrade, multiply by 5 and divide by 4.

To convert degrees of Reaumur into those of Fahrenheit, multiply by 9, divide by 4, and add 32.

In De Lisle's thermometer, used in Russia, the graduation begins at boiling point, which is marked *Zero*, and the freezing point is 150.

EFFECTS OF TEMPERATURE.

Deg. of Fahr.

8696 Cast iron melts (Morveau.)
2200 Gold melts (Kane,) 2518 (Morveau.)
1996 Copper melts (Kane,) 2548 (Daniell.)
2233 Silver melts (Daniell.)
1869 Brass melts (Daniell.)
1000 Iron bright cherry red (Poillet.)
980 Red heat, visible in daylight (Daniell.)
941 Zinc begins to burn (Daniell.)
793 Zinc melts (Gmelin,) 648 (Daniell.)
644 Mercury boils (Daniell,) 662 (Graham.)
630 Whale oil boils (Graham.)
612 Pure lead melts (Parkes,) 609 (Daniell.)
600 Linseed oil boils.
545 Sulphuric acid boils (Phillips,) 620 (Graham.)
518 Bismuth melts (Gmelin,) 476 (Phillips.)
442 Tin melts.
380 Arsenious acid volatilizes.
356 Metallic arsenic sublimes.
315 Oil of turpentine boils (Kane.)
302 Ætherification ends.
256 Sat. sol. of acetate of soda boils.
257 " sal ammoniac boils (Taylor.)
248 " nitric acid 1·42 boils, and sol. soda 1·44.
238 " nitre boils.
232 Sulphur melts (Turner,) 226 (Fownes.)
221 Sat. sol. of salt boils (Paris Codex.)
220 " alum, carb. soda, and sulph. zinc boil.
218 " chlorate, and prussiate of potash boil.
216 " sulph. of iron, sulph. of copper, nitrate of lead, boil.
214 " acetate of lead, sulph. and bitartrate of potash boil.
213 Water begins to boil in glass (or 213·5.)
212 Water boils in metal, barometer at 30°.
211 Alloy of 5 bismuth, 3 tin, 2 lead, melts.
201 " 8 bismuth, 5 lead, 3 tin, melts (Kane.)
194 Sodium begins to melt.

Deg. of Fahr.

185 Nitric acid 1·52 boils.
180 Starch dissolves in water.
176 Rectified spirit boils, benzole distils.
173 Alcohol (sp. gr. ·796 to ·800) boils.
151 Bees'-wax melts (Kane,) 142 (Lepage.)
150 Pyroxylic spirit boils (Scanlan.)
140 Chloroform, and ammonia of ·945, boil.
136 Potassium melts (Daniell.)
132 Acetone (Pyroacetic spirit) boils (Kane.)
122 Mutton suet, and styracine, melt.
116 Bisulphuret of carbon boils (Graham.)
115 Pure tallow melts (Lepage,) 92 (Thomson.)
112 Spermaceti and stearine of lard melt.
99 Phosphorus melts.
98 Ether (·720) boils. Temperature of the blood.
88 Acetous fermentation ceases, water boils *in vacuo.*
77 Vinous ferm. ends, acetous ferm. begins.
62 Oil of anise liquefies, congeals at 60.
59 Gay Lussac's *Alcoomètre* graduated at.
55 Syrups to be kept at.
42 Sulphuric acid, sp. gr. 1·741, congeals or (41.)
36 Olive oil freezes.
32 Water freezes.
30 Milk freezes.
28 Vinegar freezes.
20 Wine freezes.
0 Cold produced by snow and salt.
—7 Brandy freezes.
—39–40 Mercury freezes.

Gentle Heat of London and United States pharmacopœias, and *Inferior Heat* of Dub. ph., from 90 to 100°
Medium Heat, Dub. ph., from 100 to 200°
Superior Heat, Dub. ph., from 200 to 212°
Maceration, Dub. ph., to be performed at 60 to 90°
Digestion, Dub. ph., at 90 to 100°
Specific Gravities, taken at 60° Lond. ph.; at 62° Ed. ph.

SPECIFIC GRAVITIES.

1. *Solids.* *Water* 1·000.

Platinum, 20·980; Gold, 19·250; Mercury, 13·560; Lead, 11·350; Silver, 10·500; Bismuth, 9·822; Copper, 8·895; Cadmium, 8·604; Cobalt, 8·538; Nickel, 8·279; Iron, 7·788; Tin, 7·291; Zinc, 6·861 to 7·100; Antimony, 6·720; Sodium, ·972; Potassium, ·865; Caoutchouc, ·933; Amber, 1·078; Scammony, 1·210; Resin, 1·072; Camphor, ·988; Gum Arabic, 1·452; Bees'-wax, ·962; Spermaceti, ·943; Sulphur, 1·990; Glass, 2·540 to 2·953.

2. *Liquids.* *Water* 1·000.

Mercury, 13·560; Sulphuric acid, 1·843; Nitric acid (monohydrated,) 1·517; Pure nitric acid (Ed. and Dub. ph.,) 1·500; Nitric acid (Lond. ph.,) 1·420; Commercial nitric acid, 1·380 to 1·390; Double aqua fortis, 1·360; Single aqua fortis, 1·220; Muriatic acid (strongest,) 1·210; Muriatic acid, Lond. ph., 1·160; Ditto Ed. ph., 1·170; Ditto Dub. ph., 1·176; Solution of caustic potash (Lond. ph., containing 6·7 per cent.,) 1·063; Ditto Dub. ph., 1·068; Ditto Ed. ph., 1·072; Water of ammonia (Lond. and Ed. ph., containing 10 per cent.,) ·960; Ditto (Dub. ph., 12·7 per cent.) ·950; Stronger water of ammonia, Lond. ph. (32 per cent.,) ·882; Ditto, Ed. ph. (33 per cent.,) ·880; Ditto Dub. ph. (27 per cent.,) ·900; Saturated solution of alum, 1·033; Saturated solution of common salt, 1·200; Sat. sol. of sulphate of copper, 1·150; Sat. sol. of sulphate of magnesia, 1·218; Sea water, 1·027; Milk, 1·032; Alcohol, ·976; Rectified spirit, ·838; Proof spirit, ·920; Chloroform, 1·496 (not less than 1·480, Lond. ph.;) Bisulphuret of carbon, 1·272; Spirit of nitric ether, Lond. ph., ·834, Ed. ph., ·847; Ether (pure,) ·724; Lond. and Dub. ph., not above ·750; Ed. ph., ·735; Acetic ether, ·917; Caoutchoucine, ·680; Oil of turpentine, ·867 to ·869; Olive oil, ·9175; Spermaceti oil, ·890; Southern whale oil, ·920; Almond oil, ·917; Creasote, 1·046; Oil of wine, 1·05; Essential oil of anise, ·985; of caraway, ·938; of cinnamon, 1·008; of cloves, 1·055; of cajeput, ·911; of lemon, ·847; of rosemary, ·897; Tincture of sesquichloride of iron, ·992; Tincture of opium, ·952.

3. *Gases and vapours. Atmospheric Air* 1·000.

Hydrogen, ·690; Nitrogen, ·972; Oxygen (Graham,) 1·1056; Carbonic oxide, ·972; Carbonic acid, 1·524; Light carburetted hydrogen, ·5595; Olefiant gas, ·981; Chlorine, 2·470 (2·421 Graham;) Vapour of ether, 2·582; v. of water, ·620; v. of sulphur, 6·648 (6·617 Graham;) v. of phosphorus, 4·327; v. of iodine, 8·700.

TABLE OF CHEMICAL ELEMENTS, WITH THEIR SYMBOLS AND EQUIVALENT NUMBERS.

ELEMENTS.	SYMBOL.	HYDROGEN 1.		OXYGEN 100.
		Brande.	Turner.	Berzelius.
Aluminum . . .	Al.	14	13·7	171·17
Antimony [Stibium] .	Sb.	129	64·6	806·45
Arsenic . . .	As.	75	37·7	470·04
Barium (Phillips, 68) .	Ba.	69	68·7	856·88
Bismuth . . .	Bi.	213	71·	886·92
Boron	B.	11	10·9	136·25
Bromine . . .	Br.	78	78·4	978·31
Cadmium . . .	Cd.	56	58·8	696·77
Calcium . . .	Ca.	20	20·5	251·94
Carbon	C.	6	6·12	75·40
Cerium. . . .	Ce.	46	46·0	574·70
Chlorine . . .	Cl.	36	35·42	444·65
Chromium . . .	Cr.	28	28·	351·82
Cobalt	Co.	30	29·5	368·99
Columbium [Tantalium] .	Ta.	185	185·0	2307·43
Copper [Cuprum] . .	Cu.	32	31·6	395·70
Fluorine . . .	F.	19	18·68	233·80
Glucinum (Phillips, 27) .	G.	5	26·5	331·26
Gold [Aurum] . .	Au.	200	199·2	2486·03
Hydrogen . . .	H.	1	1·	12·4795
Iodine (Liebig, 127·1) .	I.	126	126·3	1579·50
Iridium. . . .	Ir.	99	98·8	1233·50
Iron [Ferrum] . .	Fe.	28	28·0	350·27
Lead [Plumbum] . .	Pb.	104	103·6	1294·50
Lithium (Graham, 6·43) .	L.	7	6·	80·33
Magnesium . . .	Mg.	12	12·7	158·35
Manganese . . .	Mn.	28	27·7	345·89
Mercury (Phillips, 200) .	Hg.	100	202·	1265·82
Molybdenum . . .	Mo.	48	47·5	598·52
Nickel (Phillips, 30) .	Ni.	28	29·5	369·68
Nitrogen . . .	N.	14	14·15	177·04
Osmium . . .	Os.	100	99·7	1244·49
Oxygen . . .	O.	8	8·	100·00
Palladium (Phillips, 53) .	Pd.	54	53·3	655·90
Phosphorus (Schrötter, 31)	P.	32	15·7	196·14

Table of Chemical Elements, &c.—continued.

Elements.	Symbol.	Hydrogen 1.		Oxygen 100.
		Brande.	Turner.	Berzelius.
Platinum . . .	Pl.	99	98·8	1233·50
Potassium [Kalium] .	K.	40	39·15	489·92
Rhodium . . .	R.	52	52·2	651·39
Selenium . . .	Se.	40	39·6	494·58
Silicium, or Silicon .	Si.	15	22·5	277·31
Silver [Argentum] .	Ag.	108	108·	1351·61
Sodium [Natrium] .	Na.	24	23·3	290·90
Strontium . . .	Sr.	44	43·8	547·29
Sulphur . . .	S.	16	16·1	200·80
Tellurium . . .	Te.	64	64·2	801·76
Thorium . . .	Th.	60	59·6	744·90
Tin [Stannum] . .	Sn.	59	57·9	735·29
Titanium . . .	Ti.	24	24·3	303·66
Tungstan Wolfram .	W.	100	99·7	1246·25
Vanadium . . .	V.	68	68·5	856·86
Uranium . . .	U.	60	217·	2711·36
Yttrium . . .	Y.	32	32·2	402·51
Zinc	Zn.	32	32·3	403·23
Zirconium (Phillips, 22)	Zr.	23	33·7	420·20

Remarks.—The first column of figures shows the equivalent numbers adopted by Prout, Brande, Dumas, Phillips, and other chemists, who regard all equivalent numbers as simple multiples of that of Hydrogen, which they adopt as unity.

In the second column are those of Turner and others, who adopt Hydrogen as unity, but do not consider that the other equivalents are exact multiples of it.

In the third column are the numbers of Berzelius, &c., who adopt Oxygen as unity, or rather, as 100.

Besides the difference in the numbers arising from the adoption of a different standard, there are others which arise from discordant views of the composition of the compounds from which the equivalents are determined. Some Continental chemists also make a distinction between the equivalents and *Atomic weights*, supposing the equivalents of certain elements to consist of two atoms. But this distinction is not adopted by English chemists.

The newly-discovered metals, Didymium, Erbium, Lanthanum, Niobium, Norium, Pelopium, Ruthenium, and Terbium, require further investigation. The following numbers on the Hydrogen Scale have been assigned to some of them:—Lanthanum 48 (Graham,) Didymium 49·6 (Marignac,) Ruthenium 52.

Composition, equivalent numbers, and symbols of some of the more important compounds employed in Pharmacy and the Arts.

[The numbers here adopted for the elements are those of the first column of the preceding table.]

	Symbols.	Equiv.
Acetone . . .	$C_3\ H_3\ O$	29
Acid, Acetic (anhydrous)	$C_4\ H_3,\ O_3$ *or*, $\bar{A}$ . .	51
— Acetic, glacial . .	$\bar{A}$, HO	60
— Arsenious . . .	$As\ O_3$	99
— Arsenic . . .	$As\ O_5$	115
— Benzoic . . .	$C_{14}\ A_5\ O_3$ . . .	113
—— Cryst. . . .	$C_{14}\ H_5\ O_3$, HO . .	122
— Boracic . . .	$Bo\ O_3$	35
—— Cryst. . . .	$Bo\ O_3$, HO . . .	62
— Carbonic . . .	$C\ O_2$, *or*, $\ddot{C}$ . . .	22
— Chromic . . .	$Cr\ O_3$	52
— Citric (dry) . .	$C_{12}\ H_5\ O_{11}$ . . .	165
—— Cryst. (commercial)	$\bar{C}$, 4 HO . . .	201
— Hydrochloric . .	H Cl	37
— Hydrocyanic . .	C_2 N H, *or*, H Cy . .	27
— Hydrosulphuric . .	S H	17
— Iodic . . .	$I\ O_5$	166
— Nitric (dry) . .	$N\ O_5$	54
— Nitric sp. gr. 1·5 .	$N\ O_5$, HO . . .	63
— Nitrous . . .	NO_4	46
— Oxalic (dry) . .	$C_2\ O_3$, *or* $\bar{O}$ . . .	36
— Oxalic, cryst. . .	$C_2\ O_3$, 3 HO . . .	63
— Phosphoric . .	$P\ O_5$	72
— Sulphuric . . .	SO_3	40
— Sulphuric liquid .	SO_3, HO . . .	49
— Tartaric . . .	$C_4\ O_5\ H_2$, *or*, $\bar{T}$ . .	66
— Tartaric, cryst. . .	$\bar{T}$, HO	75
— Chromic . . .	$Cr\ O_3$	52
Alcohol . . .	$C_4\ H_6\ O_2$	46
Alumina . . .	$Al_2\ O_3$	52

	Symbols.	Equiv.
Alum, cryst . . .	$Al_2 O_3$, 3 (SO_3;) KO, SO_3 + 24 HO .	476
Ammonium . . .	NH_4	18
Amidogen . . .	NH_2	16
Ammonia . . .	NH_3	17
— Hydrochlorate . .	NH_3, H Cl . . .	54
— Sulphate, cr. . .	NH_3, SO_3, 2 HO . .	75
— Sesquicarb. . .	2 NH_3, 3 CO_2 2 HO .	118
— Hydrated bicarbonate	NH_3, 2 CO_2, 2 HO . .	79
Antimony, sesquioxide .	Sb O_3	153
— Sesqui, *or*, ter-sulph. .	Sb S_3	177
— potassio-tartrate .	KO, $\overline{T}$, Sb O_3, $\overline{T}$, 3 HO .	360
Baryta	Ba O	77
— Carbonate . .	Ba O, CO_2	99
— Sulphate . . .	Ba O, SO_3	117
Barium, chloride . .	Ba Cl	105
Bismuth, oxide . .	Bi O_3	237
— Nitrate (dry) . .	Bi O_3, NO_5 . . .	291
Borax	Na O, 2 BO_3, 10 HO .	192
Calcium, chloride . .	Ca Cl	56
— Chloride, crys . .	Ca Cl, 6 HO . . .	110
— Oxide (Lime) . .	Ca O	28
Chloroform . . .	C_2 H Cl_3	121
Cinchonia . . .	C_{20} H_{12} NO . . .	154
Copper, oxide . .	Cu O	40
— Dinoxide . . .	Cu_2 O	72
— Sulphate . . .	Cu O, SO_3	80
Sulphate, cryst . .	Cu O, SO_3, 5 HO . .	125
— Nitrate . . .	Cu O, NO_5	94
— Nitrate, cr. . .	Cu O, NO_5, 3 HO . .	121
— Acetate, cr. . .	Cu O, $\overline{A}$, HO . . .	100
Cyanogen . . .	C_2 N, (or Cy) . . .	26
Ether	C_4 H_5 O	37
Ethule	C_4 H_5	29
Glycerine, anhydrous .	C_6 H_7 O_5	83
Gum	C_{12} H_{11} O_{11} . . .	171
Iron, protoxide . .	Fe O	36
— Black oxide . .	Fe_3 O_4	116

	Symbols.	Equiv.
Iron, sesquioxide	$Fe_2 O_3$	30
—— (Phillips)	$Fe O_{1\frac{1}{2}}$ (or $\frac{1}{2} Fe_2 O_3$)	40
— Chloride	Fe Cl	64
— Sesquichloride	$Fe_2 Cl_3$	164
—— (Phillips)	$Fe Cl_{1\frac{1}{2}}$ (or $\frac{1}{2} Fe_2 Cl_3$)	82
— Iodide (dry)	Fe I	154
— Sulphate	$Fe O, SO_3$	76
— Sulphate, crys.	$Fe O, SO_3$, 7 HO	139
— Potassio-tartrate	$\overline{T}$ KO, $Fe_2 O_3$, $\overline{T}$	260
Lead, Acetate, cr.	Pb O, $\overline{A}$, 3 HO	190
— Diacetate	2 (Pb O) $\overline{A}$	275
— Protoxide	Pb O	112
— Carbonate	$Pb O, CO_2$	134
— Iodide	Pb I	230
— Chloride	Pb Cl	140
— Sulphate	$Pb O, SO_3$	152
— Nitrate, cr.	$Pb O, NO_5$	166
Lime, Carbonate	$Ca O, CO_2$	50
— Hydrate	Ca O, HO	37
— Sulphate	$Ca O, SO_3$	68
— Phosphate (bone-earth)	$3 Ca O, PO_5$	156
Magnesia	Mg O	20
— Com. carbonate	$5 Mg O, 4 CO_2$, 6 HO	242
— Sulphate	$Mg O, SO_3$	60
— Sulphate, crys.	$Mg O, SO_3$, 7 HO	123
Manganese, binoxide	$Mn O_2$	44
— Chloride	Mn Cl	64
— Sulphate	$Mn O, SO_3$	76
Mannite	$C_6 H_7 O_6$	91
* Mercury, chloride	Hg Cl	236
— Bichloride	$Hg Cl_2$	272
— Protoxide	Hg O	208

* Mr. Brande has now adopted 100 as the equivalent of mercury, with Dr. Kane and others; but we have here retained the old symbols and equivalents, which are those of Phillips, as the change would necessitate an alteration in the pharmacopœial and established names of the several mercurial compounds. Two must be added to each of these numbers, if mercury be 202, as stated by Turner. The ammonio-chloride, containing 2 eq. of mercury, will be 526.

	Symbols.	Equiv.
Mercury, binoxide	$Hg\ O_2$	216
— Iodide	$Hg\ I$	326
— Biniodide	$Hg\ I_2$	452
— Ammonio-chloride	$Hg\ O_2$, $Hg\ Cl_2$, $2\ NH_3$ (?)	522
— Nitrate (proto)	$Hg\ O$, NO_5	262
— Nitrate, crys.	$Hg\ O$, NO_5, 2 HO	280
— Bipersulphate	$Hg\ O_2$, $2\ SO_3$	296
— Bisulphuret	$Hg\ S_2$	232
Morphia, dry	$H_{20}\ C_{35}\ NO_6$	292
— Crystallized	$H_{20}\ C_{35}\ NO_6$, 2 HO	310
— Acetate, cr	$H_{20}\ C_{35}\ NO_6$, $\overline{Ac}$, HO	352
— Muriate, cr	$H_{20}\ C_{35}\ NO_6$, H, Cl, 6 HO	383
— Sulphate, cr	$H_{20}\ C_{35}\ NO_6$, SO_3, 6 HO	386
Platinum, chloride	$Pl\ Cl_2$	171
— Ammonio-bichloride	$Pl\ Cl_2$, NH_3, H Cl	225
Potash, dry	KO	48
Potash, hydrate	KO, HO	57
— Acetate, dry	KO, $\overline{A}$	99
— Carbonate	KO, CO_2	70
— Carbonate, hydrated	KO, CO_2 $1\frac{1}{2}$ HO	$83\frac{1}{2}$
— Bicarbonate, cr.	KO, $2\ CO_2$, HO	101
— Chlorate	KO, $Cl\ O_5$	124
— Chromate	KO, $Cr\ O_3$	100
— Bichromate	KO, $2\ Cr\ O_3$	152
— Nitrate	KO, NO_5	102
— Sulphate	KO, SO_3	88
— Bisulphate, crys.	KO, $2\ SO_3 + 2$ HO	146
— Tartrate	KO, $\overline{T}$	114
— Bitartrate	KO, 2 $\overline{T}$, HO	189
Potassium, Bromide	K Br	118
— Chloride	K Cl	76
— Iodide	K I	166
Proteine	$C_{46}\ H_{36}\ N_6 O_{14}$	520
Quina	$C_{20}\ H_{12}\ NO_2$	162
— Disulphate, crys.	$2(C_{20}H_{12}NO_2,)SO_3$, 8 HO	436
— Neutral sulphate	$C_{20}\ H_{12}\ NO_2$, SO_3, HO	274
— Hydrochlorate	$2(C_{20}H_{12}NO_2,)$ H Cl, 3 HO	388
Silver, oxide	Ag O	116

	Symbols.	Equiv.
Silver, chloride	Ag Cl	144
— Iodide	Ag I	234
— Cyanide	Ag Cy	134
— Nitrate	Ag O, NO_5	170
Soda	Na O	32
— Carbonate	Na O, CO_2	54
— Carbonate, crys	Na O, CO_2, 10 HO	144
— Bicarbonate	Na O, 2 CO_2 HO	85
— Sesquicarbonate	Na, $1\frac{1}{2}$ CO_2, 2 HO	83
— Sulphate, dry	Na O, SO_3	72
— Sulphate, crys.	Na O, SO_3, 10 HO	162
— Bisulphate	Na O, 2 SO_3	112
— Phosphate	2 Na O, PO_5, 25 HO	361
— Potassio-tartrate, crys.	Na O, KO, 2 $\bar{T}$, 10 HO	302
Sodium, chloride,	Na Cl	60
Starch (anhydrous)	C_{12} H_{10} O_{10}	162
Strychnia	C_{44} H_{24} O_4 N_2	348
Sugar (anhydrous)	B_{12} H_9 O_9	153
— Cryst.	C_{12} H_{11} O_{10}	171
Sulphuretted hydrogen	SH	15
Veratria	C_{34} H_{22} NO_6	288
Water	HO	9
— Oxygenated	HO_2	17
Zinc, oxide	Zn O	40
— Carbonate	Zn O, CO_2	62
— Sulphate, cr.	Zn O, SO_3, 7 HO	143
— Chloride	Zn Cl	68

Table of the Neutralizing Proportions of some of the Acids and Alkaline Carbonates, omitting minute fractions. The best commercial preparations are intended.

Tartaric Acid.	Citric Acid.	Lemon Juice.	Cr. Subcarb. of Soda.	Sesqui or bicarb. of Soda and Subcarb. of Potash.	Bicarbonate of Potash.	Carbonate of Magnesia.	Sesquicarbonate of Ammonia.	Bicarbonate of Ammonia.
Grs.	Grs.	ʒ	Grs.	Grs.	Grs.	Grs.	Grs.	Grs.
10	9¼	2⅙	19	11	13½	6½	8¼	10½
10¾	10	2⅓	20½	12	14½	7	8½	11½
13	12	2⅘	25	14½	17½	8¼	10	13½
15	14	3¼	29	17	20⅓	9½	12	16
15½	14½	3⅓	30	17¼	21	10	12¼	16½
18	17	4	34½	20	24¼	11½	14	19
20	18½	4⅓	38½	22⅓	27	12¾	15½	21
20½	19	4½	40	23	27½	13	16	21½
26	24	5½	50	29	35	16½	28¼	27
27	25	5⅚	52	30	36	17	21	28½
32	30	7	61	36	43	20½	25	33½
36	33½	7⅚	69	40	48½	23	28	38
47	44	10¼	90	52½	63	30	37	49½
52	48½	11⅓	100	58	70	33	41	55
62	58	13½	120	69	84	40	49	65½
73	68	15⅚	140	82	98	46½	57	77
75	70	16¼	144	84	101	48½	59	79
90	84	19½	172	101	121	57½	71	94½
92	86	20	177	103	124	59	72	97
100	93	21⅔	192	112	134	64	78	105½
108	100	23⅓	206	120	145	69	84	113
180	168	39⅕	344	202	242	115	141	190

We have estimated the equivalent of subcarbonate of potash (Potassæ Carbonas of the Pharmacopœia,) and of sesquicarbonate of soda, at 84 each. Mr. PHILLIPS makes the former 83·5; but ·5 may be allowed for impurity and extra moisture: the sesquicarbonate of soda he makes 83, but the composition of the best commercial specimens approaches nearer to the bicarbonate, which is 85.

Table of the Relation between the Principal Areometers for liquids lighter than water.

[The first five columns are from SOUBEIRAN, the last from Dr. CHRISTISON and Mr. REDWOOD. The degrees of GAY-LUSSAC's alcohometer indicate the per-centage by measure of pure alcohol; but are not quite exact as here given, the fractions being neglected.]

Baumé.	Cartier.	Pharm. Batava.	Specific Gravity.	Gay-Lussac.	Sykes.
					Under proof.
10	10	0	1000	0	100
11	10·92	1	993	5	93·5
12	11·84	2	987	10	83·5
13	12·76	3	979	17	73·5
14	13·67	4	973	23	62
15	14·59	5	966	29	51
16	15·51	6	960	34	42
17	16·43	7	953	39	32
18	17·35	8	947	43	25
19	18·26	9	941	47	20
20	19·18	10	935	50	14
21	20·10	11	929	53	8
22	21·02	12	923	56	3
					Over proof.
23	21·94	13	917	59	2
24	22·85	14	911	61	7·5
25	23·77	15	905	64	11·5
26	24·69	16	900	66	15
27	25·61	17	894	69	20
28	26·53	18	888	71	25
29	27·44	19	883	73	28·5
30	28·38	20	878	75	32
31	29·29	21	872	77	38
32	30·31	22	867	79	41
33	31·13	23	862	81	44
34	32·04	24	857	83	45·5
35	32·96	25	852	84	48
36	33·88	26	847	86	51
37	34·80	27	842	88	54
38	35·72	28	837	89	56·5
39	36·63	29	832	91	59
40	37·65	30	827	92	61·5
41	38·46	31	823	93	
42	39·40	32	818	94	
43	40·31	33	813	96	
44	41·22	34	809	97	
45	42·14	35	804	98	
46	43·06	36	800	99	
47	43·19	37	795	100	
48	44·90	38	791		

Specific gravities corresponding with the degrees of BAUME's *Areometer for liquids heavier than water.*—[Pharmacopœia Batava.]

Degrees.	Sp. gr.	Degrees.	Sp. gr.
0	1000	39	1372
1	1007	40	1384
2	1014	41	1398
3	1022	42	1412
4	1029	43	1426
5	1036	44	1440
6	1044	45	1454
7	1052	46	1470
8	1060	47	1485
9	1067	48	1501
10	1075	49	1516
11	1083	50	1532
12	1091	51	1549
13	1100	52	1566
14	1108	53	1583
15	1116	54	1601
16	1125	55	1618
17	1134	56	1637
18	1143	57	1656
19	1152	58	1676
20	1161	59	1695
21	1171	60	1715
22	1180	61	1736
23	1190	62	1758
24	1199	63	1779
25	1210	64	1801
26	1221	65	1823
27	1231	66	1847
28	1242	67	1872
29	1252	68	1897
30	1261	69	1921
31	1275	70	1946
32	1286	71	1974
33	1298	72	2000
34	1309	73	2031
35	1321	74	2059
36	1334	75	2087
37	1346	76	2116
38	1359		

INDEX.

Observe: For Medicines for Horses, Cattle, &c., see the VETERINARY INDEX *at the end.*

INDEX

TO THE

VETERINARY FORMULARY.

[The Veterinary Materia Medica being alphabetically arranged it is not considered necessary to include the Drugs, whose uses and doses are there stated, in this Index.

Abbreviations employed in this list; *c.* Cattle; *s.* Sheep; *d.* Dogs; *sw.* Swine. The Horse Medicines have no mark of distinction.]

THE END.

www.ingramcontent.com/pod-product-compliance
Lightning Source LLC
LaVergne TN
LVHW020918110826
845150LV00004B/714

* 9 7 8 1 4 2 5 5 5 5 0 9 2 *